Novel Medicine

Novel Medicine

HEALING, LITERATURE, AND POPULAR
KNOWLEDGE IN EARLY MODERN CHINA

Andrew Schonebaum

A Robert B. Heilman Book

UNIVERSITY OF WASHINGTON PRESS *Seattle and London*

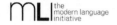

THIS BOOK IS MADE POSSIBLE BY A COLLABORATIVE GRANT
FROM THE ANDREW W. MELLON FOUNDATION.

Novel Medicine is published with additional support
from a generous bequest established by Robert
B. Heilman, distinguished scholar and chair of the
University of Washington English Department from
1948 to 1971. The Heilman Book Fund assists in the
publication of books in the humanities.

University of Washington Press
www.washington.edu/uwpress

Library of Congress Cataloging-in-Publication Data

Names: Schonebaum, Andrew, 1975–
Title: Novel medicine : healing, literature, and
    popular knowledge in early modern China /
    Andrew Schonebaum.
Description: Seattle : University of Washington Press,
    2016. | Includes bibliographical references and
    index.
Identifiers: LCCN 2015038296 | ISBN 9780295995182
    (hardcover : acid-free paper)
Subjects: LCSH: Chinese fiction—Ming dynasty,
    1368–1644—History and criticism. | Chinese
    fiction—Qing dynasty, 1644–1912—History
    and criticism. | Healing in literature | Medicine
    in literature. | Diseases in literature. | Medical
    literature—China—History. | Literature and
    society—China—History. | Books and reading—
    Social aspects—China—History. | Popular
    culture—China—History. | Knowledge, Sociology
    of—History.
Classification: LCC PL2436 .S35 2016 | DDC
    895.13/409—dc23
LC record available at http://lccn.loc.gov/2015038296

CONTENTS

Acknowledgments   vii

Introduction   3

1. Beginning to Read: Some Methods and Background   14

2. Reading Medically: Novel Illnesses, Novel Cures   47

3. Vernacular Curiosities: Medical Entertainments
   and Memory   73

4. Diseases of Sex: Medical and Literary Views
   of Contagion and Retribution   122

5. Diseases of *Qing*: Medical and Literary Views of Depletion   148

6. Contagious Texts: Inherited Maladies and the Invention
   of Tuberculosis   173

   Chinese Character Glossary   201
   Notes   213
   Bibliography   257
   Index   281

ACKNOWLEDGMENTS

I would like to thank Marta Hanson, Dore Levy, Shang Wei, and Yi-Li Wu for taking the time to read the entire manuscript and for providing me with their invaluable comments and support. Thanks to Margaret Wong for her devotion to teaching the Chinese language to me and to many, many other high schoolers. Dore Levy introduced me to the study of Chinese literature—its rigors and its pleasures—for whom and for which I am extremely grateful. I owe a great deal of gratitude to David Rolston, whose thoroughness in commenting on the manuscript helped me to make connections, excise tangents, and saved me from making numerous embarrassing errors. I learned from him an enormous amount about Chinese fiction and about my own topic. I also am indebted to David Wang, Charlotte Furth, Carlos Rojas, Paize Kuelemans, Anthony Yu, Volker Shied, Yenna Wu, and Kirk Denton for their suggestions on the various articles and talks that make up parts of this book. Nathan Sivin, Hsiu-Fen Chen, Chang Che Chia, Angela Leung, Bob Hymes, Charles Stone, and Paul Unschuld also gave generously of their time in answering my many e-mail queries. Guiling Hu helped me to locate and fix errors of pinyin and Chinese. Thank you to the editors of *Modern Chinese Literature and Culture* for allowing me to reprint parts of my article "Vectors of Contagion and Tuberculosis in Modern Chinese Literature" from their spring 2011 volume. This work was aided by a grant from the American Philosophical Society. I am grateful for the institutional support of Columbia University and the Heyman Center for Humanities, SUNY New Paltz, Bard College, and the University of Maryland. The staff at the National Library of Medicine, Starr Library, Gest Library, Staatsbibliothek zu Berlin, the Wellcome Library, Academia Sinica, McKeldin Library, Hornbake Library, and

Library of Congress have all been enormously helpful in their willingness to help me track down materials. My colleagues Michele Mason, Bob Ramsey, and Eric Zakim gave sound guidance at various stages of development. I am grateful to the two anonymous readers of my manuscript—their suggestions were extremely helpful. Thanks also to Lorri Hagman of the University of Washington Press. Richard C. Y. Chung was very helpful and a good friend. Pat Hui has been a great facilitator and an inspiration for my studies of Chinese culture all along. Most of all, I would like also to thank Angus Worthing, Eugene Poon-Kaneko, Andy Auseon, my parents, and especially Chava Brandriss, Ella, Maggie, and Molly for their support and expertise. I love you.

Novel Medicine

Introduction

It was the summer of 1843, and in Tai County the okra flowers had just bloomed. Lu Yitian's aunt, Madame Zhou, enjoyed making medical concoctions and people came from all around seeking her treatment. There was a man who had been severely scalded, so that his body was covered in festering sores, and no one had been able to affect a cure. He came to beg for a prescription of Ms. Zhou. She thus consulted the novel *Flowers in the Mirror* (Jinghua yuan, 1818) by Li Ruzhen (1763?–1830) because she knew that it "used a great deal of well-documented and extensive evidence" (*zhengyin haobo*) and because the "medical prescriptions work very well" (*zhibing douxiao*). She found in this satirical fantasy of adventures to strange lands a prescription for burns that called for okra flowers soaked in sesame oil to be applied topically. Ms. Zhou followed the prescription, and the patient recovered quickly. Thereupon, she picked all of the okra blossoms in the area, put them in bottles of sesame oil, and distributed them. According to Lu's cousin, who related this story to him, there were none who, having received this medicine, were not cured with it.[1]

The ways that novels and medicine illuminated each other in the last decades of imperial rule in China may seem like an unusual topic, but this passage provides some clues about what can be gained from such an investigation. The aunt of a medical expert (or, rather, a literate medical amateur, author, and official) gets a prescription from a novel, and her nephew incorporates it into his store of medical knowledge. He then records the story and the prescription in his medical text and his collection of notes, which further circulates the prescription, its source, and use. This story and its dissemination raise questions of intended and actual audience and of what texts written in the vernacular are meant to "do," especially considering the explicit fictionality of some of the sources used by healers. This sort of reading that focused on gathering useful knowledge for daily life disregarded the nature of the text in which it was found—a manner of reading that was possible precisely because there was so much medical information circulating by the late Qing in various forms. That a medical amateur's reading of a novel was reprinted in *Medical Discourses from Cold Hut* (Lenglu yihua, 1858) gives some indication that the authority surrounding practices like reading and healing were becoming diffuse.[2] Lu Yitian's passage suggests that readers were as interested in the nonnarrative, encyclopedia-like aspects of the novel as their authors were in filling novels with displays of every kind of knowledge.[3] Madame Zhou was able to separate the fantastical plots and hyperbolic descriptions in the novel from what she believed to be the very real and useful knowledge that they contained. But story and knowledge are not mutually exclusive. Fantastical plots helped to sell, literally and figuratively, the useful knowledge included in these novels. Moreover, novels were an efficient way to transmit this kind of knowledge, particularly, as many believed, if the author was hoping to accumulate merit by spreading useful (and secret) pharmaceutical recipes to as many people as possible. In any case, Ms. Zhou consulted *Flowers in the Mirror* rather than some other, more strictly medical text such as the *Systematic Materia Medica* (Bencao gangmu, 1596), a text known to all who practiced the most orthodox, elite medicine, and from which the prescription was likely taken.[4] She even participated in the tradition of transmitting prescriptions, modeling herself on the protagonist Tang Ao (and author Li Ruzhen?) who disseminated prescriptions as acts of charity. Perhaps she trusted *Flowers* because Tang Ao is a model practitioner of medical virtue. Or maybe it was because *Flowers* had been published only a few years earlier that Ms. Zhou considered the knowledge in it to be up-to-date, or to have some other quality she deemed valuable. Or perhaps Ms. Zhou trusted the novel to cure her neighbors because *Flowers* contained so many different kinds of pragmatic knowledge—about flood control, mathematics, navigation, poetry, and even linguistics—that it seemed a reliable encyclopedia.[5]

A world of change faced literate men in late imperial China. It was harder to gain official employment than it ever had been before.

The civil service examinations that determined the amount of official responsibility and compensation had become so crowded with
candidates that passing them was virtually impossible. Odds of
securing employment were also reduced by increasing graft and the
practice of purchasing office by those rich merchants who, despite
their wealth, were otherwise looked down upon. Literati had been
turning to other professions, such as tutor, doctor, editor, or author,
for a few centuries, in greater numbers near the end of the Ming
dynasty (1368–1644) and in still greater numbers during the Qing
(1644–1911) when Manchu rulers were even less inclined to appoint
Han Chinese to office.

This was the time that the novel began to establish itself as a new
and important genre in China. The situation of literati, turning their
esteemed hobbies into mundane, practical professions, is likely one
of the reasons why the Chinese novel (*xiaoshuo*) has a particularly
encyclopedic nature. After spending their youth memorizing philosophical and historical texts, literati who failed the official exams
that were the sole determinant of official employment had to ply a
trade—and tutoring, writing, and practicing medicine were among
the most popular of these. This context gave rise to the "scholar-
novel," identified by unity of plot, structural coherence, and single
authorship, in contradistinction to folk novels, with their patchwork
of traditional stories, incorporated a broad range of practical knowledge. Many novelists in China turned to vernacular literature in part
to display their knowledge of medicine, science, architecture, mathematics, poetry, and myriad other areas of inquiry. The new genre
accommodated (and later served as) encyclopedic texts as much as it
portrayed quotidian life, entertained the reader with complex plots,
and enabled literati to comment on their increasingly nebulous place
in society.

The account of Ms. Zhou's practice, even if it is apocryphal, illustrates that medical belief and practice were intersecting with fiction
in early modern China. Educated doctors who read the literature of
elite medicine by day and entertainment literature by night encoun-
tered these intersections, as did lay practitioners and readers. Literate
people, an increasingly diverse group who read and produced diverse
texts, understood the world and their bodies' place in it through a
frame of both elite and vernacular knowledge. When ill, we want to
know not just the etiology of our disease but what our disease *means*.
In China, as elsewhere, the experience of disease was conditioned

by peculiarities of culture. What is more, the meanings of disease defined by popular entertainments affected thinking about etiology, and a complex discourse evolved between novelistic and medical texts. Practitioners were evaluated in the pages of fictional texts, and their representation in novels resonates with doctors' recorded cases and autobiographies written at the same time. Literate patients were also amateur practitioners; they wanted to know how to treat themselves, their sick family members, and neighbors. They availed themselves of all kinds of popular guidebooks and practical medical texts, and even novels. Through a sustained analysis of early modern fictional and medical texts, as well as fiction commentary, criticism, newspaper advertisements, medical manuscripts, essays, collectanea, biographies, oral tales, performance literature, and more, this book examines how vernacular knowledge of medicine and the body was created and transmitted, and how much of it persisted into the modern era.

Each chapter of this book is organized roughly according to chronology, but because the materials used to investigate each thematic topic are different, discussions of historical context necessitate moving back in time to differing degrees in each. Many of the texts discussed have no publication date, little publication data, or were never published, which means that precise dating of the creation or consumption of these texts must yield to logical approximations. In this study, the terms "early modern China" and "late imperial China" are not incompatible. The "early modern" period of China here refers to the seventeenth through nineteenth centuries—the *longue durée* period extending across the dynastic boundary between Ming and Qing. I am more concerned with understanding the relationships of medicine and fiction in this period than in situating them in a strict, diachronic history of belief or practice. It is, however, important to understand the late Ming and Qing as "early modern," since China's modernity has a domestic history, as this study demonstrates with regard to medical knowledge.[6] This is not to say that belief and practice in the seventeenth through nineteenth centuries were *only* early modern. The chapters in this book each culminate in the last decades of the nineteenth century or the first decades of the twentieth, but this is not meant to suggest that their investigations are all entwined, mutually influential, or products of one cultural moment.

Illness and the body are complex topics that demand interdisciplinary approaches. Vernacular entertainments, themselves complex, polygeneric, and interdisciplinary texts, are also a vast cache of depictions and explanations of the quotidian and popular knowledge. They illuminate how illness and the body were understood in individual works and as trends in literary history. As complex texts that are both narrative and instructive, written by and for literati, scholarly novels of early modern China share much with medical compendia and case histories, and even materia medica produced in the same period. Fictional texts were used or imagined as medical texts, but medical texts increasingly looked like fiction and drama—containing a great deal of narrative and dialogue, and drawing upon a wide range of sources, including poetry and fictional literature, as evidence to back their claims. Studying these kinds of texts together also makes sense because they were being published in great numbers for the first time starting in the sixteenth century, often sharing the same publishing houses, editors, readers, and, sometimes, authors.[7] Metaphor and figurative language are powerful forces that alter how people understand their bodies and their world, but they also codify complex notions, and resist change. The flourishing of these texts marked a watershed moment in publishing and reading culture, and they exerted long-term effects on the public imaginary with both their content and their form.

NOVEL MEDICINE AND POPULAR KNOWLEDGE

"Novel medicine" refers here to medicine found in novels, as well as works of drama and short stories, which shared the same kind of readers.[8] "Novel" medicine is also meant as a corrective to the emphasis put on the "medicine of systematic correspondence," the paradigm emphasized more than any other in scholarship on Chinese medicine (which focuses on *yinyang* and five phases correlations that underlie relations between particular medicines and bodily dysfunctions), and in contradistinction to which many widely held beliefs and common practices seem "strange" or "unorthodox." Novels also presented and represented elite medicine, but vernacular literature was one of the few printed sources that recorded these "other," vernacular traditions of healing practice. Medicine, or, more precisely, healing, included all phenomena that affected the body: hard masses and strong emotions, miasmas and wind, ejaculation and diarrhea, corpse worms (*shichong*) and ghosts, and a multitude of other pathogenic factors. Novel medicine also implicates the ways in which medicine illuminates vernacular literature. We cannot understand how early modern Chinese readers comprehended fiction without investigating the history of medicine and the body of the period. But we cannot fully appreciate how bodies were understood without trying to access the most popular and important representations of the body—those found in entertainment literature—and the literary logic that undergirded those representations.

"Popular knowledge" refers to vernacular or common knowledge, and to ways of knowing that lie in the lived practice of everyday individuals, outside "official," elite, or formal discourse or modes of education.[9] Much of medical knowledge at that time lay outside elite medical practice; employed local, folk, or apotropaic remedies; or was transmitted through texts written in the vernacular and likely intended for mass consumption. But "popular knowledge" also refers to ways of knowing and strategies of transmission that employed narrative technique, metaphor, metonymy, linguistic correlation, and other kinds of logic found in entertainment literature. Much of what nonelite healers knew about medicine came from vernacular sources—novels, dramatic literature, household manuals, encyclopedias, and almanacs.

In English, the word "medicine" commonly refers to a specialized form of healing codified in and accessible through written literature and thus holding privileged orthodox status.[10] "Healing," by contrast, is encompassing in its inclusion of medical theory and practical reality. In Chinese the word *yi* can refer to any variety of healing practice but is most commonly used to identify the practices of elite medicine, or perhaps acupuncture or moxa (historically the purview of more lowly specialists). Healers in imperial China could be graduates of the imperial medical academy or other diverse types of doctors, shamans or spirit mediums (*wu*), "remedy masters" or magicians (*fangshi*), or other kinds of caregivers. The differences between these practitioners and the beliefs that undergirded their practice were not always clear.

There were essentially three strata of medical practitioner in early modern China: those who responded to a command (court physicians), those who responded to an invitation, and those who solicited business.[11] Court physicians, or physicians-in-waiting (usually known as *yuyi, neiyi, taiyi,* or *daiyi*), served only the court and were paid a fixed salary. Other doctors, often known as "business physicians" or "city physicians" (*shiyi*), practiced medicine in a fixed location in town and made house calls in response to a call from a family, who then paid them an examination fee (*zhenjin*). These physicians constituted the largest number among all medical practitioners, and historically were those who represented literate medicine, though this was a diverse group jostling for authority and prestige in a field without much regulation. This group could also include local mid-wives, shamans, astrologers, and others who were amateurs or part-time practitioners. Local physicians are prominent among healers in fiction. Doctors who solicited customers tended to wander between small towns and villages in the countryside and treat those who did not otherwise have access to medicine. Commonly known as "bell doctors" (*ling yi*), "grass and marshes doctors" (*caoze yi*), "wander-ing doctors" (*zoufang yi*), "doctors [who pass] over rivers and lakes" (*jianghu yi*), and "common doctors" (*yong yi*), they were figures of city marketplaces as well, since many urban dwellers lacked the finan-cial resources to pay the fees of a regular doctor. This group also encompassed monks and nuns; peddlers of nostrums, aphrodisiacs, and abortifacients; and dentists and surgeons. Although each strata of medical practice was represented by a diverse group of practitio-ners, with differing medical and educational backgrounds, they were separated by mobility, with one group fixed as local doctors, and another as itinerant ones. It was these city excursions that brought mainstream doctors into contact with traveling doctors, and these points of contact inspired the vitriol and disdain of one group toward the other.

Beginning with the Yuan (1260–1368) and Ming dynasties, notes on itinerant physicians began to appear more frequently in medical literature, voicing both praise and criticism. Mostly, these are case histories recording the successful conclusion of a treatment after a faulty approach by some itinerant physician. It seems that only in the Qing did itinerant doctors begin to constitute a group that was perceived to have its own medical tradition.[12] Some writings contain prompt notes for use by itinerant physicians. These provide lengthy discourses on the origins of disease and therapeutic practice with points clearly meant to punctuate a sales pitch. This performance was meant not to educate but to befuddle and to sell medicine. The earli-est extant text by an itinerant doctor was published in 1593, though the text detailing the practices and knowledge of wandering doctors that caused a great stir among "city physicians" was that recorded in Zhao Xuemin's (ca. 1730–1805) *Strings of Refined [Therapies]* (Chuanya, 1759).[13] Zhao explains that he excised the prompt notes for pitching nostrums and other tricks of the trade because he did not want to spread immoral or illegal knowledge.[14] Based on a large collection of medical manuscripts held in the Berlin library, the practice of willfully cheating patients was not uncommon. Many of these manuscripts reveal strategies to persuade reluctant patients to purchase treatment, or to pay high prices for medicine.[15] The linguistic talent of these itinerant physicians is summed up in one manuscript: "To sell medications and to predict one's fate—this entirely depends on rhetoric."[16] The manuscripts also show that in the late Qing there was a good deal of competition within the group of itinerant healers.

Suspicion of doctors dates back to at least the first century CE and the earliest extant biography of a doctor, in which the Prince of Huan warns, "Physicians, fond of profit, try to gain credit by [treating] those who are not ill."[17] Evaluations like this one were reiterated, often in fiction, until the modern period, and point to a consistent ambivalence regarding the status of medicine and its practitioners. The most common way of representing doctors in traditional Chinese fiction was as comedic quacks. Given the absence of licensing laws and formal medical instruction in the Ming and Qing, and the long-standing suspicion of any profession practiced for money (usually classified as craftsmen [gong] or technical specialists [ji]), doctors vied with each other for legitimacy.[18] Doctors also contributed to their profession's own bad reputation by frequently bemoaning the proliferation of quacks generally, or attacking specific medical groups or individual practitioners. Both elites and hereditary doctors (shiyi) sought to appropriate some of the others' legitimacy, but hereditary physicians and scholar-physicians wanted to distinguish themselves from folk healers, mendicants, women practitioners, and peddlers of medicine.[19]

Those who sought to legitimize the practice of medicine relied to some extent on the Confucian values of humaneness, benevolence, and rightness. They defined these as the qualities of the ideal doctor, a "literati-physician," "scholar-physician," or "Confucian-physician" (ruyi). Early uses of the term ruyi (twelfth century) refer to hereditary physicians with Confucian (ru) values. The term also applied to men from families of ruling elites who eschewed government service to practice medicine, though it is more likely that they turned to the medical profession once their path to officialdom became blocked.[20] Scholar physicians are significant marginal figures—their scholarliness elevating them above common doctors, their medical practice excluding them from the category of scholar-officials.[21] That is to say, even physicians of the higher order were still not quite gentle-men.[22] These elite outsiders, who were elevating the practice of medicine—in status, at least, if not in efficacy—play a part in the history of fiction and drama, just as authors of fiction and drama were similarly seeking to establish those genres as legitimate prac-tices of educated gentlemen.

Ruyi status identified people who read—texts, the body, and pat-terns (*li*). *The Golden Mirror of the Medical Lineage* (Yizong jinjian), published for use as a teaching manual at the Qing Imperial Academy (Taiyi Yuan), stated, "If physicians are not intimately familiar with books, they will not understand principle [*li*]. If they do not under-stand principle, they will not be able to recognize the situation clearly. Then when they go to treat illness, they will vacillate and be indeci-sive, their medicines will not accord with the sickness, and it will be difficult to obtain an efficacious result."[23] Those who claimed status as *ruyi* created for themselves a new lineage of texts, and vilified the old one that relied on transmission of knowledge from one person to another as a tainted heredity that could not discern patterns.

Which practice, practitioner, or idea is esteemed over others as "medical" is often a point of contestation between elite and popular texts. Complicating the situation, the knowledge and ability of lit-erate medical amateurs overlapped with those of professional physi-cians, yet early modern observers clearly considered certain people to be doctors and others not.[24] Ms. Zhou, who consulted *Flowers in the Mirror* for a prescription, was a healer, and her nephew Lu Yitian was not a physician in the strict sense but a literate medical amateur, yet he claimed authority for himself by publishing medical texts. More-over, that Ms. Zhou herself was a literate healer reflects an increasing access to textual medicine and the degree to which medical publish-ing incorporated popular methods of healing.[25] Popular medicine increasingly was communicated through published works as literacy rates increased and many medical texts in the late Ming–and Qing–contained useful medical knowledge. Before the late imperial period, most of these were books published by renowned physicians to engage their peers on topics of medical theory. These texts were reprinted in the great imperial collections and discussed by other famous physi-cians down through the centuries. They remained elite but were no longer the only textual sources of medical knowledge.

Medicine had been elite because of its written status, and the sta-tus of its practitioners, who were officials or scholar-physicians (*yi*, *ruyi*), was privileged over that of the "illiterate" healers—shamans, laymen, midwives, nuns, and countless others. In the Ming and Qing periods, that status was challenged, complicated, and subverted by all manner of printed texts propagating the kind of vernacular knowledge that had once been the purview primarily of medical outsiders.[26] Increasing literacy and the growth of printing gave many of these outsiders access to a panoply of medical texts. Clashing schools of thought, such as "warm-epidemic" and "cold-harm," sought to draw more and more followers to their camp.[27] Part of that strategy included publishing texts that were accessible to a broader audience. Additionally, elite medicine was incorporating literary forms (narrative and dialogue) familiar to a less-elite readership and content useful for amateur practitioners (prescriptions, incantations, and therapies) previously eschewed by the literate medical tradition. Other kinds of printed texts contained practical and theoretical medical knowledge but were not primarily or explicitly concerned with medicine and healing, or did not advertise themselves as such. Vernacular knowledge of the body was thus expanding to include what had formerly been confined to elite medical texts.

Many of the "medical texts" that inform this study would not merit that term by historians of medicine. In this context, the term refers to texts that claim to be useful, true, or verified, as opposed to works that by virtue of their form (drama, libretto, etc.) or content (fantastic tales) are clearly meant to entertain but that also contain a great deal of medical knowledge. Most of the medical texts discussed here meet one or both of these criteria: they were produced for popular consumption (including, or particularly, texts that had commercial value), and they lent themselves to being used as guides for direct action by nonexperts, even if their intended audience included experts (e.g., "If you have this symptom, take this drug."). "Vernacular" medical texts, like published medical case collections (*yi'an*), collections of medical recipes (*fangshu*), and pharmacopeia (*bencao*), are of primary interest, as these were appealing to a broader audience in late imperial China and often represent healing practices not found in elite medical texts—demonology, apotropaic medicine, sexual therapy, and so on.[28] These vernacular medical texts merit the designation because they were meant to be used and because every aspect of practice is represented there. Thus they, like fictional texts, are revealing in their depiction of how people thought about their bodies in relation to the world. From elite medical use of prescriptions to talismanic rituals to folk remedies to astrological prognostication, fiction and vernacular medical texts represent these practices and the varied beliefs that undergirded them.

Vernacular medicine encompasses many traditions, but one of them is usually characterized by historians of medicine as "magic."[29] Some have discussed these magical medical beliefs as falling into two categories: homeopathic magic, in which linguistic or other resemblances give power to a treatment (walnuts nourish the brain because they look like little brains), and contact magic, in which a part stands for a whole (a fingernail or a hair can be used to steal the soul of the person from which they came). These medical concepts are not only similar to but dependent upon literary devices and figurative language such as metaphor and metonymy. I call these kinds of correspondences, upon which much vernacular medicine is based, "literary logic."[30] Foundational medical texts such as the *Systematic Materia Medica* use literary logic as the basis of common sense. Ironically, practical medical texts also employ stories, particularly fantastic stories, as evidence for their claims of efficacy.

Clues to the way people read novels and other entertainment literature can be found in newspapers, published notebooks (*biji*), commentary, and other paratexts, and, importantly, in a treasure trove of hand-copied medical manuscripts from the nineteenth and early twentieth centuries by people who practiced medicine. These manuscripts are records of how people practiced medicine and how they read the variety of texts that fall under that rubric.[31] They, like novels, practical medical texts, and other guidebooks, reflect a robust belief system of competing and complementary treatments, but they also reveal the degree to which literature was a part of those practices.

CHAPTER I

Beginning to Read

Some Methods and Background

Consider how behavior is altered by medical concepts. Those who have a biomedical understanding of the body may open doors with their feet, sneeze into their elbows, and wash hands after greeting a friend. Their daily rituals—using the bathroom, preparing and consuming food, wearing clothes, and interactions with others—are all conditioned by the knowledge that invisible things move from one body to another and cause illness. So, how did those who believe in avenging ghosts as a cause of illness behave? If you know that changes in the flow of vital breath cause illness, what do you do when the temperature drops, or you smell something foul? How do you interact with others knowing that violent swings of emotion can be fatal? How do you read if you know that it can destroy health? Fiction represented these actual practices, but also critiqued, recommended, or explained them. In doing so, fiction reveals its intrinsic interconnectedness with the debates and concerns of its time. But it is also an agent of its time, a vector of transmission that entertains and affects its readers, conditions and instructs them. By capturing these robust practices, fiction is one of the very few kinds of sources that aid the historian of daily life. Yet fiction is fiction, and its fantastical, critical, or hyperbolic representation of healing practices reveal much about readers who would blithely employ or imitate them as if they were reading a medical manual. To rely on fiction as historical source material requires comparison with other kinds of texts to evaluate how authentic, logical, or unique are descriptions found in fiction. Readers' commentary on fictional and medical texts, published notebooks (*biji*), accounts in newspapers and gaz-etteers, medical practitioners' handwritten manuscripts, historical encyclopedia, guides to daily life, biographies, and medical case histories help to evaluate how fiction was used and, at the same time, provide examples of popular medical knowledge.

Chinese medicine really is a classical scheme of knowing. In addition to the circulation and balance in the body, and between the body and the universe, of blood, essence, and qi, Chinese medicine is based on a theory of systematic correspondences. The health of the state functions like the health of the body (a metaphor that has pervaded medical discourse in China since *Huang Di's Inner Classics* of the first or second century BCE). Harmony can be disturbed by excessive desire or gluttony; by external conditions, such as a change in temperature or environment; or by the invasion of evil influences or spirits. Harmony is achieved though the maintenance of the flow of blood, essence, and qi through the body—and, in the case of qi, through immediate and extended environments.

In a syncretic worldview, all appearances belong to two opposite yet complementary poles, yin and yang, which are constantly changing into and out of each other. Early thinkers in the *yinyang* school considered all phenomena to be interconnected and constantly transforming—day into night into day, high tide to low to high, and so on. A similar school of thought saw the world's dynamics as based on the interactions of five phases (*wuxing*) or five categories of all things material and immaterial. Wood, water, fire, earth, and metal represented more than the physical elements—they were also phases, each with their own set of characteristics, and related to each other in a cycle of conquest and generation. Applied to the human body, five-phases theory explained the dynamic relationships and affinities of five basic bodily systems, loosely associated with liver, heart, spleen, lung, and kidneys. The liver stored the blood; the heart regulated the movement of the blood and governed consciousness; the spleen stored and regulated energy from food; the lung regulated the qi of breath and also kept internal and external energy in their proper channels; and the kidneys governed reproductive function and the stores of primordial qi, the original source of life.[1] The *yinyang* and five-phases schools were synthesized during the first or second century BCE and came to characterize Chinese medicine. The body, with its organs and processes, functioned like the natural and social environments surrounding it (fig. 1.1).

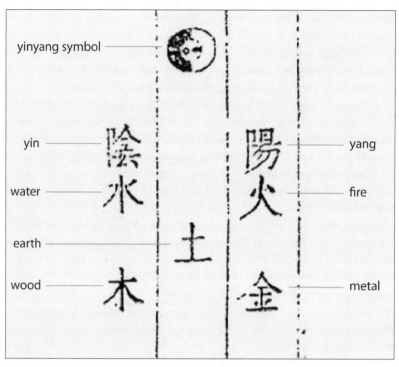

Figure 1.1.   Diagram of yin and yang and the five phases. From Xu
Dachun, *Yiguan bian*. Courtesy of Waseda University.

Everyone has a body, and everyone gets sick, but these things
are culturally conditioned and construed. Some scholars of Chinese
medicine routinely capitalize words such as "Blood" or "Liver" to
remind readers that these universals have significant differences in
their respective medical paradigms.[2] Modern blood is not the same
as premodern blood, and blood in early modern Europe is not the
same as blood in early modern China. This is true also of diseases.
While modern biomedicine posits that disease spreads by invisible
pathogens, and that the syphilis contracted in Lisbon in the sixteenth
century was the same disease contracted in Canton, we cannot ignore
the cultural beliefs about a disease—how it was contracted, how it
spread, how to treat it, and what it meant—in a given time or place.
For convenience, familiar European terms for maladies are often used
here. For example, for diseases that affect the genital region or are
somehow associated with sex, "venereal disease," which has fallen
out of favor among modern doctors, is used precisely because it is old

and imprecise. It retains the meaning "related to sex," and for this reason is useful both to discuss meaningful disease categories, and to remind the reader that the topic under discussion is not specifically biomedical syphilis or any other disease that might be diagnosed in the modern West. The fusty, premodern term "consumption" does not correlate directly to biomedical "tuberculosis," and its symptom set—coughing blood, weight loss, and weakness—is similar to depletion and taxation disorders in premodern China. Moreover, since it is often the result of excessive emotion or passion, with the implications of heat and the consumption of bodily resources, the translated term captures some of the illness mechanism, although not every implication of that classical malady in Europe coincides with instances in China. Such terms are not used for detailed analysis of these differences (i.e., the disease Marguerite Gautier suffers from is not exactly that of Lin Daiyu).

The use of imprecise terms is also warranted because vernacular medicine has different nosological systems than elite medicine, with which it overlaps. For instance, elite Chinese medicine most commonly identified nocturnal emission as caused by a deficient condition of the heart, a deficient condition of the kidney, an invasion of pathogenic humidity or heat, or an evanescence of vital essence. Vernacular medicine would also include among the causes of nocturnal emission excessive melancholy damaging the heart or bewitchment by fox spirits.[3] Vernacular knowledge sometimes coincided with or encompassed elite knowledge, but at times, the two remained distinct. For instance, the belief that bugs (*chong*) and demons (*gui*) played a decisive role in the generation of disease was an accepted conceptual basis of elite health care prior to the medicine of systematic correspondences that rose to prominence in the second century BCE. After that period, bugs were largely neglected by the sorts of elite medical texts collected in the *Complete Library of the Four Treasuries* (Siku quanshu) as possible pathological agents until modern Western bacteriology entered China in the late nineteenth century.[4] The important role played by bugs and demons in the creation and transmission of disease was, however, a fact continuously repeated in much of the materia medica literature, formularies, recipes, manuscripts, and practical medical texts produced in the past two millennia.[5] Medical authors who recorded a variety of treatments for their own practice also recorded a much more robust world of belief than those found in traditional treatises. Formularies and fiction, popular texts starting at the end of the sixteenth century, point to a world of belief that had previously existed outside of printed margins. Elite medicine, the practice of which was usually confined to pulse palpitation and the prescription of medicine based on systematic correlations, was "elite" by virtue of its dominant position in printed texts for centuries. The robust, heterogeneous world of vernacular healing—including bugs and ghosts, and apotropaic and other kinds of medicine—are well represented in the fiction, encyclopedias, and practical medical texts of the Ming and Qing, and reflect the diversity and diffusion of healing practice.

LITERARY TEXTS AND ENTERTAINMENT LITERATURE

One way of knowing the world was through poetry. Poetry, in particular rhapsodies (*fu*), became critical to the post-Ming development of natural history and medicine. The genre of rhapsodies lent itself to works of natural history because it was always heavily descriptive (rather than lyrical) and became more so over time. But poetry was generally part of the natural history of things, and poems were regularly included in texts describing the known world. Scholars used poems, particularly famous or ancient ones, as evidence. Informational texts of every variety, including practical medical texts, use the phrase "there is a poem as proof" (*you shi wei zheng*).[6] The authority of poems was predicated on a respect for the genre, which took emotional truth if not historical fact as its basis. Poetry also carried the hefty weight of esteemed literary tradition, and for that reason as well may have been perceived as a record of empirical evidence regarding the natural world. Another way of knowing was through telling stories. In all kinds of guidebooks we see authors citing a story as precedent, or even a conversation with someone else as evidence for a claim. For many, the only way to learn something new in the premodern period was from texts or word of mouth. Few conducted their own investigations, as did Li Shizhen (1518–1593), the author-compiler of the *Systematic Materia Medica*. Many essays record accounts of others and cite them as they would a poem. Poetry and stories also reinforced linguistic correlation—the sense that things in the real world that share names or that are related somehow through language have an actual corresponding relationship.[7] These linguistic correlations undergird many medical interactions. Knowing in premodern China involved a literary logic, and texts that sought to communicate knowledge, particularly novels, recipe books, and medical compendia, employed this logic extensively.

Today, the hegemony of biomedicine is so complete that anything else is, to many, "alternative." The scientific method is so enshrined as the only *real* way of knowing that poetry and stories seem poor resources compared to empirical observation, proof, method, and data. Moderns tend to judge therapies based on their effectiveness, not on their accordance with the logic of the universe as it has been known for millennia. It is difficult to imagine the world before biomedicine and scientific inquiry. Ghosts were a fact of life in premodern China. The heart produced thought. Wind flowed into meridians and produced six different pulses in each wrist. Historians of science, religion, myth, and social life all cite texts such as the *Systematic Materia Medica* to show how common certain beliefs were. But those diverse studies tend to obfuscate the fact that some of the most popular medical texts in China included everything all at once, without any disciplinary or generic distinctions. While the term "medical text" can mean anything from works on a particular group of disorders to instructional texts on palpating pulses to recipe books to apotropaic manuals, few medical texts represent the gamut of medical belief. Those that do represent a broad range of beliefs tend to be practical rather than theoretical. But practical medical texts are not syncretic; they are a collection of effective remedies, or simply a record of reading and life experience. In this regard practical medical texts rivaled novels in representing the complexity of the world.

Chinese novels and practical medical texts were not syncretic and did not make fast distinctions between strata of practice. Elite medicine commingled with popular healing practice in these texts. In novels and materia medica for instance, ghost-influx disorder could be treated with herbs, as could soul loss. Venereal diseases could be blamed on miasma as well as heredity. Pregnancy was aided by pharmaceutical drugs, eating placenta, prayer, sacrifice, and drinking the ashes of written talismans mixed with wine.

SOME USES OF *XIAOSHUO*

Historically, the literary genre *xiaoshuo* commonly translated as "novel," shifted within and between traditional bibliographies and literary taxonomies. Literally meaning "small talk" or "trivial discourse," in its earliest uses (Han dynasty, 206 BCE—220 CE) *xiaoshuo* meant something along the lines of "miscellany." Only as late as the late sixteenth century did *xiaoshuo* come into common use as a term for full-length prose fiction. *Xiaoshuo* still includes a variety of genres of different lengths and levels of language that are distinguished from each other by modifying terms.[8] However, the lack of a precise generic term for the premodern Chinese novel does not mean that the genre was poorly understood. Generally speaking, in China, the novel grew out of the historical tradition, which itself included not only battles and dynastic conquests but also exemplary people and "accounts of the strange" (*zhiguai*). In fact, works of vernacular fiction were sometimes called, and served as, "unofficial histories" (*waishi*).

These premodern novels include a great degree of classical-language poetry that coexists with the surrounding vernacular narrative.[9] This likely shows the influence of traditional Chinese dramatic art, which also fuses vernacular narrative and classical lyric. The novel and serious drama in China had a great degree of mutual influence; sharing the same narrative structures and motifs, as well as the same readers, publishers, and, often, authors. Poetry in novels, like arias in operas, stopped narrative time and focused on a certain character, point, scene, or experience.[10] This lyrical interlude provided background information or foreshadowed coming events. In part, the poetry in Chinese novels creates an interaction and tension between high and low diction, literati and popular culture. In this regard, poetry marks the novel in China, even more than drama, as a hybrid genre. The great works of vernacular fiction self-consciously exploit this intrinsic hybridity by playing with generic and linguistic differences to achieve ironic disjunctions or harmonious visions.[11]

The novel in China grew out of particular historical conditions in the sixteenth and seventeenth centuries. Contributing to the appearance of the novel in China and represented in them were increased urbanization and population shifts to urban centers of the Yangzi River Delta region, increased printing and literacy, the shift to an economy based on silver bullion, overseas colonization and trade, and incipient industrialization. *Xiaoshuo* displays a shift in class affinity away from the old elite and the pretensions of classical literature toward a broader, more generously encompassing literature. The new literary form presented subject matter that appealed to a wide audience, namely depictions of the quotidian, mundane settings, and middlebrow characters. It also suggested a resistance to or subversive stance toward those political and cultural forces that had previously kept these strata of life from being represented. The representation of *things* in the Chinese novel, particularly in those more domestic works, both reflects a literati fascination with material culture in the "poetry of useful things" and presents the reader with a recognizable world of sights, smells, and sounds. Many of the novels from the eighteenth century in particular serve historians of China with their repositories of meticulously documented stuff of daily life.

Most of the novels discussed in this study were written by literati for literati to entertain their friends, relatives, and, in some cases, wives.[12] Most were not intended for publication—not so much because they would not be profitable, as indeed they were, but primarily because the writing of fiction was not a highly respected endeavor. Reading novels was something to be done in private, and writing them was a game by which the author might showcase his education and cleverness to his peers, for fun. It was not until the nineteenth century that many of the great classic novels were even attributed to particular authors—and that some writers became comfortable enough with the genre's popularity to claim authorship of their own works.[13]

The novels considered to be "masterworks," written by and for the most educated members of Chinese society, display an overwhelming degree of intertextuality. In referencing, borrowing from, and incorporating all manner of texts, the Chinese novel is virtually unparalleled in its complexity. Novels are hybrid texts, and *xiaoshuo* even more so, with their incessant borrowing from all genres. Additionally, most literati novels were published with commentary, multiple prefaces, and other paratexts that make some links to preexisting texts explicit. They also map out the logic and structure of the work. The hybrid, polygeneric nature of *xiaoshuo* and the many *other* texts in these texts shows that literati authors of fiction and their presumed readers read everything. But many kinds of readers consumed novels, and they did so using a great range of approaches. Literati novels are usually defined in contradistinction to "popular" novels, but literati novels became popular—they were read by lots of people who were not "men of letters," and who read differently from one another. It is important to remember that the literati, while representing a small (roughly 2 to 5) percentage of the population, were a diverse group—in origin, employment, education, connections, and so on—as reflected in the quality of writings they produced. In the late Ming, literati faced a number of crises that further blurred the boundaries separating their group from the likes of increasingly wealthy and literate merchants. These "other" readers were the ones who used novels as compendia of elite knowledge and culture, and it was also these "other" readers who constituted a large cohort of medical practitioners.[14]

Basically defined, "literati" (*wenren* or *shi*) in Ming and Qing China were those of the "gentry" who were educated and who maintained their status as cultural elites primarily through classical scholarship, knowledge of lineage ritual, and literary publication.[15] But the literati were not an undifferentiated group. Who was and who was not a literatus was not always clear, especially at a time of such great underemployment and increasing literacy rates, and many wanted to make an argument for themselves. In general, the increased publication and readership of these polygeneric texts contributed to the formation of a common discourse. Novels helped to create a popular vision of Confucian identity through language that is mixed with or complemented by values and wisdom drawn from many sources. Novels lent themselves to synchronicity—to a blending of philosophical stances, and easy movement between popular, official, and inherited registers of knowledge. Novels talked about daily life in a way that was both imperative and indicative; they provided a stable structure of values with which the reader could make sense of the world, and in this sense also participated in the construction of reality.

Most consumers read *xiaoshuo* in commentated editions, with printed and sometimes handwritten commentary by previous readers in the margins, between lines, or at the ends of chapters. Standard, sanctioned classical texts were read in commentary editions almost exclusively for centuries, but now readers (and sometimes authors) supplied their own commentary to novels. Commentary and novel paratexts literally and figuratively taught the reader how to read that particular novel. They also claimed to be teaching how to read novels in general. As such, *xiaoshuo* became a literary site for creative reading and interpretation that revealed trends in scholarship, literati life, and even medicine. Some commentaries, such as Zhang Xinzhi's 1881 commentary on Cao Xueqin's famous novel *Story of the Stone* (Shitou ji, 1791–92; also known as *Dream of the Red Chamber* [Honglou meng]), insist that the numerology, *yinyang* cosmology, and medicine of systematic correspondence is the key to understanding the entire work; others make more modest claims that a prescription is useful or that the author was engaging in physician bashing.[16]

Fiction represented and commented on life, and fiction commentary evaluated the authenticity and meaning of fictional representation. Commentators legitimized writing and reading novels as the work of fellow scholars, connected the work at hand to those of the past, and also corrected what was written.

Some of the most important medical texts of this late imperial period, such as the *Systematic Materia Medica*, were primarily commentary meant to collect and evaluate what had been previously written on a topic. Compendia of pharmaceuticals, prescriptions, and medical handbooks shared a similar discursive space, as did *xiaoshuo*, in that neither kind of text was a part of the elite forms of medical or literary practice, yet both enhanced their own popularity and utility by incorporating knowledge from diverse realms. Medical cases adopted many narrative strategies from fiction, and fiction incorporated all kinds of medical knowledge.[17] Readers treated medical texts in much the same way they treated novels (or rather, both were increasingly treated like the classics). They added commentary, explained intertexts, and compiled, quoted, and even followed up medical case histories and materia medica with sequels.[18] Literati had been engaging in these reading practices for centuries, and now they were subjecting fiction and medicine to the same kind of scrutiny. The addition of these texts to the canon of those deserving commentary signaled a shift in intellectual history, and was reflective of a desire to consider vernacular texts and practical knowledge as capable of sustaining that kind of inquiry.

SOURCES OF VERNACULAR KNOWLEDGE: ENCYCLOPEDIAS, ALMANACS, NEWSPAPERS, AND FICTION

By many accounts, the most popular published books in the late Ming dynasty (1506–1644) were medical works, encyclopedias, and fiction.[19] These books were newly popular and appealed to a similar readership. Guides to passing the social service exams and other texts related to the Confucian classics were still among the most printed texts, but they commanded a much smaller share of the market than in the early Ming (1368–1505) and earlier.[20] That all three genres were becoming exponentially more popular in the Ming—more popular than the classics, philology, biographies, and other genres—was not a coincidence, nor was that fact that they often shared editors and printing houses.[21] Practical medical texts, fiction, *xiaoshuo*, and daily-use encyclopedias, aside from all being classed as "philosophy" (*zi*), had much in common.[22] Publishers were not only editing and printing a variety of useful and entertainment literature; they were also creating it.[23] Members of publishing families and editors wrote medical works and novels, which explains some of the similarities in form and content among genres.[24]

Since the Song dynasty (960–1279), official bibliographic works referenced an independent category of texts generally translated as "encyclopedias" (lit., "books topically arranged"). The *leishu* category encompassed a variety of books, including collections of examination literature, instructions for carrying out family rituals, biographical dictionaries, primers on reading classical literature, handbooks on letter writing, pharmacopoeias, geographical surveys, administrative and procedural manuals, and dictionaries of quotations. In the Ming, *leishu* for the first time referred to works that were truly encyclopedic in their scope that functioned as guidebooks to daily life (*riyong leishu*). Although these had begun in the Yuan (1271–1368) with works such as the *Essentials of Domestic Living* (Jujia biyong shilei quanji), in the Ming daily-use encyclopedias flourished, with new compilations, reprintings, and new editions. A large portion of the extant editions of late-Ming encyclopedias for daily use originated in Jianyang County in Fujian, one of the late-Ming print centers, long known for its production of books of low quality in enormous quantity, with correspondingly modest prices.[25]

These guides to daily life concerned themselves to a considerable degree with medicine. While the word "medicine" (*yi*) does not appear at all in the table of contents of the *Essentials of Domestic Living*, the section on "guarding life" (*weisheng*) contains well over 200 do-it-yourself prescriptions for treating maladies, including everything from hot soup burns (*tanghuo shaodang*) to consumptive disorders (*laozhai*). Sections in this encyclopedia, such as "protecting the body" (*jinshen*), also contain many prescriptions, as well as guidelines concerning damage from emotions, and prescribed amounts of sexual intercourse, food, and drink. Ming encyclopedias commonly featured chapters on medicine (*yixue* or *yilin*), nourishing life (*yangsheng*), and expelling disease (*fabing* or *qubing*). In popular encyclopedias of the late Ming, such as *Ye Jia's Newly Cut Complete Book of Myriad Treasures* (Xinke yejia xincai wanbao quanshu, 1599), and *Santai's Orthodox Instructions for Myriad Uses for the Convenient Perusal of All People under Heaven* (Xinke tianxia simin bianlan santai wanyong zhengzong, 1614), chapters are devoted to medicine, as is an entire chapter on smallpox (*douzhen*). Chapters on pregnancy, birth, and children (*taichan, zhongzi, huyou,* or *quanying*) take medical issues as the primary focus, providing prescriptions, advice, and guidance on palpating the pulses (*maijue*). Chapters on livestock and husbandry (*niuma* or *majing*) are also largely concerned with medical matters. Chapters on "teachers and scholars" (*shiru*) feature subsections titled "Tried and True Prescriptions" (Jingyan liangfang), as do chapters relating to sex, such as "Young Men" (Zidi) or "Romance" (Fengyue), which provide aphrodisiac prescriptions, including "good prescriptions for sexual desire" (*seyu liangfang*), "medicine for thoughts of love" (*chunyi yao*), and tips for enhancing virility. Fair to say, these encyclopedias and others popular in the late Ming and Qing dynasties were substantially concerned with the practice of medicine and the transmission of medical knowledge high and low.

Traditional Chinese almanacs, too (*tongsheng, tongshu, lishu, lipu,* or *rishu*), included considerable medical guidance and medical prescriptions. Virtually every household in premodern China used almanacs, and instances in which they were consulted abound in fiction.[26] Almanacs listed all types of human activities and gave guidance about selecting the most suitable days on which to perform them. They advised on matters of travel, marriage, buying and selling, opening a business, weaning a baby, pacifying the kitchen god, starting construction, burying a corpse, preparing wine, and all manner of quotidian activities. The most fundamental relationship between almanacs and medicine had to do with interpreting certain physical and emotional changes as omens or signs. Almanacs then gave guidance about how to interpret the meanings of quick-eye movements, ringing in the ear, heat in the face, trembling in the flesh, anxiety, sneezing, and so on. The meaning of each bodily or emotional change was different, depending on the hour of the day. For instance, if the twitching eyelid change occurs at noon, if it is the left eye, that person will soon enjoy good food and wine. If it is the right eye that has a twitching eyelid, that person will soon have a terrible experience.[27] The section on "dispelling illness" (*fabing* or *qubing*) commonly found in daily-use encyclopedias was very much like an almanac in this regard. *Fabing*, which literally means "statutory diseases," were diseases caused by demons or ghosts, and were tied to the calendar. For each day one of the month a different demon was responsible for causing a different disease, and each of those diseases was treated by a different means. Like encyclopedias, almanacs included a great many talismans to treat particular illnesses, to be copied out, burned, and the ashes taken with some wine. Encyclopedias and almanacs drew on similar sources—perhaps each other—in reproducing these talismans. Almanacs also often had a section titled "Finding Doctors and Curing Illness" (Qiuyi zhibing) that gave guidance on when to consult with doctors and what means of diagnosis should or should not be employed at certain times. Almanacs also, like encyclopedias, provided a number of parallel couplets to copy and put on the wall or doorframe to prevent malevolent influences from entering, or to entice curative ones to come in.

By the early Qing, many almanacs devoted sections to "medicine" (*yixue*) or "guarding life" (*weisheng*). Some almanacs that date from at least the early nineteenth century contain a long section titled "Methods for Producing Children" (Zhongzi fangfa), which provided explicit information for women and men concerning menstruation, times for and frequency of sexual intercourse, preparations for pregnancy, and so forth. These included prescriptions for regulating menstruation, strengthening vital essence (*jing*), and supporting pregnancy. Although the majority of almanacs' content indicates that much of life is preordained, it also made it clear that human action could still influence events. For instance, if a husband and wife wanted a healthy male child, they should be rested before having intercourse, choose a quiet time on a yang day and at a yang hour, and avoid eating dog meat. After intercourse, the woman should lie on her left (yang) side. These sections also tended to have a highly moralistic tone, repeating the same sentiments as famous doctors such as Zhu Zhenheng (aka Zhu Danxi, 1281–1358), who emphasized moderation and self-restraint. The *Complete Almanac* (Daquan tongshu) for 1819, for instance, informed husbands that they must curb their selfish desires if their wives were to have healthy children. They should not force themselves upon their spouses, have intercourse too frequently, or engage in sexual activity while drunk.[28] Extant medical manuscripts include sections hand-copied from encyclopedias and almanacs showing that medical practitioners found this information useful. Some authors even thought their medical manuscripts worthy of inclusion, as shown by the title "Broad Records in a Jade Casket with Contents Worthy to be Selected for an Almanac" (Xuanze tongshu guang yuxia ji, Daoguang [1821–1850] period).[29]

Late Qing and early Republican-era medical manuscripts also include medical prescriptions copied from newspapers.[30] Some people intending to pass on medical recipes as an act of merit or gratitude took out ads and published them in newspapers. Such publicized recipes often aimed at remedying acute diseases, such as sore throat, "leg-hoisting sand disease" (*diaojiaosha*), injuries from dogs and poisonous snake bites, intrusion into the abdomen by centipedes, scalding, and accidental swallowing of metal needles. Many of these were clearly intended to garner merit, since they are prescriptions that treat life-threatening maladies. One 1874 manuscript lists prescriptions the author intended to publish in newspapers. Other medical manuscripts from that period copied prescriptions from the newspapers *Shangbao, Xibao, Shenbao, Jingbao,* and *Shibao,* and these are copied next to excerpts from (mostly contemporary) printed medical texts.[31] The practice of publishing prescriptions in newspapers continued at least through the 1930s, and medical manuscripts from that period often drew heavily on them.[32] In the last decades of the nineteenth century, it was common to find newspaper articles and advertisements recommending simple medicines, but over time, these gave way to ready-made prescriptions, commonly recommended for supplementing depletions.[33] In the twentieth century, prescriptions in newspapers that included Chinese and Western ingredients became increasingly common, and medical manuscripts informed by newspapers reflected this change as well.[34]

Practical, vernacular medical texts, in their broad range of collected knowledge, resembled encyclopedias and novels, from which they gathered information. In the late Ming, novels began to display a dizzying degree of intertextuality, which coincided with their increase in popularity.[35] *Plum in the Golden Vase* (Jinping mei, 1618 or shortly after), for instance, was not just encyclopedic in its range of contents but was an encyclopedia.[36] In its copied source texts, *Plum in the Golden Vase* collects and assimilates virtually the entire spectrum of Ming dynasty literature.[37] Almost all the major categories of materials that make up contemporary miscellanies and guides to daily life find their way into this work.[38] Why the author chose to incorporate this kind of practical knowledge into his novel is not entirely clear. From a literary standpoint, it complicates the narrative discourse and adds a great deal of robustness to the varieties of vernacular language in the novel. The novel was also a venue for displaying mastery of many topics, but there is evidence that *Plum in the Golden Vase*'s author copied source texts word for word, as if he were assembling a personal encyclopedia, like those who made manuscripts for their own use.[39] The whole spectrum of medical knowledge is presented, albeit with considerable bias. The motive for working material into the novel is often ironic. At times, it seems authors were either commenting on the original source or having a character misread a passage to humorous effect.[40] Such novels became troves of information that were given the weight of popular response, legitimized through the story context, and disseminated to the point that they became common knowledge.

Medical, fictional, and encyclopedic books newly popular in the late Ming shared a readership. Relatively cheap editions of each were widely available for purchase.[41] An episode in the seventeenth-century novel *Marriage Destinies to Awaken the World* (Xingshi yinyuan zhuan, 1661) suggests a potential owner and use of these various texts. Chao Yuan, a dissolute young man who frequents brothels and marries a prostitute, calls for the lusty quack Dr. Yang to treat him when he falls ill.[42] The doctor calls for a book to prop Chao's arm so that he can palpate his pulses. The maid has a terrible time locating a book, and finally comes up with the sex manual *Secret Games for Spring Nights, Illustrated* (Chunxiao mixi tu), which she found next to his pillow. The doctor thinks this will make Chao's pulse race, so he calls for another book, and the maid brings him the erotic novel *The Lord of Perfect Satisfaction* (Ruyijun zhuan), which the doctor also rejects. Finally they locate a sufficient book for propping an arm: the daily-use encyclopedia *Seeking No Help from Others for Myriad Things* (Wanshi buqiuren).[43] Chao, for all that his collection insinuates, at least is a reader interested in the practical knowledge found in guidebooks, encyclopedias, and novels.

Fiction, practical medical texts, and encyclopedias were all written in the vernacular or a simple classical language.[44] All three kinds of texts were also "vernacular" in that they were generally not included in officially sponsored collections. For instance, the 1772 imperial edict concerning the criteria of inclusion for books in the Qianlong Emperor's (r. 1736–1796) "Complete Library of the Four Treasuries" (*Siku quanshu*) clearly states that books like daily-use encyclopedias would not make the cut. This virtually defined daily-use encyclopedias as having no cultural value for the scholarly elite and categorized them as popular compendia of vernacular knowledge.[45]

Since the Yuan dynasty at least, large numbers of scholars who failed in the imperial civil examinations subsequently turned to medicine as an alternative career choice.[46] Many printed books served as introductions to the field. Readers often copied selections of these, along with other printed materials, into manuscripts for regular use. These medical manuscripts may have been created because their copyists could not afford printed texts or because copying was such a time-tested way of acquiring knowledge. Copyists would add their own knowledge by commenting on the source text and copying other texts side by side. These medical manuscripts are, in essence, personally created medical encyclopedias for daily use. While the manuscripts were mostly unpublished, the majority of their contents are copied from printed sources, and as such they constitute records of reading practice—a kind of commentary based on what was selected from practical texts, and what was left out.

Almost all medical manuscripts contain recipes, and some are focused on them.[47] Collections of recipes, like pharmaceutical texts, imply a much broader conception of medicine than do the medical classics or other treatises. Since the manuscripts focus on practical knowledge, when they draw on official medical texts, they select the most useful chapters. The official medical text most commonly excerpted by the medical manuscripts is the *Imperially Compiled Golden Mirror of Medical Learning* (Yuzuan Yizong jinjian), but the sections copied are invariably those on acupuncture, pox, women's ailments, pediatrics, and external medicine, the aspects of medicine most commonly addressed in practical texts.[48] The manuscripts very rarely draw on works that elucidate or debate medical theory, and look more often to formularies, materia medica, almanacs, encyclopedias, religious texts, medical cases, and reports of local practitioners. As such, these medical manuscripts give real insight into what kinds of information were thought to be important for practitioners of medicine, and what they believed. Reading through their contents, we get a view of therapeutic practice that is broadly encompassing, a vernacular tradition that is focused on expediency and unconcerned with the often contrasting or competing beliefs undergirding coexisting treatments.

TRADITIONS OF MEDICINE IN FICTION

Medicine and healing as depicted in vernacular fiction reveals the tension between the needs of readers and the dictates of fiction: sometimes graphically real, at other times hyperbolic and cliché.[49] In many cases, the use of medicine in novels reveals a distinction between middlebrow literati novels and lower-brow "popular" fiction. Authors of literati fiction allotted more space to describing diseases and doctors than did those who wrote popular fiction. Popular fiction is usually centered on action, which probably explains its general lack of detailed descriptions of or meditations on disease. This pattern is so distinct that "there is a direct correlation between the educational level of the author and the attention given to medical matters."[50] But only a few literati authors direct particular, extended, and explicit attention to medicine. Among them are Li Yu (1610–1680), who gave special consideration to sexual function and dysfunction in stories and novels; Li Ruzhen, who included over twenty-five prescriptions in his novel *Flowers in the Mirror*; and Xia Jingqu (1705–1787), who described medical expertise as one of the characteristics of the ideal Confucian gentleman in his eighteenth-century novel *Humble Words of an Old Rustic* (Yesou puyan, first published 1881, but written over a century earlier).

In all kinds of fiction, high or low, disease was a common element, but it was not usually discussed at length or depicted in detail. Fiction before *Plum in the Golden Vase* was not very interested in describing the minutiae of daily life, generally, and therefore sickness in early fiction was mostly a device to kill off a character, rather than a literary device that revealed something about that character. Interestingly, there is very little representation of epidemic disease in traditional fiction, even in popular works.[51] Perhaps epidemics did not lend themselves to metaphor well, or authors shied away from such a gruesome topic, despite the fact that many lived through major epidemics in the late Ming and Qing. In all kinds of fiction, though, people tended to fall ill while traveling. These man-out-of-place illnesses are typically attributed to unpleasant weather conditions, accidents, or passing into a different geographic area. This leads the patient to stay at an inn or temple to recuperate, where he is helped (or robbed) by a stranger, monk, or Daoist.[52]

Literati fiction also treats the theme of possession more commonly than does popular fiction. This is particularly common in novels where retribution (*bao*) is the structuring morality, and the victim of possession is being haunted by a person they have wronged or killed. Although in medical texts there are many treatments for "ghost infection" (*guizhu*) and "ghost stroke" (*guiji*), in fiction there is rarely a cure for possession, and the victim usually dies in a fit of madness.[53] Madness unto death can also happen when a victim, usually a young woman, is possessed by a fox or monkey spirit, or is seduced by one on repeated occasions. In this case, the sprit has to be exorcised to save the weakened victim from continued depletion. Professional exorcists are usually not as successful at exorcising these demons as are examination graduates and lovers. Long novels from the seventeenth and eighteenth centuries in particular liked to treat the theme of possession,[54] presumably because it fit so well with a literati obsession with bodily depletion, loss of essence or semen (*jing*), desire, sentiment (*qing*), longing, and retribution.[55]

Loss of semen and vaginal secretions gets a great deal of attention in these literati novels, which recast recreational sex and masturbation as dangerously depleting activities.[56] In fiction, aphrodisiacs, which are among the most commonly discussed drugs in medical formularies, were markers of foolish men about to die an excruciating death.[57] Adepts at using intercourse to rob the vital energy of others were likely to be defeated in this same manner by a more skillful practitioner of that art.[58] The victors are usually roving monks, Daoists, or nuns, and the narrative usually instructs readers (sometimes by addressing them directly) to avoid such people. Medical texts of the Ming period argued strongly against the possibility of prolonging life by nourishing the vital essence—the practice of having intercourse but not ejaculating so as to reabsorb that essence into the body—but they rarely fail to address the topic, which suggests that these notions were persistently on the minds of the literate. Neither medical nor literary texts questioned the power or danger inherent in the sex act. The theme of depletion was popular in part because it helped to define and distinguish *qing*, sentiment, passion, and desire—all distinct literati endeavors—from mere lust, to which the other, lesser, classes were also subject. But the concern with loss and depletion was also tied up with the literati fascination with obsession—their interest in and wariness of losing oneself in the pleasures and details of an act.[59]

A related malady important to literati fiction, lovesickness, is usually described without much reference to medical theory. Commonly women, but sometimes men, fall ill after being separated from someone for whom they may or may not have declared their love. When described, the symptoms are weakness, listlessness, and loss of appetite, sometimes accompanied by coughing and weight loss. Doctors may be called in, but only being or expecting to be reunited brings recovery, which is usually quick, particularly via sex or marriage. If however, the union is frustrated, one or both lovers die. This lovesickness theme is frequent and not limited to fiction. Yuan and Ming drama present many such lovesick cases. Lovesickness is the more refined parallel to seminal loss; the former is caused by unrestrained emotion, the latter by unrestrained carnal lust. Authors of literati fiction represented both but differentiated between sympathetic lovesickness and base depletion due to lust. They also drew upon a notion found in medical texts and popular fiction—namely, that one emotion can be used to cure another.[60]

As for those who would attempt to effect cures, doctors in popular fiction are usually called in to treat characters that have been poisoned; they rarely treat illnesses.[61] Most long works of domestic fiction, by virtue of being detailed accounts of daily life, include a doctor in their cast of characters, though these usually play a minor role. Fiction high and low featured three or four quacks for every talented doctor, which presumably reflected prevailing attitudes toward and suspicions about that profession. In the Ming and Qing, there was a tendency to valorize "lower-class" characters from iffy professions who upheld Confucian values as a way to shame their social betters who did not uphold standards of loyalty, honor, or humaneness. These included professional storytellers and courtesans as well as doctors. Portrayals of charlatans also established effective medical knowledge as something both rare and virtuous.

As for drugs, poisonous and beneficial, one of the more common medicinals discussed in fiction is human flesh. Dangerous monks try to kill pregnant women or otherwise obtain the fetus for use in some kind of magical medicine. Demons and villains particularly desire to eat the flesh of devout or virile characters for its medical properties. If trying to eat human flesh characterized villains, trying to get a sick relative to eat one's own flesh, usually in a medicinal soup and without their knowledge, marked a great filial sacrifice of a noble Confucian. This was potent human medicine indeed, and it rarely failed to cure the patient.[62]

In both popular and literati fiction, good medicine works immediately, its potency often indicated by its rarity or repugnancy. Authors rarely mention therapies other than medicinal prescriptions or apotropaic medicine. When authors discuss therapies such as massage, acupuncture, and moxibustion, they designate them as the practices of unlearned medical hacks. Writers may have excluded them from fiction because they are therapies, and the demands of plot require a cure. Therapies are also likely absent because illness in fiction is usually not chronic, only poorly treated. There is a general belief that an "upright person" (*zheng ren*) is immune to demons and less likely to fall ill than others; the corollary is the foolish person ruining his health and inviting disaster with immoderate living or otherwise tempting fate. Novelists rarely mention healing through prayer, although many families made copies of sutras for free distribution to accrue merit that might be used to fight off illness. In both popular and literati fiction one of the most desirable kinds of medicine is fictional—a miraculous pill of unknown composition.

LITERARY LOGIC AND REGISTERS OF MEDICINE

When medical texts told stories it was to prove a point. In practical medical texts, anecdotes were facts that served as evidence, even in the absence of a logical explanation. The mechanism is different than that of the poetry employed throughout the *Systematic Materia Medica*, for instance, which relies either on the authority of the well-known poet or poem, or on the sort of daily-use logic that is found in practical poems. In the *Materia Medica*, poems were usually included in the "explanation of names" (*shiming*) or "collected notes" (*jijie*) section of each drug's description that explained which names a drug was known by and why, and what its properties were. To cite just one of many references to poetry, Li Shizhen discusses the properties of *xiebai*, the stem of green onion:

> Poet Du Fu wrote a poem about the long-stamen onion:
>
> "In the color of green hay
> With a round head like hairpin of jade
> Warm as it is
> It works to warm the cold in chest."
>
> What the poem says is in conformity with the record in the classics. So what Su Song said in his *Tujing Bencao* [about *xiebai* being] 'cold and tonifying' is not correct."[63]

For Li Shizhen at least, poetry was an authoritative source for knowing the natural world and the properties of objects in it. Stories were usually included in the "indications" (*zhuzhi*), "explications" (*faming*), or "prescriptions" (*fufang*) section of a given drug entry. If poems verified a drug's properties, stories provided a literary logic or pattern of precedents to convince readers that the medicine was effective.

Claims made in the *Systematic Materia Medica* were legitimized by citing geographic provenance (knowledge originating in a city), experience (tried and true, personally witnessed), or text (famous poet, weighty text), but vernacular medicine in a fictional framework persuaded through narrative logic or familiarity taken for truth. Vernacular medicine encompasses many traditions, one of which is usually characterized by historians of medicine as "magic." In the *Systematic Materia Medica* many drugs are deemed effective because of precedent, no matter how far-fetched the story of the precedent may seem to modern readers. Such stories often present an argument for the drug's literal action based on the logic of metaphor. That fish are averse to vinegar makes vinegar the perfect cure for hallucinations brought on by having eaten too much fish, for instance.[64] If there was no such logic based on homonyms or etymology, the medical author had no recourse but to cite a story with a familiar structure (many ineffective prescriptions followed by a miraculous one) as evidence for his claims.

Since delineations between apotropaic and elite medicine were age-old, we might expect them to employ different systems of logic, as there were many different ways of thinking about the body and its relation to the cosmos. Yet, as doctors in the Ming and Qing increasingly adopted vernacular practices and folded them into the more orthodox traditions, we see that these systems of logic could coexist if not exactly overlap.[65] This was certainly the case in fiction. Authors of fiction may have found certain apotropaic practices lent themselves to literary use more readily than those of elite medicine, but these were practices observed in real life too. The 1736 Zhejiang provincial gazetteer discusses at least twenty-six cases of magical medicine in its "Filial Devotion and Friendliness" (Xiaoyou) section. In most of these, an adult male seeks to cure a sick parent by medicine and prayer, offering up his own life if all else fails. The magical healing usually takes the form of a god appearing in a dream to grant the wish, the devoted son cutting his thigh or liver to make medicinal soup, or the natural world responding to extreme grief or devotion during mourning and restoring the patient to life.[66]

The term "literary logic" is a way of explaining the causal relationship between a therapy and its effects. "Magical" correspondences can also be understood as literary correspondences. The logic of metaphor, the logic of homophones, symbolic correlation, metonymy, and the meaning inherent in Chinese characters—derived from component parts of a character, its etymology, and its polysemy—all fall under the rubric of literary logic. For instance, peach blossoms kill demons that have infected the body, because arrow shafts were made of peach wood and killed things outside of the body.[67] The logic of homophones is a major part of knowing the uses and properties of objects in the natural world dating back at least to the *Classic of Mountains and Seas* (Shanhai jing, 4th–1st century BCE). This is the sort of thinking that asserted that a patient would not be lost or confused (*mi*) if he wore some lost-mulberry (*migu*) in the belt. Although not strictly a book of pharmaceutical medicines, the *Classic of Mountains and Seas* employs literary logic to illustrate the tie between the nature of the drug and the disease it treats—the best-known example of this being the claim that eating hermaphroditic animals will cure jealousy, because such an animal presumably does not require a mate.[68] These kinds of logic lie outside of the *yinyang* and five-phases systems of correspondence and were all well represented in materia medica, almanacs, and encyclopedias.

Early Qing medical scholars produced a corpus of diverse and complex new knowledge that absorbed folk or popular medicine into the elite canon.[69] Although demonology was, by most accounts, the most influential system of healing in China, literati physicians did not traditionally practice it.[70] The late Ming and Qing periods marked a change in the tradition, in part because medical authors became keen on incorporating demonology, which had existed independently of Confucian doctrine, into systematic correspondence. This period saw a flourishing of literate doctors who were deeply invested in pharmaceutical treatments as well as demonological, apotropaic, and magical medicine. Virtually all of the best-known authors of Ming and Qing medical works, including Yu Bo (fl. 1515), Li Shizhen, Li Ting (fl. 1570), Xu Chunfu (fl. 1570), Gong Tingxian (fl. 1615), Xu Dachun (1693–1771), and Sun Derun (fl. 1826), along with a host of less-well-known medical authors, acknowledged the pathogenic influence of demons as a self-evident fact, though they also frequently declined to offer up treatments for those maladies. Belief in the existence of luck, of evil spirits, and in a cosmos that is tied together in mysterious ways was not at all limited to the lower or uneducated segments of the population. Historians of medicine in China have made it clear that both kinds of healing practice—elite medicine and "other" kinds of healing (folk, popular, and apotropaic)—very frequently coexisted in practice, if less often in printed medical texts.

Among the more symbolic of the apotropaic cures in the *Systematic Materia Medica*, old mirrors (*gujing*) are particularly effective in repelling demons. Li Shizhen says that mirrors are the essence of gold and water. They are bright (*ming*) on the inside and dark (*an*) on the outside. Like ancient swords, ancient mirrors are capable of dispelling malevolent spirits, evil, and disobedient demons (*bixie meiwu e*). Li quotes Ge Hong's (283–343) *Master Who Embraces Simplicity* (Baopu zi, 317, revised 330), saying that ancient creatures can take the shape of a human, but that mirrors reveal their true forms. This is why Daoists hang mirrors on their backs when walking in the mountains, because when a demon sees his own true form, he will be frightened and run away. In the *Materia Medica* and elsewhere, stories abound of people looking into mirrors to see things that would ordinarily be hidden.[71] For this reason (and because they are also able to dispel a child's night crying), Li recommends that "every family should hang a big mirror up to prevent invasion by devils and evils."[72]

In fiction, mirrors are a figure for individual subjectivity, and in both fictional and medical literature, mirrors cure demons and illusions. In *The Story of the Stone*, Jia Rui is told to look at the back of a mirror depicting a skeleton as a way of curing him of an illness brought on by longing and depletion. The skeleton is either that of Jia Rui himself or the object of his desire, and thus a (Buddhist) reminder that life and desire are ephemeral. This act of looking into the back of the mirror also points the reflective surface of the mirror away from himself, and therefore Jia Rui is unwittingly also fending off demons tempted to infect him or carry off his soul because of his physical depletion and moral transgressions. The mirror, after all, is said to cure "diseases of rushing indiscriminately into action because of evil thoughts" (*xiesi wangdong zhi zheng*), a term that can simply mean "illnesses that come from impure mental activity," or, if taken literally, a disease caused by the demons that rush into those who overexert themselves with thinking.

The *Systematic Materia Medica* details many treatments for illnesses such as demonic influence (*guizhu*, or sex with demons), demons (*guimei*), evil (heteropathic) qi (*xieqi* or *e'qi*), ghost/demon qi (*guiqi*), and ghost essence (*guijing*). Apotropaic medicine employs a metaphorical logic, but it also subverts metaphorical readings in fiction. To differing degrees for different people, demons were real, and the way they were read in fiction would have been meaningfully different based on that degree of belief. Readers might consider the demons in fiction to be "personal demons" or character flaws, or they just as easily could view them as real demons that punish character flaws with illness. To mention just one more example from *Story of*

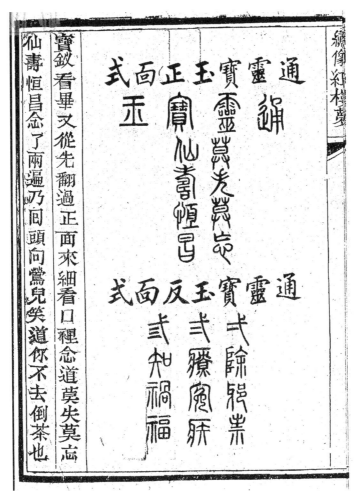

Figure 1.2.   One example of Baoyu's talisman from a late eighteenth-century edition of *The Story of the Stone*. From Cao Xueqin,
Honglou meng yibai ershi hui, call number D8653500, University
of Tokyo Library.

the Stone, Baoyu's jade is literally a talisman that he wears around his
neck. It does (or claims to do) almost everything apotropaic medicine
seeks to achieve: guard against evil spirits (*chu xiesui*), cure retributory illnesses (*liao yuanji*), and predict disaster and fortune (*zhi
huofu*) (fig. 1.2).[73]

When Baoyu loses his jade talisman, he exhibits all of the symptoms
of soul loss.[74] It was commonly thought that a person had two souls—a

spiritual soul (*hun*), which governs the higher faculties of mind and heart and corresponds to yang forces, and a bodily soul (*po*), which is tied to yin and governs physical senses and bodily functions.[75] The spiritual soul, light and volatile, can easily be separated from a living person. This separation can happen during sleep, be caused by fright or shock, or be the work of soul-stealing demons or magicians.[76] It results in a state characterized by trances and madness, and leads to death.[77] The condition is cured with a ritual known as "calling back the soul" (*zhaohun, shouhun,* or *jiaohun*).[78] Baoyu's fits of delirium are caused by the bewitching of a specialist hired by Aunt Zhao; by being frightened when the maid Nightingale teasingly tells Baoyu that his love, Lin Daiyu, is returning home to the south; and by the loss of his jade, which is repeatedly referred to as his "very soul" by characters and commentators alike. Apotropaic medicine is described when Baoyu loses his jade and falls ill because of it (chapter 113), when exorcising demons from the garden (chapter 102), when repelling demons that have come to take his friend Qin Zhong to hell (chapter 16), when keeping demons at bay during Qin Shi's funeral (chapter 14), and when combating the spell put on Baoyu and Wang Xifeng (chapter 25).[79] Distinguishing between healing and metaphor in fiction requires more than a disambiguation between represented reality and metaphorical magic, since magic was a part of the real world.

FAMILIAR FANTASTIC STORIES

Stories in medical texts normalize the weird and bring treatments that skeptical readers find incredible down to earth. Authors of such texts most often resorted to textual precedent to bolster their claims, but they also referred to stories from cases or personal experience. Medical manuscripts in particular show a good deal of concern with veracity, or at least with how to lay claim to it. A prescription frequently is followed by the comment "has been effective" (*yanguo*) or "has been effective *x* times" (*yanguo x ci*). Sometimes, as in medical case histories, prescriptions include details, such as the names and addresses of the patients who were successfully treated. This gives claims of the prescription's efficacy the appearance of fact. Other times, folk recipes are accompanied by remarks such as "passed on from Beijing" (*Beijing chuanlai*) and "transmitted from Wei county" (*Weixian chuanlai*), details meant to convey the authority of knowledge that comes from a major city or county center.

Pharmaceutical and recipe books encompassed a much broader definition of medicine than more traditional texts, often citing fantastic or miraculous stories that illustrated the miraculous effectiveness of some medicine. A typical example is the story attached to the prescription "barefoot great immortal's recipe of pills with a fish's swim bladder to seed sons" (*chijiao daxian yubiao zhongzi wanfang*). The story features a sixty-year-old man named Zhou who had one wife and nine concubines but no sons. His "body was weak, his essence cool and his marrow cold, and his original yang unstable," and therefore it was difficult for him to beget a son. Since he was distressed to be without male offspring, he traveled to a famous mountain where he met a Daoist master. The immortal, impressed with Zhou's sincerity, gave him a good recipe that "strengthens muscles and bones, adds to the essence, and supplements marrow. It nourishes the yin, and stabilizes the foundations." Zhou respectfully received the medicine, followed the Daoist's recommendations, and felt his body regain strength and vigor. His bones became firm, and his eyes became clear. His hair turned black. Subsequently he fathered seven sons; his clan expanded enormously. Zhou died at the age of ninety-seven.[80] There are no details in this story that point to historical truth. We are not provided with Zhou's full name or the name of the Daoist, nor of the prescription, its ingredients, effects, or indications, or anything else about it. This made the story useful for arguing the effectiveness of any aphrodisiac the physician cared to prescribe. The story is listed under the prescription for "black goat pills" (*wuyang wan*) in one manuscript, and could easily fit under any number of prescription recipes. There are many such stories, and many versions of the same story. They must have been convincing for them to have been so often repeated. In materia medica and pharmaceutical literature, these sorts of fantastic stories are usually found under the sections in each entry for a drug that discusses the author's own experience with it. Stories were most commonly attached to drugs relating to sex and procreation, but they were also appended to drugs whose origins and effects are not clearly linked to their names or to symbolic properties.

Medical case histories, told from one doctor's perspective, became a subspecialty of Chinese medical literature, and were collected and published as stand-alone volumes for the first time in the late Ming, and commonly in the Qing.[81] Cases told stories of effective doctors, described symptoms as a narrator does, showed doctors in dialogue with the patient, and ultimately ended with the doctor demonstrating

superior knowledge of medicine by curing the patient when others
were unable to do so. Many extant manuscripts from the late Qing
and Republican periods either quote from published collections of
medical case histories or record case histories from the practices of
their teachers or friends, or of their own practice. Recorded cases presumably served as models or teaching texts for novice doctors, and
perhaps also as arrows added to the quiver of a shady medicine peddler.[82] In addition to approximating the form of legal cases (gong'an
or yanyu) and court-case fiction (gong'an xiaoshuo), medical cases
have been compared to "tales of the strange" (zhiguai) and "unofficial
histories" (yeshi), and are characterized by brief anecdotal accounts
of events purportedly witnessed or heard about by the author. These
are written in simple prose and mainly unadorned by literary techniques such as allusion or metaphor.[83]

The employment of a drug in medical cases implied a reading,
a diagnosis. The following example illustrates how medical cases
shared linguistic codes and structures with detective fiction, the
graphic details of novels, and the secret and miraculous events of
"stories of the strange." This case comes from Xu Dachun's *Medical Cases of Huixi* (Huixi yi'an), written in the mid-eighteenth century, and published posthumously in 1855, with commentary by the
prominent Qing physician Wang Mengying (1808–1867). In this case
of "lower chancres" (xiagan), a common designation for syphilis or
similar venereal disease, Dr. Xu narrates,

> Shen Weide of Puyuan, terrible lower lesions, his penis down to
> the root had completely rotted off, and he urinated through a slit
> between bones, which caused him to cry out with pain. His anus
> was also festering to a depth of half an inch. He had been taken to
> the Yu family, where he had been told that he would be lucky if his
> life could be saved. [Doctor] Yu had never seen such an illness and
> was reluctant to try to cure it. He gave him pills to remove the poi-
> son and strengthen the blood, and a topical medicine to relieve the
> pain. After a few applications, it got to the point where it no lon-
> ger hurt. After two months, it formed a scar and [Shen] was able to
> walk. But all that remained of his penis was the root. [At that time]
> Yu by chance was reading a secret book. In it was a prescription to
> grow a penis. The prescription called for a dog fetus. The Yu family
> dog had just given birth to three puppies. They took one, covered it
> in mud, and baked it. They added it to other things. Two years later
> [Weide] unexpectedly had a son. His entire extended family was in an
> uproar: without a male member, how could he conceive a son? This
> was probably because Weide had family wealth and the beneficiaries

had covetous feelings. His parents-in-law made secret inquires to me. Shen said, "After I took the medicine, my member grew back. How can you doubt my having a son?" I then gathered Shen's family together to see it, and the penis had completely grown back, but the member only had joints and no skin [like bamboo]. After that, he had another son. The many who heard this [story], both near and far, took it as an extraordinary event. Even today, those who hear it consider it remarkable.[84]

As in the discussion of stories attached to aphrodisiac prescriptions, that this story is fantastical is simply brushed aside by saying that those who hear it consider it "remarkable." It is this deviation from the norm that purportedly somehow makes the story more believable, but this deviation also called for the story's telling in narrative form.

Li Shizhen in the *Systematic Materia Medica* relates another remarkable story of a drug found in Hong Mai's (1123–1202) compendium of anomalous events, the *Record of the Listener* (Yijian zhi):

Mr. Lu Ying, official title Jinshi of Xiuchuan, suddenly vomited blood profusely, with spasms and contractions, fright, and maniacal manner. Late at night, the patient wanted to jump out of the window. This was repeated the next night. Drugs of all kinds had been tried to no avail. He dreamed of seeing Guanyin [Goddess of Mercy], who told him a secret prescription—one dose of which would root out the ailment. The scholar remembered the prescription and managed to have it filled and prepared. He recovered after taking it. The prescription is as follows . . . [85]

Dreams in which people encounter immortals or bodhisattvas are often authoritative sources for prescriptions in the variety of materia medica literature.

Relying on a literary logic and archetypal plot structure normalizes the miraculous. Stories also account for what does not fit into an orderly cosmos. The tremendous number of prescriptions handed down by immortals, bodhisattvas, dreams, and accident all amount to a deus ex machina in a chaotic world of disease and illness left unattended by emperor and officials.[86] In the absence of imperially sponsored medicine, and given a vast sea of medical knowledge transmitted by word of mouth, the precedent provided by stories, as well as the literary logic imposed on that knowledge, helped to distinguish efficacy from chaos.

Some medical recipes have much in common with, or perhaps were influenced by, anomalous accounts, such as Pu Songling's (1640–1715) "Liaozhai's Records of the Strange" (Liaozhai zhiyi). One example comes from a late-Qing medical manuscript titled "A Convenient Overview of Medical Formulas" (Yifang bianlan), one of the few works of ordinary medical literature to record a "recipe to treat bewitchment by coquettish fox [spirits]" (zhi humei fang):

> Whenever a fox seduces a male or female, it sucks with its mouth human semen during daylight and engages in sexual intercourse like a human person at night. Smear tung tree oil [tongyou] on the genitals, and the [fox spirit] leaves by itself. Or rub them with pearl orchid root [zhulan gen],[87] and the animal will die. Dry the animal's meat, grind it to powder, and ingest it. This is even better.[88]

Another medical manuscript records the same prescription: "To treat persons confused by a fox spirit, regardless whether male or female. Smear genuine tung tree oil [an emetic] into the vagina or onto the penis. The fox will vomit severely and then leave."[89] These are mundane prescriptions compared to many more elaborate apotropaic remedies to expel or protect against demons that require talismans, special objects or times of year, incantations, and so on. The first recipe suggests that the patient ingest the powder of the dead fox in a sympathetic gesture that uses the virility of the fox as a tonifying (buyang) drug that can undo the depletive harm caused by the fox.[90] Mundane cures for fantastic illnesses place the weird in a nosology that is a logical extension of knowledge (in this case, sympathetic medicine—"like cures like") found in fiction and medicine.

The range of medical belief and practice is particularly wide in these manuscripts. Although the prescription to treat bewitchment by fox spirits is uncommon, the range of implied medical belief in the manuscript that contains it is not. This manuscript, for example, contains a lengthy section titled "Strange Illnesses, Strange Cures" (Qizheng qizhifa) with some particularly bizarre prescriptions—syphilis is treated with "black gold paper" (wujin zhi) and red silk that has been used by a married woman. Some of these strange prescriptions were copied from Li Lou's Extraordinary Recipes for Unusual Pathoconditions (Guaizheng qifang, 1592). The manuscript combines the strange with the mundane, with a great number of practical prescriptions and a large section with long quotes from several printed books on external medicine. This section focuses on recipes to cure syphilis (yangmei) and includes extensive theoretical and etiological discourses on syphilis taken from doctors such as Zhu Danxi, Xue Lizhai, and Wang Ren'an.[91] Following this are sections on "apotropaic remedies," (jinyao), as recorded in Zhao Xuemin's Qing dynasty

work *Strings of Refined [Therapies]* (Chuanya, 1759).[92] The manuscript takes information from other, presumably similar, sources relating the knowledge and experience of itinerant healers. Prescriptions
are culled from both published works and regional sources. Although
more than three quarters of this manuscript are devoted to medicine,
like many other medical manuscripts, it also includes tangential or
unrelated information. It lists several methods of writing invisibly,
and of making invisible writings appear, as well as directions on how
to write on difficult surfaces such as oilpaper and water. It explains
how to breed animals and how to prevent them from growing, such
as "how to raise dwarf chickens" and "how to raise dwarf dogs," as
well as "how to raise turtles with green fur," "how to raise pigs and
have them become fat easily," and "how to raise colored chickens."
Furthermore, the text gives advice on cosmetics, on pharmaceutical
substances that will protect a fetus, and on how to give up smoking
opium.[93] Another manuscript, which quotes many of the same recipes,
adds a section on gynecology, discourses copied from *Instructions on
the [Movements in the] Vessels in [Verses of] Four Characters* (Siyan
maijue, Song dynasty) with commentary, and a section on talismans
(*shufu*).[94] Some of these talismans are recommended for gynecological
problems and abscesses, while others are for "expelling evil" (*bixie*),
"suppressing ghosts" (*zhenguai*), and "protecting the body" (*hushen*).
This comingling of the practical and the fantastical is reminiscent of
tales of strange events, as well as the *Classic of Mountains and Seas*.[95]

Many of the stories draw on a familiar literary or sympathetic
logic, and they are not set off by introductory remarks that suggest that they are anything less than factual. The world implied by
these medical manuscripts and by pharmaceutical literature is full of
strange creatures and things that are primarily useful and only sec-
ondarily curious. One prescription, for example, a "recipe to treat
choking disease" (*zhi yebing fang*), was supposedly "transmitted by a
strange priest" (*yiseng suochuan*):

> To drink fresh goose blood several times will bring the cure. Once
> there was a priest named Zijiu of the Xianhua temple outside the
> small south gate of Wuchang. He suffered from a choking disease,
> and no drug was effective. When he was about to die, he said to a
> disciple, "As I suffer like this, I should think that there is an object [in
> me] that deserves to be held in high esteem. After I have passed on,
> dissect me before you encoffin me." The disciple did as he was told
> and found [in the priest's throat] a bone shaped like a hairpin. He
> took it and placed it on the table with the sacred scriptures, where it

remained for many years. [One day], a priest from the Rong people
happened to visit the temple. When [Zijiu's] disciple set out to slaughter a goose and was just about to cut the animal's throat, he suddenly
saw the bone. He took it and pierced the animal so that its blood
spurted out. The bone melted. When Zijiu's disciple himself began
to suffer from choking disease, he concluded that goose blood could
bring the cure. He drank it several times and was healed. He gave this
recipe to many people, and it was effective in all cases.[96]

There is a distinct aversion to questioning serendipity in these stories
copied into manuscripts, as seen in figure 1.3, below. They record
effective treatments, and the proof of their efficacy relies on the fact
that the medicine has a story. Eyebrows should have been raised at a
story that includes dissection (which was frowned upon by Confu-
cians as a violation of filial piety) and happenstance, but the logic
that goose blood could dissolve a [presumably goose] bone is powerful. The logic of that story imputes *why* a certain cure is effective, no
matter how fantastical.

Li Shizhen, in his *Systematic Materia Medica*, was a bit more skeptical. He evaluated claims of efficacy and found many to be wanting.
Ge Hong claims, in his *Master Who Embraces Simplicity*, that spi-
ders and leeches could be used to make a pill that allowed a person
to live under water. Li points out, "These fantastical accounts of the
remedy masters cannot be believed."[97] But it is clear from his penchant to cite all kinds of miraculous tales that it is only some tales,
perhaps only those of the remedy masters that should not be believed.
Not only did Li cite fantastic tales, he also cited books in the genre
"tales of the strange" *as* proof:

> Urine from a white horse has proven effective in curing diseases [aris-
> ing from] obstruction in the belly. According to *Zu Taizhi's Records
> of the Strange* [Zu Taizhi zhiguai]: Once, a man and his servant both
> suffered from a painful illness of the heart and stomach. When the
> servant died, the man cut open his body and found a white turtle
> [bie] with red eyes, still alive. The man stuffed all manner of drugs
> into the turtle's mouth, but it still would not die. Another man riding
> by on a white horse noticed this. His horse urinated on the turtle, and
> the turtle's head started to shrink. The turtle was given horse urine to
> drink, and soon the turtle dissolved into water. At this point, the man
> realized that taking a white horse's urine would cure his illness. This
> proves the efficacy of the drug.[98]

The structure of the horse urine story and the goose blood story is
repeated in hundreds of stories in materia medica and recipe books

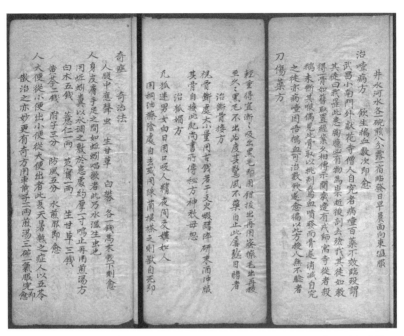

Figure 1.3. From a late-Qing manuscript, "An Easy View of Medical Formulas" (Yifang bianlan), showing (*left*) a section on "strange illnesses, strange cures"; (*center*) a prescription for curing "bewitchment by coquettish fox spirits" (which is *not* one of the strange illnesses or cures); (*right*) a cure for choking disease. Staatsbibliothek zu Berlin—Preußischer Kulturbesitz, East Asia Department Slg. Unschuld 8453.

(*fangshu*). Symptoms of an illness are described, a cause is discovered by investigation or observation (often involving dissection or some other taboo violation), something odd or miraculous happens, a connection is made to a cure, it is said to be effective, and the matter is thus proved. No questions are asked about *why* horse urine works to cure abdominal blockages or *how* a turtle got into the servant's belly, let alone that of the master. Various "turtle" (*bie*) illnesses are discussed in the *Systematic Material Medica*, most of which describe the malady as a blockage caused by a turtle [-shaped] conglomeration—that is, a blockage in the shape of a turtle. Here, as often happens in fiction, a medical notion that depends on metaphor or figurative language paradoxically becomes literalized in the tale. Li does not question the provenance of this story, coming as it did from a collection of records of strange occurrences. In the last paragraph of Li Shizhen's voluminous work, he writes about human anomalies and in so doing explains his underlying principle with regard to the fantastic:

> The evolution and transformation of the Heaven and Earth are boundless. Human beings also have endless changes. . . . All changes are based on the condition of the qi. When a person who is not well-versed says that such things in strange forms and odd shapes are unbelievable, it means he has not learned that all things are subject to infinite changes in infinite time. How can it be said "It is impossible?"[99]

Which is to say, the more learning a person has, the more he has read, the more familiar the fantastic becomes.

CHAPTER 2

Reading Medically

Novel Illnesses, Novel Cures

The well-known Qing poet Yue Jun (1766—1814) writes about a "foolish woman" (*chinüzi*) in a passage from his 1794 collection *Fodder for the Ears* (Ershi lü), volume 2, published just two years after *The Story of the Stone*.[1] He tells of a young woman who died from reading *Story of the Stone* "like all those who died from reading *The Peony Pavilion*." She had obtained a copy of the novel from her older brother's desk and could not stop reading it. She was so enthralled she neglected food and sleep. When she came to a beautiful passage, she would stop and contemplate it and then continue reading as she wept. She would read the passage over and over again, ten or a hundred times, not necessarily even finishing the chapter. Reading thus, she fell ill. Fearing that it was the book that had caused their daughter's illness, her father and mother quickly consigned it to the flames. The young woman cried out, "How can you burn Baoyu and Daiyu!" She fell into a pathetic delusion and would talk without rhyme or reason, always calling out to Baoyu in the middle of her dreaming sleep. Shamans and doctors recommended a hundred cures, but none had any effect. One night, staring at the lamp by the side of her bed, she muttered, "Baoyu is here, Baoyu is here," and following that drank her tears and died.[2]

This young woman manifests the symptoms of one obsessed—forgetting to eat or sleep, exhibiting passionate appreciation, and repeating actions over and over. Going beyond obsessive engagement with the novel, she becomes deluded and mistakes fiction for reality. But her story is complicated, since Yue Jun disavows the veracity of this

tale.[3] The story about a woman who *really* dies from reading fiction
and mistaking it for reality is perhaps itself fictional. Yet, she suffers
from a passionate empathy for the lovesick protagonist just like all
of those young women who died from reading *The Peony Pavilion*
(Mudan ting, 1598), a phenomenon that was so well known it also
became the subject of entertainment literature.[4] The truth of the story
may be in doubt, but Yue Jun adds commentary to it that makes death
by novel seem like a given:

> Someone said, "*The Story of the Stone* is a book of illusion. Baoyu
> is made up; he does not really exist. For the girl to die for him, that
> would be foolish in the extreme." Alas! Under heaven who is not
> made up, who really exists? The foolish die; does that mean that
> those who are not foolish live long? Moreover, as for the death of the
> girl, it was for *qing*, not for Baoyu.[5]

These women were perceived to have died because they were foolish readers; they could not prevent the novel from provoking in them
extreme emotion. They could not preserve a distinction between fiction and reality.

DEATH BY READING

Reading vernacular literature in the late Ming and early Qing dynasties was a danger to health, and women readers were particularly at
risk. Stories of women readers who so identified with the plight of
beautiful and talented female protagonists that they themselves fell ill
and died were common. The famously beautiful concubine, poet, and
commentator Xiaoqing (1595–1612) and two of the three wives of Wu
Wushan, Chen Tong (d. 1665) and Tan Ze (d. 1674),[6] for instance, are
just a few of several young women whose deaths were said to have
been caused by reading *Peony Pavilion*.[7] These women all read and
commented on the play, passionately engaging with it despite becoming increasingly sick, and refusing to put it down until they died. The
heroine of that play, Du Liniang, dies from lovesickness and melancholy brought on by desire conceived in a dream, and her figure
sparked a rage among young women readers.[8] *The Peony Pavilion*
had repeatedly found "discerning and sympathetic readers among the
fair sex, who intensely identified with Du Liniang."[9] Due to its length
and complexity, *Peony Pavilion* was a play as often read as viewed.[10]
Viewing the play was considered dangerous, but reading it was even
more so.[11] The misreading of the play unto death follows the same

pattern of Yue Jun's foolish young woman, and their deaths in turn further obfuscated the fictionality of the play.[12] Xiaoqing's commentary on the play was burned in a fire (caused by a jealous wife), but her life and poems were the subject of many poems by women, and the three wives' commentary was a popular edition of the text. Their commentary was concrete evidence that they had painstakingly read these works and interacted with them.[13] These women's illnesses and deaths, now made into texts, circulated among other women readers who became as obsessed with the texts as the heroines that came before them.

Scholars have suggested that the recurrent cultural myths about the deaths of the readers and commentators who come in contact with *Peony Pavilion* point to an infectious danger emanating from the play.[14] They argue that it was the affective power of the play that caused a fatal response in women readers.[15] While it was true that only masterworks of literature could kill, it was equally true that it was primarily beautiful and intelligent young women who were susceptible to death by reading.[16] A well-known story about a young Xiaoqing says that a Buddhist nun, after testing her with the heart sutra pronounces her brilliant and says that she will live longer if she never learns to read.[17] A widespread belief during this period in the Qing held that literacy and writing posed a grave danger to the health and happiness of talented young women and, in extreme cases, could even be blamed for their deaths.[18]

Concern for the health of beautiful young women was not confined to stories. Medical texts from the seventeenth century to the mid-nineteenth century depicted women as the "sickly sex," particularly vulnerable to blood loss and bodily depletion,[19] symptoms that were most commonly brought on by a womanly predisposition to overemotionality, and, more precisely, oversentimentality.[20] Ming physicians paid much more attention to the unrestrained emotions of unmarried women than had their predecessors.[21] For example, the physician Wang Ji's (1463–1539) medical case histories suggested that women are prone to suffering from mournful or apprehensive thoughts.[22] Another sixteenth-century physician, Gong Xin, also pointed out that sexually frustrated women—in particular nuns, widows, unmarried women, and scholars' and merchants' wives—"easily become pensive and jealous. They are melancholic whenever encountering things against their will. Their anger is full and qi blocked; their blood depleting and qi replete. That is why they suffer from yin fighting with yang, periodic fevers, loss of appetite, a weak appearance, and other disorders."[23] Weather and emotions were by far the most important causes of illness in premodern China.[24] These affected both sexes, but medical case histories and literati fiction tend to be more fascinated with the emotional plight of women, who were susceptible to passionate extremes, and the literature that could provoke them.

This development in the discourse of women's medicine coincided with a literati fascination—even obsession—with sentimentality, desire, and emotion associated with the "cult of *qing*."[25] The dangers of excessive emotion were recognized very early in the medical tradition, and remained a major concern of physicians throughout the Qing. Xu Dachun, writing in the Qing, echoed the oft-repeated notion that all of the illnesses man might suffer from are related either to the seven emotions[26] or to the six excesses.[27] Excessive emotion had from very early on been conceived as *the* primary internal cause of illness. Excessive emotions were dangerous because they resulted in the depletion of bodily resources. Excess and depletion were linked and discussed in many medical treatises and manuscripts under the common formulation "depletion and repletion" (*xushi*). Though they are paired opposites, one leads to the other: excess (emotion, sex) leads to depletion, and depletion similarly leads to excess (depleted yin, which is cool, leads to excessive heat in the body). Depletion of blood (yin), essence (yang), and qi could happen through loss (outflow from the body, particularly regarding blood and essence) or by being consumed through exertion or taxation. Depleted conditions were susceptible to invasion by wind, miasmas, demons, or other pathogenic influences. Depletion enabled exogenous forces to enter the body, and also permitted the lighter of two souls residing in every body to escape, resulting in "soul loss," which manifested as a state of confusion, hallucination, or even insanity.[28] Excessive emotions directly consumed bodily resources, just as excessive sex resulted in their loss.[29]

The medical case history narratives collected by Wang Ji, arguably the most successful and prolific physician of his time, focused on depletion and excess. Some scholars read his frequent diagnoses of male corporeal depletion as an extension of his era's moral concern about the excesses of pleasure and consumption.[30] Wang treated depletion disorders in his male patients that were brought on by the immoral behaviors and high social aspirations of the newly emergent merchant class in his native Huizhou region. He advocated warming and replenishing drugs to boost the protective system he thought his upwardly mobile male clients had worn down through excessive sex, food, and wine. Wang also quoted Zhu Zhenheng to more clearly draw a line between "depleted men" and "emotional women" in an essay titled "On Women's Disorders No. 89," which focuses on female susceptibility to emotions: "Women's temperament is to hold on to the emotions; they are not able to release them and are more often [than men] damaged by the seven emotions."[31]

Stories of women dying from excessive emotion were often retold, seemingly with relish. Chinese literati of the seventeenth century displayed a morbid fascination with the death of young women, often in their teens, who read fiction and poetry and who were moved to write commentary or poetry.[32] By the mid-Qing death from reading became entangled with an obsession with chastity, and with maladies resulting from repressed passion or love. An example from *Story of the Stone* illustrates this conflation. Lin Daiyu, the ailing, beautiful young heroine, reads and memorizes passages from romantic dramas, constantly demonstrates her intelligence with clever banter, writes poetry and commentaries, and in many ways shares a pathology with Xiaoqing, the three wives, and other female readers. One of the first things the reader of *Story of the Stone* learns about Lin Daiyu is that she is congenitally sick because of sadness, and that sadness is tied to her debt of tears from a previous incarnation. She dies of consumption resulting from yin depletion brought on by desire, a predisposition to sadness, and her obsession with risqué works of fiction and drama.[33] She created a fervor of her own among readers, with "every languishing young lady imagining herself a Daiyu," as seen in the case of the young woman discussed by Yue Jun.[34] Fictional characters modeled bad reading for their own female readers.[35] It was not reading per se that was dangerous, but the presumed inability of young women to avoid the excesses of emotion that fiction could provoke in the unsophisticated. Their youth, their naïveté, and their inexperience ultimately caused the resulting death by reading vernacular literature.[36] One of the earliest accounts of death by reading plays concerns an unmarried girl named Miss Yu (Yu Niang), who is said to have composed a commentary on *Peony Pavilion* shortly before she died at the age of seventeen. Two poems by the play's author, Tang Xianzu, lament her untimely death.[37] The tragic and inevitable image of the dying young woman obsessively reading about dying young women reading was a popular one for male readers, the self-appointed guardians of sentimentality, true feeling and fictional practice, who by discussing these charming, emotional women were also establishing their purview over reading fiction.

Such deaths were caused not by the affective power of the work; rather, the reader was sensitive enough to be deeply affected by the work but not sophisticated enough to withstand harm. Women who died from reading proved that they were rebellious, sensitive, and charmingly inexperienced readers. It was a mark of refined sensibilities that a woman died from reading, and a mark of refined sensibilities in both men and women to appreciate such a death.

MISREADING AND LOSS

The problem with novels was that they encouraged confusion. Readers mistook fiction for reality.[38] Li Ruding, in his 1666 preface to Li Guochang's *Essentials of Self-Cultivation* (Chongxiu zhiyao), complained,

> Even worse than [copies of exam themes] are licentious sayings and love songs, the fictitious "histories," romances, and novels that are published and circulated. Thus, after *Outlaws of the Marsh* [Shuihu zhuan] was published, villains frequently gathered in the greenwood, and after *Plum in the Golden Vase* came out, there were nightly elopements from the women's quarters.[39] Such works are the means of instructing thieves and licentious women. . . . They really do great harm to the manners, morals, and minds of the people.[40]

Novels taught, but they taught the wrong things to the wrong people.[41]

Those who died from reading *Story of the Stone* felt for the foolish romantics who populate the novel and became them through misreading fiction for reality and patterning themselves after negative models, as in this 1805 account:

> *Peony Pavilion*'s Du Liniang died because of a dream, *Jealousy-curing Soup*'s [Liaodu geng] Xiaoqing died because of jealousy,[42] but these two [deaths] are really nothing more than *qing*—from matters that they experienced themselves. I met Gui Yuqian in Jiangning, and he implored me to never read *Story of the Stone*. I asked him why. [By way of answering], he related the words of Zang Yongtang from Changzhou, [who said], "There was a scholar, who read *Stone* voraciously. Whenever he reached a passage full of emotion, he would close the book and contemplate it, or heave a long sigh, or shed tears and wail plaintively. He lost all interest in food and drink. In the course of one month, he read the novel seven times. It got to the point where his state of mind was completely distracted,

his heart's blood was used up [*xinxue haojin*], and he died." He also
said that there was a girl, Miss Someone-or-other, who read *Stone*,
and then coughed blood, and died. I said, "You could call these [cases
of] 'scratching your feet with boots on'; [there is nothing you can do
about] those who feel anxiety on the behalf of others."[43]

The readers, real people, here are criticized because they died not
from their own experience of *qing* but from reading about the *qing*
of fictional (or fictionalized) characters who experienced emotion
firsthand. Wang Fuzhi (1619–1692) might have disagreed with Gui
Yuqian's concerns: "That which one has personally experienced, that
which one has personally seen, that is a gate of iron limiting us."[44]
After all, the "investigation of things" (*gewu*), one of the major intellectual trends that was rewriting the interpretation of the Confucian
classics at the time, was often an intuitive and text-based pursuit.
Interest in things outside oneself commonly was investigation not so
much of the other as of the self in the other.[45] Gui Yuqian seems to
believe that the menace of fiction is that it obscures the boundary
between self and other, and that it compels its reader to do so.

The accounts of death by novel differ somewhat along gender lines.
In these accounts, the two young women, Miss Yu and Miss Someone-or-other, become Lin Daiyu, one in love with Baoyu, and one
coughing blood unto death. The scholar, by contrast, read *Story of
the Stone* seven times in one month and died shortly afterwards from
melancholy. All die from obsessive reading, yet, according to their
sex, the women die from a wasting consumption, and the scholar
from protracted and extreme melancholy. It is expected that young
women have a hard time preventing damage to their health from
excessive emotionality, just as young men have trouble guarding their
physical resources. Reading *Story of the Stone* seven times in one
month is a picture of excess, taxing not only emotional resources but
also physical ones.[46] The man who dies from reading *Stone*, like the
two women, unwittingly models one of its characters. In the novel,
Jia Rui's misreading costs him his life.[47] He is obsessed with the beautiful Wang Xifeng, who considers him so far below her station as to
be insulted by his affections. She teases and torments him, his health
deteriorates, and he becomes bedridden. Doctors are unable to help.
Jia Rui remains infatuated and engages in constant masturbation,
which brings his health to a crisis. At this point, a Daoist shows up
saying that he can cure "retributory illnesses" (*yuannie zhi zheng*).[48]
The monk says that medicine cannot cure Jia Rui. Instead, he lends

him the Mirror for the Romantic (Fengyue Baojian), which was created by the fairy Disenchantment herself. It is meant to serve as an
antidote to the ill effects of impure thinking and rash actions, and it
works through sympathetic correlation. Contemplating its truth will
cure the illness brought on by lustful thoughts. Jia Rui is supposed to
look only at the back of the mirror, which portrays a skeleton, but he
violates the Daoist's command and looks into the front of the mirror,
in the reflections of which he sees Xifeng beckoning to him. He enters
the mirror, where he has intercourse with her, after which she sees
him out. He finds himself back in bed, having had a wet dream and
sweating profusely. The mirror has turned itself around in his hand,
showing him once more the skeleton. He repeats this process three or
four times, after which demons prevent him from leaving the mirror.[49]
They drag him away screaming, "Let me take the mirror with me!"
He is found dead, in a puddle of icy semen on the bed. He dies from
lovesickness, but the mechanism is really obsession and taxation, the
overspending of bodily resources, a particularly male problem.[50]

Magic mirrors have a long tradition in Chinese literature, going
back at least to the Tang dynasty (618–907). They represent truth and
falsehood, love and death, self-knowledge and self-deception, and so
on. Jia Rui is given an instrument to cure an illness of desire, of mental
and emotional attachment, but he uses it incorrectly, not according to
instructions. Looking into the mirror, for Jia Rui, is a kind of reading
that parallels reading a novel, and *Mirror for the Romantic* was one
of the alternate titles of *The Story of the Stone*.[51] Seduction by what
one encounters there is unhealthy. The reader may sympathize with a
negative role model or may become too attached to a character. Savvy
readers will understand that with all fiction a detached and objective
reading allows enjoyment of the literary construction without literally or figuratively getting sucked in.[52] Readers who died from reading *Story of the Stone* lacked this understanding. It was a charming
but tragic naïveté in young women that led to their demise; in men, it
was an unenlightened philistinism, an inability to do the most fundamental thing that educated men did—read.[53] In each of the stories of
women who died from reading *Story of the Stone*, the family immediately burns the book that caused the death. Jia Rui's family similarly
tries to burn the mirror, but the Daoist rescues it and then accuses
the family of confusing the real with the unreal.[54] That is, the family has mistaken the proximal cause of death, the book, for the ultimate one: the excessive repression or expression of desire caused by

the improper reading of fiction as truth. That Jia Rui actually, physically, dies from uncontrolled seminal emission, one of the most feared
maladies of men, oft-discussed and oft-prescribed in medical literature high and low in the Qing, shows just how dangerous this kind
of misreading is. It also links Jia Rui's misreading to that of Baoyu in
chapter 5 who, while dreaming, mistakes the disillusionment that his
dream sexual encounter was supposed to provide for an introduction
to pleasures of the flesh. The result was involuntary emission. The
Jia Rui episode is a warning about literati obsession and misreading:
foolishly overspending his essence through an attachment to fiction,
Jia Rui, like the obsessed young man reading him, ends up being a
spendthrift of his own corporeal reserves.

In contemporary medical texts, particularly recipe books, there
are many formulas specifically for scholars who read too much,
though what they read was presumably not fiction.[55] One example is
the widely renowned "celestial king's elixir to supplement the heart/
mind" (*tianwang buxin dan*).[56] Wang Ang (1615–ca. 1699) described
the pathogenesis of the symptoms associated with this formula thus:
"Both the essence and will of humans are stored in the kidneys. When
the essence is insufficient, the will and qi become weak and are unable
to communicate above with the heart. This leads to erratic emotions
and forgetfulness." Wang recommended that those who read or study
a lot take the pill regularly.[57] In other words, dying from reading was
not simply a metaphor—it had a very clear pathology.

PLUM IN THE GOLDEN VASE: POISON AND ANTIDOTE

The ability to engender unenlightened and obsessive reading
in those who consumed them marked novels as dangerous texts
almost from the beginning. The story behind the creation of one
of the first novels in China to focus on domestic life illustrates
this danger. *Plum in the Golden Vase* describes, in great detail,
the downfall of the Ximen household. The story centers on Ximen
Qing, a corrupt social climber and lustful merchant with six wives
who vie with one another for power and control of Ximen. The
most lascivious of these, Pan Jinlian, ultimately gives him an overdose of an aphrodisiac while he is exhausted and drunk, leading to
his gruesome death by sexual intercourse, in which he unceasingly
ejaculates semen and then blood and then qi. *Plum in the Golden
Vase* itself acts like this aphrodisiac.

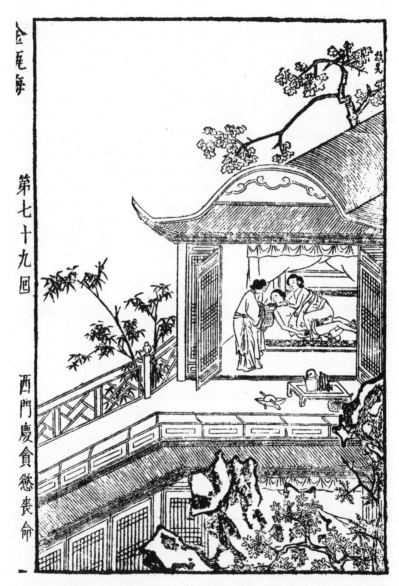

Figure 2.1   In the novel *Plum in the Golden Vase*, Ximen Qing dies from an overdose of aphrodisiac and excessive intercourse. Note the mortar and pestle in foreground. Xiaoxiaosheng, Jinping mei cihua.

Those who viewed fiction as dangerous emphasized the need to read objectively. In the preface to his *Sequel to Plum in the Golden Vase* (Xu Jinping mei, 1660), Ding Yaokang (1599–1669) writes, "There are people who do not know how to read *Plum* correctly. The book intends to abstain from the obsession with desire, yet it turns them toward such an obsession. The book intends to abstain from licentiousness, yet it turns them toward licentiousness."[58] Ding wrote his sequel to teach people how to read the novel correctly, to force them to identify the proper themes, and to resist being led into immoral ways by misreading social criticism and "turning it into a guidebook for debauchery."[59] The preface by Xihu Diaoshi claims, "Only those who do not know how to read will label [*Plum in the Golden Vase*] as being weirdly supernatural, violent, or licentious and think they have violated the way of the sages. It is beyond their comprehension that novels are powerful enough to enhance the influence of the teachings of the sages and the classics."[60] The language of apology for these early novels describes their danger as a potent medicine—when used correctly, it is as powerfully fortifying as the Confucian classics, but for those who use it carelessly, it can do a great deal of harm.

The paratexts attached to printed novels disagree about the mechanisms by which they provided moral instruction or harm. One of the prefatory pieces to Zhang Zhupo's (1670–1698) commentary edition of *Plum in the Golden Vase* (1695) suggested that fiction was a vector for literal and metaphorical poison. In "The Bitterness of Filial Piety" (Kuxiao shuo), the author claims that it was none other than Wang Shizhen (1526–1590), the leading poet and essayist of his time, who wrote *Plum in the Golden Vase*, and that he did so to avenge his father's death.[61] The story goes that Wang's father was executed by the diabolical minister Yan Song (1481–1568) for selling him what he was told was an original version of a famous painting but that turned out to be a copy. Yan Song died in 1568, so Wang set his sights on Yan's son, Yan Shifan (1513?–1565), who had risen in rank and was a model of corruption. While Yan was cunning and managed to escape many of the assassination plots directed against him by Wang, Yan's fatal weakness was his penchant for licentious literature. Wang thus wrote a novel that would be of interest to Yan. When he finished, he soaked the pages in poison and hired a merchant to sell the book to Yan. Yan, falling prey to his base inclinations, bought the book, and as he licked his fingers to turn pages over the course of the long novel, he eventually ingested enough of the poison to fall ill and die. More remarkable than this most assuredly apocryphal account is the fact that it circulated until to the modern period.⁶² Taking the poison as a metaphor for toxic topics or words, the author participates in the tradition of "selling the sickness" (*maibing*), whereby an ill person writes the name of his sickness on a piece of paper and leaves it out for someone else to find. He who reads the name of the illness then falls ill with it, and the author is thereby cured. Often the contagious words had to be left in a basket with food or money to entice passersby into reading them—a gesture not unlike hiding poison in the pages of a licentious book.⁶³ In this case, reading transmits disease.

Even more precisely, Wang engages in a literary version of *gu* poisoning. *Gu* 蠱, emblematized visually by the component parts of the character three "worms" over a vessel, was a poison believed to be created by filling a container with various poisonous insects, worms, or snakes, which after a period of time (usually one hundred days) destroy or devour each other until only one remains. This last worm was believed to have absorbed all of the concentrated poison of the others. This creature is the *gu*, a manifestation of the *gu* demon, which requires a human host to reproduce.⁶⁴ The *gu* is slipped into food, and as soon as someone consumes this poison, the seeds develop into worms resembling their parents, which gnaw on the viscera of the victim, producing pain, a swollen abdomen, progressive emaciation, and ultimately, death. The proof of *gu* poisoning was visible after death, when worms crawled out from orifices in the corpse. As a reward for providing the *gu* with a host in which the seeds can mature, the *gu* demon presents the human agent with all of the possessions of the deceased victim. If the person who initiates this process is unable to find a host for the *gu* in a timely fashion, he is killed by the *gu* demon. For this reason he may even find himself forced to select a relative from his own household as the victim. The actor's obligation to the *gu* demon could be transferred to another by enticing a stranger to take home the *gu* worm by hiding it in a basket of treasure, such as silk, silver, or gold, left at a crossroads or other public place.⁶⁵ Poisoning by *gu* was explicitly forbidden in Ming and Qing legal codes, and was a topic of great interest to authors of medical texts.⁶⁶

Wang, in an effort to relieve himself of the debt of vengeance, pours the accumulated poison into a novel in the form of detailed descriptions of the sex act, jealous wives, and all manner of debauchery, knowing that it will entice Yan to take it home, where he will be poisoned with it and will not only die, but in doing so, will relieve Wang of his burden. Wang was not motivated by greed, though, as agents of *gu* were, and thus prefatory essays argue that his novel was an instrument of filial revenge. The novel is also like *gu* in that it appealed to the highbrow and lowbrow alike in its incorporation of all registers of knowledge. *Gu* did so by comingling the universal encounter with parasite infection and demonological concepts. The result was a convincing explanatory model for both disease transmission and retributory illness that fascinated and terrified the educated and uneducated alike for centuries, up until the early twentieth century.[67] The endurance of *Plum in the Golden Vase*'s creation myth as an instrument of Wang's revenge drew on the same mix of high- and lowbrow logic as *gu* poison and selling the sickness.

It may have been this story of poison and filial revenge that spurred readers to discuss *Plum in the Golden Vase* with medically minded language borrowed from commentary on the classics. Not only was *Plum in the Golden Vase* one of the first (if not *the* first) novels in China to focus on domestic matters, it was also the work of a single author who did not retell or piece together known stories.[68] Perhaps this formal cohesion (the novel was intricately structured like a body), or the novel's concern with daily life (diseases and doctors were a prominent fact of life), or the seeming contradiction between its content and form (poison and antidote) warranted or demanded use of medical language by commentators. The Xinxinzi preface to the earliest existing text of *Plum in the Golden Vase* alludes to the function of the novel as a bodily system and makes the connection between moral and medical effects:

> From its beginning to its end the strands of the plot are as intricately articulated as the conduits of the circulatory system. . . . It is scarcely to be denied that in this work the language encroaches on the vulgar and the atmosphere is redolent of rouge and powder. But I would assert that such allegations miss the point. The first song in *The Book of Songs* [Shijing] has been characterized by Confucius as expressing "pleasure that does not extend to wantonness and sorrow that does not lead to injury." Sorrow and resentment are sentiments that man dislikes, but few are able to experience them without injury to themselves.[69]

The phrase "the threads of the plot are as intricately articulated as the conduits and arteries" (*mailuo guantong*) comes from Zhu Xi's preface to his commentary on the *Doctrine of the Mean* (Zhongyong, 1189).[70] This preface would have been familiar to every educated reader of the sixteenth through eighteenth centuries, since the *Doctrine of the Mean* is one of the Four Books that formed the core of Confucian education during the Ming and Qing dynasties, and Zhu Xi's commentary editions were the standard texts. Xinxinzi was not the first to take these medical terms out of classical commentary and apply them to fiction, but he goes further in drawing a parallel between the bodily structure of the novel and its emotional effects on the reader's body.[71] Prefatory pieces to the Zhang Zhupo edition of *Plum in the Golden Vase* employ the phrase "threaded together like qi and channels" (*guantong qimai*) to describe the intricacies of the plot, and Zhang bolsters that image with his phrase "channels that connect widely separated [plot] elements" (*qianli fumai*), saying that the marvelous quality of *Plum in the Golden Vase* is the way in which it conceals them.[72]

While it is true that these phrases were a part of the standard lexicon for literary critics, and therefore do not merit undue emphasis, they were oft-repeated comments about *Plum in the Golden Vase* and the novels that followed it. Zhang Zhupo writes, "Only if you take several days and read *Plum* all the way through will you perceive the connecting nerves and arteries that act like a single thread upon which the author has strung together his succession of rising and falling actions." He says "From the prologue in the first chapter one can see how the arteries and veins [*xuemai jingluo*] of the entire book are finely interconnected [*guan tong qi mo*]."[73] The careful reader must uncover the literary and rhetorical devices, as a skilled doctor would carefully detect the meaning of palpitations in the pulse.[74]

Circulation was a concept and pulse taking a practice central to elite medicine. The relation of medicine to the circulatory system (*mailuo*) or pulse taking (*qiemai*) lies in the belief that most diseases stem from the improper flow of blood and qi through the body. Applied to literature, the concept of circulation highlights not only the complexity of the work but also its harmony and its health.[75] But the critics did not limit themselves to the language of elite medicine. Just as often, for instance, Zhang Zhupo refers to acupuncture, a practice that was usually relegated to nonelite healers, itinerant physicians, or women, claiming that "the author's acupuncture [*zhenbian*] uses satiric barbs instead of regular needles." The Woxian Caotang commentator on *Unofficial History of the Scholars* writes, "Here the author's acupuncture is aimed at curing just such people."[76] Novelists were representing complex worlds, and commentators drew on the language of medical practice high and low to discuss it.[77]

EMOTIONAL MEDICINE

The saying that "one does not need to pay with his life if he angers a person to death" (*qisiren bu changming*) may derive from the *Romance of the Three Kingdoms* story of Zhuge Liang, minister of the state of Shu, tricking General Zhou Yu of Wu three times until he finally died of anger.[78] The *Unofficial History of the Scholars* features a similarly well-known story of Fan Jin, who, hearing that he had passed the provincial imperial examinations after many years of disappointment, became so overjoyed that he went crazy.[79] Traditionally, medical texts located maladies due to emotional excess under the rubric "wind disorders" (*feng*), a broad grouping based on one of the six external causes of disease. An innovation in the late imperial era was a more specific category found in medical texts, usually termed simply "emotions" (*qingzhi*).

Examination of Medical Prescriptions (Yifang kao) by Wu Kun, written in 1584, is one of the earliest texts with this grouping, and it features many cases assembled to illustrate the use of emotions to treat disorders caused by emotion.[80] From the *Yellow Emperor's Basic Questions of the Inner Canon* (Huang Di neijing suwen) to this period, most illnesses with emotion at the root were believed to result from blockages in the flow of qi caused by those emotions and were to be dispersed with pills or medicinal broths. The late imperial period put forth a new kind of treatment: emotional counter-therapy. As Wu writes,

> When emotion is overwhelmingly excessive, no drug can cure [the resulting disorder]; it must be overcome by emotion. Thus it is said that "anger damages the hepatic system, but sorrow overcomes anger; joy damages the cardiac system, but apprehension overcomes joy; worry damages the splenetic system, but anger overcomes worry; sorrow damages the pulmonary system, but joy overcomes sorrow; apprehension damages the renal system, but worry overcomes apprehension."[81]

The renowned Yuan doctor Zhu Zhenheng was once sent to see a married woman. For half a year, she had been ill with a loss of appetite, frequently lying in bed, facing the north. Her husband had been away for five years, traveling on business. Zhu asserted that her qi was stagnated in the spleen. Her ailments, he claimed, all came from her "wanting a man but not being able to get one" (*si nanzi bu de*).[82] Zhu suggested that the only way to treat the woman's qi blockage was to drive her to the point of rage. Zhu gave the patient three slaps on the face and accused her of having affairs with other men, causing her to cry out in righteous indignation. Afterward, she felt hungry and asked to eat some food. Zhu told her father secretly that despite her improved condition, the best treatment would be to bring her joy. They deceitfully told her that her husband had informed them by a letter that he would return soon. Three months later, her husband finally came back, and she completely recovered.

Novels could lead readers to injure themselves with excessive sentiment, but they could also serve as counter-therapy to the illnesses caused by real-world vexations. Excessive sorrow and resentment could cause people to act as if drunk or stupid, speak in absurdities, and suffer hallucinations.[83] These are also the emotions that the preface to *Plum in the Golden Vase* claims are present in the novel, and because of which many readers cause themselves injury. Of course, sympathetic illness brought on by reading *Story of the Stone* also plays into a motif of Cao Xueqin's novel: that fiction becomes real when it is true. When it resonates with the reader, stirs emotions, and causes the reader to believe, then it is not fiction. In this regard, readers' deaths make the fiction real. Moreover, these stories of death from reading the novel, which draw so clearly on the medical theory and trends of the day, not only imitate the repeating cycle of paired opposites, repletion and depletion (*xushi*), but draw on that bodily image to establish and perpetuate the motif of realistic fiction and fictive truth (*xushi*).

There was an appreciation for the aesthetics of illness in late imperial China. The famous poet and critic Yuan Hongdao (1568–1610) wrote, "There is nothing more melancholic than illness. . . . There are times when [the songs of] grieving men and lovelorn women are superior to [the poetry of] scholars and literati, and oftentimes that which comes from groaning is more pleasing than everyday [sounds]."[84] At least in the popular imaginary, men tended to suffer from melancholy and resentment. The preface to *Plum in the Golden Vase* defines melancholy as a particular literati illness:

> Of the seven feelings natural to mankind, melancholy [*youyu*] is the most intractable. For such men of superior wisdom as may occasionally appear in the natural course of evolution, the fogs and ice that melancholy engenders disperse and splinter of their own accord, so there is no need to speak of such as these. Even those of lesser endowment know how to dispel melancholy with the aid of reason so that it

may be prevented from encumbering them. Among the many who fall
short of this, however, who have been unable to achieve enlightenment in their hearts, and who do not have access to the riches of the
classic tradition to alleviate their melancholy, those who do not fall
ill are few. . . . It is in consideration of this fact that my friend, the
Scoffing Scholar, has poured the accumulated wisdom of a lifetime
into the composition of this work, consisting of one hundred chapters
in all. So enticingly are the effects accomplished that the reader may,
perhaps, be beguiled into forgetting his melancholy with a smile.[85]

It was a given that literati suffer from melancholy. Yet the novel is
capable of engendering joy, which dispels melancholy according to
counter-therapy, and therefore is an antidote to the literati illness.
This class of literati so disposed to melancholy is evoked in the anecdote about Wang Yan (256–311), a reference to which occurs on the
first page of the first chapter of *Plum in the Golden Vase*, when a
friend comes to offer condolences after the death of Wang's infant
son. His friend asks why Wang is so filled with grief, since the child
was only an infant. Wang replies, "Sages may be able to forget their
feelings, and the lower order of men may lack feeling altogether. It is
people just like ourselves who are most affected by emotion (*qing*)."[86]
The novel is intended for the average best reader, or the class of literati
that is most sensitive and least able to effectively deal with the melancholy that so commonly afflicts them.

Li Yu, playwright, novelist and publisher, writes in *Causal Expressions of Idle Feeling* (Xianqing ouji) that this kind of bibliotherapy
(and the diseases it cures) is exclusively a literati endeavor:

> That which was never before seen in one's life can be taken as medi-
> cine. To want what one has never possessed is a desire all men have.
> This is like [the feeling of] men of letters toward marvelous and
> strange books . . . To allow these persons to see these objects, to
> find these especially under difficult conditions, this is the technique
> whereby to manage and control the patient . . . What I mean by "lite-
> rati" does not necessarily refer only to those with talent [but] rather
> all who are literate, who can read, who can use books as medicine.
> Stories and Unofficial Histories (*chuanqi yeshi*) are the best for expel-
> ling illness and demons.[87]

What is unspoken in Li Yu's piece about strange books and medicine
is the malady that they treat. The patient here, like Jia Baoyu in *Story
of the Stone* after he moves into the utopian realm of Prospect Garden, is overcome with melancholy. In the midst of his placid, agree-
able existence, Baoyu becomes discontented:

The garden's female population were mostly still in that age of innocence when freedom from inhibition is the fruit of ignorance. Waking
and sleeping they surrounded him, and their mindless giggling was
constantly in his ears. How could they understand the restless feelings that now consumed him? In his present mood of discontent he
was bored with the garden and its inmates; yet his attempts to find
distraction outside it ended in the same emptiness and ennui.[88]

This malady is relieved when Baoyu's servant smuggles in to him a
stack of prohibited drama and fiction—among them *The Story of the
Western Wing* (Xixiang ji, 1498). Part of this relief stems from the fact
that what Baoyu read amounted to new experiences. His reading of
these works borders on the obsessive, and *Story of the Western Wing*
becomes a guidebook for lovers—its language a code for his commu-
nication with Lin Daiyu. Obsession was equal to happiness and also
to refinement, which made it both a marker of the gentleman, and the
therapeutic counterpart to the literati illness, melancholy.[89]

Cao Xueqin claims it is not the subject but the representation itself
that makes the novel useful as medicine. The Stone defends its story
to Vanitas (Kongkong daoren):

> Surely my "number of females," whom I spent half a lifetime study-
> ing with my own eyes and ears, are preferable to [unofficial histories,
> erotic novels and talented-scholar-beautiful-maiden stories]. I do not
> claim that they are better people than the ones who appear in books
> written before my time; I am only saying that the contemplation of
> their actions and motives may relieve worry and disperse melancholy
> [*xiao chou po men*].[90]

If depressed and disenfranchised men contemplate the talented and
frail woman, it will cure him. Yet if the sensitive woman reader con-
templates her, she will sicken and die. The resolution of this gender
paradox lies in the mediating effects of representation, which moder-
ates extremes of emotion and puts at a remove from the reader those
characters that fall ill from harmful excesses of melancholy. The
appreciation of the representation, the acknowledgement of the fictionality of the novel, enables its use as medicine.

Many of the claims that the novel can cure melancholy are rhetorical, even frivolous proclamations, not meant to be taken literally.
When the Woxian Caotang commentator says of *The Unofficial History of the Scholars* that "if read when one's head gets heavy in the
middle of a long summer's day it will wake one to clarity or even cure
an illness! [*keyi shuixing keyi yubing*]," it may have been the simple

use of rhyme to add weight to praise.[91] The phrase has a lyrical flour-
ish to it, but it belies hyperbole. Melancholy in particular was linked
to other, particularly male concerns. According to the *Systematic
Materia Medica*, when excessive melancholy damages the heart, nocturnal emission occurs.[92] In medical texts, melancholy is often paired
with anxiety (*fanmen*), worry, taxation, and pent-up frustration (*silu
taiguo, silu yujie*). When these conditions are extreme, they can damage the heart and spleen, resulting in amnesia, trance, restlessness,
and insomnia. If they damage the heart and kidneys, the likely outcome will be debilitated primordial yang vital energy with white and
turbid urine and nocturnal emission with dreams of sex.[93] Melancholy is also frequently mentioned in the *Systematic Materia Medica*,
along with overstrain and excessive sexual intercourse, as resulting
in uncontrolled seminal emission.[94] This was considered a terrible
affliction, and writers of fiction and medicine virtually obsessed over
this issue throughout the Qing. Although loss of semen in novels is
more frequently a result of too much intercourse, novel prefaces that
claimed to distract the reader from his melancholy and anxiety were
not only saying that they would cheer him up but that they could prevent the most dire kind of depletion.

Reading was not unlike the practice of "bedchamber arts" (*fangzhongshu*), the purpose of which was to achieve "arousal without
emission" (*donger buxie*) to bolster health. These were practices much
written about in the late Ming medical texts that focused on absorb-
ing the bodily resources of one's sexual partner to benefit oneself.
These practices made one partner healthier while depleting the other.
Many of the medical texts and handbooks that discuss this medical-
ized view of sex refer to it as a "battle of stealing and strengthening"
(*caibu zhi zhan*).[95] For one partner to benefit from the other, usually
the other partner needed to have less training, less experience. If it
was the aestheticization of illness that enabled experienced readers
to derive joy and benefit from the novel, did their use of the novel as
medicine also depend on others being unable to distinguish between
truth and fiction? Was it essential for some to die from reading novels,
so that others could use it as medicine? Either way, the novel was an
instrument of male self-help and female destruction. Daiyu's tears are
a symbol of her depletion, and as they turn to blood, the male reader,
sympathizing but not empathizing with her fate, feels the warmth of
truth, the bitter sweet smile, and the nodding appreciation of a true
artist dispelling his own melancholy.

APHRODISIACS AND RECIPE BOOKS

Warnings about the dangers or health benefits of novels in early chapters or prefatory materials resemble similar claims in many prefaces
to medical texts, particularly those recipe books that were intended
to be used by the lay person for self-medicating. An 1873 preface by
Chen Qirong, the nineteenth-century literatus, to *Secret Formulas for
Women, from the Bamboo Grove Monastery* (Zhulinsi nüke mifang,
1852), criticizes quacks (*yongyi*) who mechanically apply ancient formulas without understanding the different manifestations that a disease might take in different people. But he also describes the text as
a guide to home treatment by medical amateurs.[96] Why did preface
writers encourage lay people to rely on prescription books but consider it unacceptable for medical practitioners to do so? The answer
lies in confidence in good readers, and in setting up an opposition
between disenfranchised literati who read widely and practiced medicine either as a hobby or as an imperative as head of house, and those
less skilled readers: professionals, hacks, and women.

Aphrodisiacs (*chunyao*) were one of the most commonly discussed
prescriptions in recipe books and in medical manuscripts copied
by practicing doctors for their own use. These were also of particular interest as contested objects in fiction, given widespread concerns about excessive sex.[97] Rural healers, for instance, copy these
prescriptions less frequently than their urban counterparts, presumably because there were fewer brothels in the country, and therefore
less need for such aphrodisiacs, and pointing to their use for recre-
ation as often as for procreation. Aphrodisiacs and tonifying medicines are often found in the recipe books of urban healers, and they
are frequently described as having the same or similar effects.[98] These
aphrodisiacs have detailed names elaborating on their effects: recipes for "preventing the golden spear from falling down" (*jinqiang
budao*), "to make an immortal [woman] take her clothes off" (*xianren zi tuoyi*), for "myriad screams of happiness" (*wanshengjiao*), for
an "erotic drug welcoming joy" (*se yaofang huanle*), for a drug to
"make a woman want to give money to her lover" (*daotiejin*), and one
to cause "long-lasting thoughts" (*chang sixiang*), but others point to
a more generic kind of enhancement, such as an "elixir to strengthen
the yang" (*zhuangyang dan*) and a "priceless treasure" (*wujia bao*).[99]

In printed medical texts, obscene elements were often edited out of
narrative explanations, but folk recipes included in manuscripts were

quite explicit, and in this regard they read like licentious fiction. Stories of sexual transgression, whether in fiction or medical texts, tend to preach a similar morality in which transgression leads to a corresponding retribution. One such story designed to prove the efficacy of an aphrodisiac formula is attached to prescriptions that have been copied into multiple, disparate practitioners' manuscripts. In one manuscript the story is attached to the "elixir to strengthen yang," and in another to "priceless pills" (*wujia wan*). The story concerns a provincial governor who was impotent and weak, and had searched all over for a cure. Eventually, he obtained a formula but died after taking the drugs. The wife of the governor heard about Ge Yu, a man of seventy-two years who suffered from the same ailment as her late husband. Not wanting to waste the formula, she gave it to Ge Yu. After Ge Yu took it, his sexual potency increased dramatically. Every night he demanded to have intercourse with his own wife more than six times. His wife concluded that this formula was too strong, so she did not let her husband take it any longer, and she told the widow of the governor what had happened. The widow could not believe it and had illicit sexual intercourse with Ge Yu, whereupon she discovered that the effects of the formula were indeed extraordinary. Subsequently, they had three sons. The relatives of the governor's widow considered this transgression intolerable, and they killed Ge Yu. As they broke Ge Yu's bones, they discovered that they were filled with marrow. Since old men were believed to suffer from kidney depletion, and as the kidneys rule the bones, their marrow was expected to be depleted too. They thus realized that this formula indeed produced miraculous effects.

This story, inasmuch as it features aphrodisiacs, sexual transgression, and retribution, sounds much like *Plum in the Golden Vase* and its descendants in speaking of fornication between a man and woman separated by age and position, excessive sex, extramarital sex, and so on. But the transgressive, like the extraordinary, in the context of practical medical texts serves to prove the efficacy of the prescription. The story stayed with the pill it described and was written out, in slightly different form, in a variety of manuscripts.[100] Why would copyists, presumably assembling medicines for their own practice, record the story in addition to the prescription? Clearly the story somehow proved the efficacy of the aphrodisiac or tonic, and the popularity of the drug perpetuated the story. The copyist must have either presumed that he would need the story to convince future patients to take the cure, or he simply viewed the story as part of the prescription. Prescriptions that lacked the authority of being in a printed text, like the many aphrodisiacs and fertility drugs found

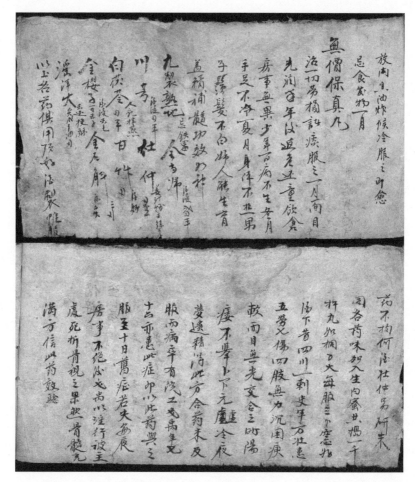

Figure 2.2.   The story of Ge Yu from a medical manuscript. Staatsbibliothek
zu Berlin—Preußischer Kulturbesitz, East Asia Department Slg. Unschuld
8429.

in these medical manuscripts, were often accompanied by stories. Stories like these, which read so similarly to popular, ribald fiction in both
form and content, may also have convinced readers of a drug's efficacy
because it was a familiar story, a well-worn exemplary tale, and through
repetition, the story created reality.

Aphrodisiacs straddled a line between health (fertility drugs that tonified the body and enhanced procreative abilities) and death (enabling
excessive expenditure of bodily resources). Presumably for this reason,

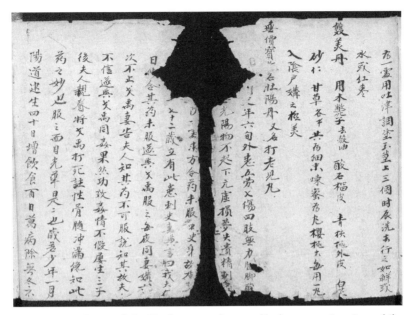

Figure 2.3. Story of Ge Yu from another medical manuscript. Staatsbibliothek zu Berlin—Preußischer Kulturbesitz, East Asia Department Slg.
Unschuld 8167.

aphrodisiacs are frequently listed next to abortifacients in recipe literature, which also hints at their semi-illicit status.[101] The Ge Yu story drew
on the logic of transgression and retribution, which may have made the
story seem true, both as proof of the medicine and as a warning against
its abuse. That the transgressor is punished added a ring of truth for
readers who believed in an orderly and just world. The functioning of retribution is borne out in fiction, since characters such as Ximen Qing who
abuse aphrodisiacs fall ill and die, while those who ingest them by mistake usually recover. The Ge Yu story warns, as does the Ximen story,
that excess and transgression will be met, eventually, with retribution.
But the story of Ge Yu also contains the same message as *Plum in the
Golden Vase*—that this medicine can strengthen and fortify if used correctly, but if one gives free reign to their desires, it becomes an instrument
of depletion.[102] It is the same as when bad readers turn the novel, with its
ability to dispel melancholy, into a guide for debauchery.

   That novels and medical texts for daily use reflected the concerns
of the city and the marketplace is not terribly strange, but that novels
portray themselves as a kind of aphrodisiac is. Few of the instances

of aphrodisiacs found in works of drama or fiction or the stories transmitted along with recipes for aphrodisiacs in medical texts have healthy outcomes. Characters in fictional literature who make reference to this kind of medicine, such as Crimson (Hongniang) in *Story of the Western Wing*, are usually lowbrow, foreign, or suspicious in some other way. The common representation of aphrodisiacs in literati fiction concerned the recurrent theme of retribution and was usually attendant upon heavy-handed moralizing. In *Plum in the Golden Vase*, Ximen Qing obtains an aphrodisiac (which itself is contained in a box shaped like a phallus) from an itinerant foreign monk who also looks like a penis.[103] The aphrodisiac, a symbol of lasciviousness and excess, and of "misreading" the sex act—taking procreation for pleasure—is contrasted with a fertility charm obtained by his dutiful, tradition-bound wife, Wu Yueniang, in another episode in *Plum in the Golden Vase* that leads, ultimately to the birth of a son.

This dual view of aphrodisiacs may reflect what was happening in the medical world at the time. Some doctors became known for prescribing aphrodisiacs and sexual techniques to attain longevity. Gong Juzhong (fl. 1630), for instance, a renowned physician at the end of the Ming dynasty, was called by some a "physician of licentiousness" (*yinyi*).[104] Gong lived during the Wanli (1573–1620) reign period, when "warming and supplementing" (*wenbu*) approaches were very popular, and it became fashionable to consume medications believed to strengthen one's yang. His *Immortals' Book on Longevity* (Wanshou xianshu, ca. 1560) advised readers on sexual techniques, prescribed sixteen recipes for aphrodisiacs, discoursed on the medicinal benefits of saliva, and introduced a section on "[bed] curtain combat" (*weizhan*).[105] Claims in the prefatory materials published in novels that despite the novel's depiction of the above acts that, for instance, "*Plum in the Golden Vase* is not a licentious novel" (Diyi qishu fei yinshu lun), draws on the properties of aphrodisiacs, emphasizing the possible tonifying benefit of reading novels with the correct purpose and in moderation.

THE CURATIVE PROPERTIES OF CHINESE FICTION

The novel could be abused in two ways—by using the novel as a guidebook to sex, or by becoming obsessed with the novel's story and characters in lieu of its artistic and intellectual qualities that stimulate a more refined kind of reader. A 1695 piece by Zhang Chao (1659–1707), titled "Biblio Materia Medica" (Shu bencao),[106] classifies books as medicinal drugs in the manner of traditional *bencao* literature. It is a playful piece, but it resonates with claims found elsewhere about the novel. It begins with the healing effects of the classics: "Four Books: There are four kinds [of this drug], one called 'great learning' one called 'doctrine of the mean' one called 'analects' and one called 'Mencius.' All are mild in nature, sweet in flavor, and nontoxic. Taking them clears the mind [heart] and increases wisdom. Nonaddictive / reduces desires. Long-term usage causes people to have a mind that is broad and a body that is ample [*xinguang tipang*]."[107] Naturally the classics are beneficial to all and have no bad side effects. The author of this piece advises against reading philosophies or works from the Buddhist and Daoist canon because of their side effects. Historical literature, he claims, can be used only by particular types of readers under certain circumstances. There are a variety of these "medicines," and "taking them broadens one's knowledge and experience. Sometimes they make people feel great anger or cause them to weep without being able to stop . . . the price of this medicine is high. . . . It is not fit for use by uncultured people." Emotion marked literati refinement, but so did being able to control that emotion. According to Zhang Chao, this ability was lacking in unrefined people. In his hierarchy, fiction constitutes the most dangerous of the textual, medical drugs:

> Fiction [*xiaoshuo chuanqi*]: The flavor of novels is sweet and their nature/effect is arid and highly toxic. This drug should be avoided because it induces insanity. It should be taken only during the summer months when suffering from overeating or melancholy [*baomen*], when bad weather makes one feel awful. It also can help those suffering from diseases caused by external factors [wind and rain]. Taking the drug can relieve anxiety and dispel stagnation [*jie fanxiaoyu*]. It can dissipate sluggishness and open up the chest. However, it ought not be taken on a prolonged basis.[108]

"Biblio Materia Medica" humorously appropriates the structure of materia medica to play a game with major genres of literature, but it also employs the same emotional counter-therapy logic as medical works.[109] The conclusion adopts the same argument to defend the novel as novel prefaces do, namely that reading them is tantamount to the skillful use of poison as medicine:

> Fei Cidu says:[110] It depends how you use medicine—if you use it correctly, even if [the medicine is from] is a snake or a scorpion, it still can be effective. Han Xin's [unconventional] battle with his back to the water, and Yue Fei's ignoring the classics on martial arts, are

examples of this. If you use medicine incorrectly, even poria [*fuling*] can kill you. Zhao Gua's reading his father's books in vain and Wang Anshi's following the *Zhou Li* are examples of this.[111] This is something that all people who use medicine should know.[112]

Books are strong medicine. If one is not a skilled reader, even histories and philosophies are dangerous, but if one is a man of talent (or, presumably a woman of advanced years and experience), one can put fiction to use. Han Xin's and Yue Fei's lack of formal training did not hinder their ability to win battles. This sort of unorthodox learning and roguish thinking is like using poison as medicine. Contrastingly, Zhao Gua's and (here) Wang Anshi's inability to understand the classics that they were reading, and their subsequent failures at practical application of knowledge, are compared to causing damage with a widely employed and gentle medicine.

The novel was pitched as preventative medicine, palliative, and cure for literati maladies. A variety of texts added reading fiction to the list of such practices as seated meditation and sexual intercourse in regard to its effects on the body. If done correctly, with the correct training, focus, and spirit, it can bring harmony to the body, but if done without the correct intention or without the proper praxis, it will do the opposite, and bring illness and harm. The novel was also an aphrodisiac, a drug that worked on the body to tonify or deplete, according to the refinement or baseness of its user. Some readers were able to perceive the meridians and the flow of qi; others caused irreparable harm by not heeding its warnings or by overdosing. In the case of both the novel and the medical handbook, literati readers appropriated the role of legitimate practitioner by claiming status as superior readers. Novels "formally enacted a sequential illness-cure regimen that simultaneously established a select circle of readers able to invoke the appropriate modal of reading. Just as illness and melancholy are functions (and discursive forms) of social and literary distinction, so too were regimens of cure and hygienic self-preservation."[113] Discussing novels in terms of medicine was a way to raise the status of the novel and of those who were able to read it well. Yet in fiction and in the marketplace for fiction, literati were also redefining an aesthetic. They savored the inability of beautiful, frail, young women to benefit from reading the novel, just as they celebrated the downfall of lechers who were unable to save themselves by reading properly. Their efforts were charming and tragic, and their inability to use novels ultimately validated a subset of literati as legitimate and talented practitioners of popular literature, be it fictional, practical, or otherwise.

Vernacular Curiosities

Medical Entertainments and Memory

The next day, the war drum of the Fan battle formation sounded like
thunder. More than half of its soldiers were women. The Han camp drew
up their troops. Shortly thereafter, Butterfly Bush Flower and Iris came
out from the Fan camp to the beat of the drums. Holding swords in each
hand, they challenged Mountain Arrowhead and Honeysuckle to come out
from the Han formation and fight. The four women commanders fought
more than twenty rounds. Suddenly, Honeysuckle slashed forth her swords
and cut Butterfly Bush Flower's horse. Rearing up in pain, the horse threw
Butterfly Bush Flower to the ground. Just then the two female immortals,
Anemarrhena Root and Fritillary Bulb, came galloping in and fought with
them in close quarters. Litharge jumped off of his Thorny Tiger to save
his sister, and Iris fled back to their camp. Immediately, Fritillary Bulb
used her Japan Stephania cane and Anemarrhena Root used her Dandelion weapon to fight with Honeysuckle. Then Anemarrhena Root went
to fight with Mountain Arrowhead. They each displayed their unique
martial skills. Anemarrhena Root suddenly took out a Gold Star Stone
to blind Honeysuckle. Although Honeysuckle quickly dodged, the stone
still hit her back and she spit up blood. Defeated, she fled. Luckily, others
came to save her and return her to camp. Seeing this, Dendrobium was
extremely worried. Privet said to him, "Marshal, ease your worries. In
my opinion, your daughter is destined to face several calamities of blood
loss, and although this wound is severe, it is not likely to take her life. I
will give you a kind of medicine known as Drynaria Root, which is also
called 'Repairs Broken Bones.' Cut it into pieces and apply them to the
wound, and she will recover in a few days." Cassia Seed overheard this and
sent some Spikemoss, also known as "Anti-death Grass" to take with it.

—*Annals of Herbs and Trees* (Caomu chunqiu yanyi), chapter 17

Annals of Herbs and Trees could very well be unique in all of world
literature as the first, if not the only, full-length novel in which all
of the characters have the names of pharmaceutical drugs. Not only
are the characters all named after medicines, but so are most of their
weapons and mounts, many of the locations in the novel, the battle

formations and tactics. Little is known about the author and nothing—save the preface—about his motives for writing such a book.
Some believe it was written prior to 1688,[1] while others consider it
a work of the Jiaqing period (1796–1820),[2] since the earliest extant
volume that can be dated to a particular year seems to be an 1818
edition.[3] There are records of least eighteen different editions printed
prior to 1916, and the Qianlong period (1735–1796) seems to be when
interest in the novel began, based on records of four printed editions
published in that period.[4] Editions were published in each subsequent
reign period, usually one apiece, until the Guangxu (1875–1908),
when four more editions were published between 1872 and 1908, and
at least another two between 1909 and 1916.[5] The preface claims that
it was the Master of Cloudy Leisure (Yunjianzi) the sobriquet of Jiang
Hong, who was responsible for "collecting and selecting" the novel,
and the Man of Happy Mountain (Leshanren) who did the "editing and compiling," but nothing is known of either. The title is a bit
strange, and somewhat rare. *Caomu chunqiu* literally means "herbs,
trees, spring, autumn," but *chunqiu*, is usually rendered "annals" to
indicate that such titles tended to record narratives of the state in
chronological fashion. Thus, the title of this work could be "Annals
of Herbs and Trees" or "Annals of Materia Medica," since *caomu*
was understood to refer to vegetation generally, or to medical drugs
in particular. Most of the medicines in the novel are herbs, plants,
and flowers, with an underrepresentation from pharmaceutical literature of stones, animals, and other objects. The *yanyi* or "historical
romance" of the title points clearly to the book's fictional narrative,
and without it, the title sounds more ambiguously like a medical text,
botanical work, or almanac.[6] *Yanyi* signifies that this work is a novel
but also suggests that it has been "novelized" or made into fiction
from a previous account of true events.

Why this novel was written is not clear. The author's preface states
that he created the *Caomu* as a work of charity:

> As for The Yellow Emperor tasting hundreds of herbs, it was to dis-
> tinguish the spicy, sweet, weak, or bitter flavor of them; the cold, hot,
> warm, or cool nature of them; if they nourish [bodies] or enhance
> flow, or moisten or dry; if they can treat man's diseases and cure ill-
> nesses. How enormous his merit is! Being influenced and moved [by
> this thought], I gathered many names of medicines and explicate
> their meanings in the form of fiction [*yanyi*] to spread it in the world.
> Although it partly seems a game, the novel contains in it metals,
> stones, grasses, trees, water, soil, birds, beasts, fish, insects, and the

like. Isn't it fitting to use these names to substitute those of heaven, earth, vessels and objects?[7]

It is possible, in the mind of the author at least, for a novel to be both a game and an act of service. The presumed entertainment value of novels serves as a delivery mechanism for this long list of medicine names. But he continues, subverting his previous claim by saying that "some ridicule this collection as depicting too much slaughter. Is it really because I hate medicine so much that I wrote it like this on purpose? I just created the novel by giving free rein to my writing brush!"[8] The preface reads like a confession of writing a guilty pleasure, an illogical entertainment, and the author even calls into question his own charitableness by suggesting that his list of drugs all fighting each other to the death might be construed as his distaste for medicine. Circulating effective remedies was an act of merit, but it is not clear why circulating an extensive list of drugs buried in narrative would be as well. Perhaps the author considered his novel to be an aid to memory that would help doctors or pharmacists. Perhaps repackaging existing knowledge in narrative form was a way of making the difficulty of understanding the properties or of differentiating between drugs less difficult. Perhaps fictional narrative was the most effective vehicle to disseminate pharmaceutical knowledge. Perhaps the author simply could not resist a lengthy display of his own knowledge. Whatever the case, the preface to *Annals of Grasses and Trees* hints at the symbiosis of and pervasive tension between the novel's entertainment value and usefulness.

RIDDLES AND GAMES

Novels and encyclopedias contained many descriptions and explanations of how to play all sorts of games, from drinking games to word games to riddles. Some of these rely on the players having a high degree of botanical knowledge. Knowing something about plants and flowers had been part of reading and writing poetry since the *Book of Songs*, but gaining such knowledge was also a practical endeavor of men and women from their youth. Starting in the Wanli period a number of porcelain objects depicted both children and adults playing a game called "herb competition" or "match my plant" (*doucao* or *doubaicao*), a game dating from at least the Tang.[9] This game is described in *Story of the Stone*, in which the participants (young female actresses) display knowledge of plants

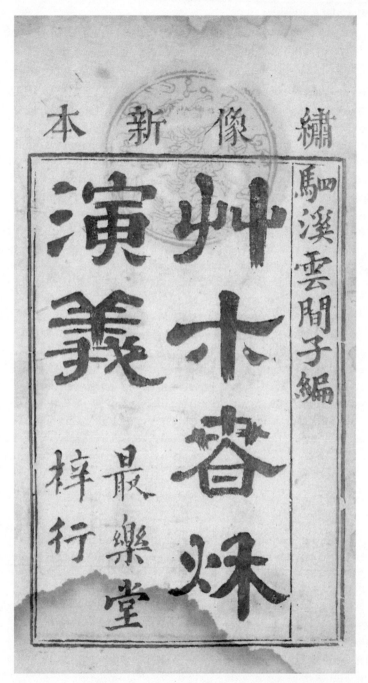

繡像新本

駉溪雲間子編

演義

艸木蓉烋

梓行 最樂堂

Figure 3.1. Perhaps the earliest edition of *Annals of Herbs and Trees*. Kangxi era (1661–1722). Columbia University Library.

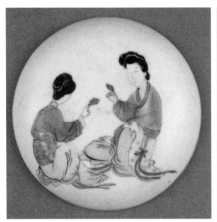 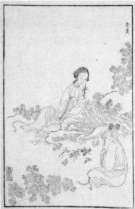

Figures 3.2a, 3.2b. (a) A scene of the game of "Match My Plant" played between two women on the cover of a porcelain box, Kangxi reign of the Qing dynasty. Collection of the Palace Museum, Beijing. (b) "Match My Plant" played between Zhen Yinglian/Xiangling (Caltrop) and others in *Story of the Stone*, chapter 61. From Gai Qi, *Pictures from* Dream of the Red Chamber, *with Encomiums* (Honglou meng tu yong), Waseda University Library, Japan.

and literacy through their performance in matching the names of plants and their symbols. One young woman says, "I've got some Guanyin willow." Another responds, "I've got some Luohan pine."[10] In this matching pair, both "willow" and "pine" are trees, while both "Guanyin" and "Luohan" are Buddhist figures. One player says, "I've got a peony [*mudan*] from *The Peony Pavilion*." Another responds, "I've got a *pipa* [loquat] from *The Story of the Lute* [Pipa ji, fourteenth century]." This version of the game "match my plant" recalls similar games played over wine. Like those drinking games (*jiuling*), the plant names are often juxtaposed in encyclopedias with other fragments of verbal literature.[11]

Verbal games were often integrated into dramatic texts and became part of the dialogue. An aria sung by Student Zhang and Crimson in *Story of the Western Wing*, for instance, is filled with medical puns and deploys them for their literary and comic effect for readers who were expected to get the joke. The play finds Student Zhang desperately ill from longing for Yingying, and other characters make numerous jokes at his expense. Doctors have been called in, but their medicine does no good. Student Zhang tells the audience that if only he could swallow a drop of his mistress's fragrant saliva, he would be cured. Crimson, Yingying's maid, arrives, telling the audience that Yingying sends young men to their deaths by making them long for her and then sending a prescription that will only make them sicker. Student Zhang admits that he knows his illness comes from lechery and that he has been invaded by a ghostly illness. Crimson offers him the prescription, explaining that each ingredient has its own use:

> (*Crimson sings:*)
> Cassia flowers sway their shade in the dead of night
> Jealousy soaks the one who "ought to return."
> (*Male lead speaks:*)
> Cassia flowers are warm by nature, "ought-to-return" vivifies the
>   blood—what is the method of their use?
> (*Crimson sings:*)
> Facing the rockery, she turned her back and hid in the shade,
> So the ingredients of this prescription are the hardest to find.
> One or two doses will make people so.
> (*Male lead speaks:*)
> What should I shun?
> (*Crimson sings:*)
> To be shunned is the "knowing mother" not yet asleep;
> To be feared is that "Crimson" might blurt it out.
> Once taken,
> It will surely "make the gentleman" "completely well."
> (*Crimson speaks:*)
> My mistress wrote this prescription out in her own hand.
> (*Male lead acts out looking at it. Bursting out with laugher, he arises.*)[12]

In this aria the names of six medicines are used in a way that plays on their vernacular names and their properties. In the first line there is a pun on the words *yaoying* (waving shadows) and *yao yinzi* (something that is added to medicine to make it more palatable). Cassia flowers (*guihua*; cinnamomum cassia) are used as both a medicine and a flavoring for medicine. "Ought-to-return" (*danggui*) of the second line is usually identified as *Angelica sinensis*, an important drug in regulating the blood and for menstruating women, which is why, according to Li Shizhen, its name indicates the longing of a husband, akin to Student Zhang's longing for Yingying.[13] Vinegar is used to treat swelling and sores but also to detoxify toxins of fish, meat, vegetables, and insects. "Vinegar" is also a common pejorative applied to young and callow students, as well as a symbol of jealousy. *Yin* ("to hide") also means a storage vessel buried in the ground. "Knowing mother" (*zhimu*) is *Anemarrhena asphodeloides*, a drug used to treat "agitation, fever caused by yin deficiency, and the wasting diseases heat [due to] depletion [*relao*], corpse transmission and pouring [*chuanshizhu*], and bone-steaming depletion [*guzhenglao*]."[14] "Crimson" (literally, "the red maiden," *hongniangzi*) is red ladybug—a constitutional tonic that makes one feel happy and vigorous. According to Li Shizhen, red ladybug is an effective treatment for the evil qi of confidantes (*xinfu xieqi*) and yin atrophy, and for bolstering vital essence or semen (*jing*) and enhancing willpower. When a boy is born whose father took a lot of this drug, the boy will develop into a man with strong sexual desire.[15] "Make the gentleman" (*shijunzi*), according to Li Shizhen, takes its name from a Mr. Gao (official title, *shijun*) who used the drug to treat infantile diseases of all kinds, though it was also good for deficiency with heat, and for killing worms. "Completely well" (*can*) pronounced differently is ginseng (*shen*), which is good for treating the five types of overstrain and seven types of injuries, deficiency with dreams in men and women, and blood loss.[16]

Given the medical knowledge expected of the reader (or audience member), the aria can be roughly paraphrased as follows:

> Cassia flowers added to the medicine for draughts deep in the night,
> Angelica root soaked in vinegar,
> Taken face-to-face from the storage pit in the rear of the false rocks–
> This is the prescription that's hardest to find.
> Don't take this powerful diuretic before you go to bed;
> I guarantee this purgative [will get rid of what's eating you] and a little
> bit of ginseng [will stimulate you].[17]

All of the medicines in this aria are related to diseases of love, longing, sex, and jealousy, which is why the Ming commentator Mao Xihe pointed out that Crimson is scolding Student Zhang with teasing language.[18] The real meaning of this aria and of Student Zhang's laughter is that Yingying is suggesting through Crimson that she is medicine for his illness. But if Wang Shifu was trying to incite laughter in his audience or in his reader, he depended on them having a ready knowledge of at least some of the most commonly used pharmaceuticals, their nicknames, and their uses. It is not just that the names of these medicines sound like something else—"knowing mother," "crimson," and "make the gentleman"—but the humor of this passage lies in the fact that these medicines, like Yingying herself, cure diseases of depletion caused by excessive longing (and sex or masturbation). Some believe that this sort of clever wordplay is part of the tradition of the early prosimetric and vernacular narratives known as "transformation texts" (*bianwen*) of the late Tang and was a common feature of the urban stage in China. Certainly it was not lost on the Ming commentator Xu Shifan (fl. late 16th century), who pointed out, "The secretly concealed six medical names are *guihua*, *danggui*, *zhimu*, *hongniang*, *shi junzi*, and *shen*," nor on Ming commentator Wang Boliang (ca. 1610) that this aria used the names figuratively; he said, "The six names of medicine all provide metaphorical meaning just like in ancient times when they used poems with names of medicine."[19] This kind of play with medical terms was not uncommon in dramatic literature, though this is a more sophisticated aria than others.[20] In this piece, though, the author does not simply rely on the audience to understand the joke; he relies on Student Zhang to understand it. Zhang has just acknowledged that his illness comes from lechery, but Yingying reveals to him through Crimson's complicated aria that she knows it too.

Poems and literary games that employ medical knowledge appear in other genres of literature in the Ming and Qing, but they tend not to add much significance to the work in which they appear. While some texts, such as *The Story of Mr. Sangji* (Sang ji sheng zhuan, late Ming), employ the names of medicinals throughout, many works simply have a few flourishes of medical knowledge.[21] In *Journey to the West* (Xiyou ji, 1592) for example, two poems feature puns on herb names. There is nothing consistent about the plants' medicinal qualities, nor are they relevant to the plot of the novel or to the themes of fighting or warfare. Some commentators were not impressed by these poems, or perhaps by any such poems. Li Zhuowu (1527–1602) writes in a marginal note, "These names of medicines are irritating."[22] Poems of a similar nature are featured in *Plum in the Golden Vase*,[23] in the form of literary games such as those in which virtually every line contains the name of a fruit, flower, drug, coin, song title, or other specialty drawn from the realm of vernacular knowledge. The earliest extant works of this kind date from the Six Dynasties period (222–589) but became increasingly common in both elite and popular literature during the Song dynasty. These seem to have no other purpose in novels than showing off either the author's talents or those of a character.[24] Superficially, *Annals of Grasses and Trees* does not seem, at least by design, to be much more than an extended version of this kind of word game. Its participation in a tradition of medical entertainments, however, suggests otherwise.

(a)   (b)

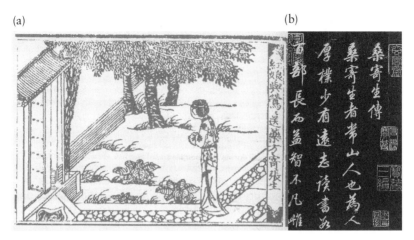

Figures 3.3a, 3.3b   (a) In *Story of the Western Wing*, Hongniang takes Yin-gying's medical prescription to Scholar Zhang; Waseda University Library. (b) Rubbing of *The Story of Mr. Sangji*; Creative Commons.

THE PLAY OF *CAOMU* LITERATURE

The period in which *Annals of Grasses and Trees* was most popular, the late Qing, saw the performance of plays (*xiqu*) that also personified drugs and had plots designed to allegorize their functions, interactions, and properties.[25] Perhaps even before the publication of that novel, but certainly afterward, a number of such operas also had the title *Caomu chunqiu*. These were read and performed well into the 1930s.[26]

Late-Qing and Republican-era medical manuscripts copy these plays with differing titles, including *An Illustration of Numerous Drugs* (Yaohuitu), *An Illustrated Study of Numerous Drugs* (Yaohui tukao), *Numerous Drugs, in Illustrations with a Musical Score* (Yaohuituqupu), *Tales of Herbs and Trees* (Bencao zhuan), *Records of Materia Medica* (Bencao ji), *Annals of Material Medica* (Bencao chunqiu), and *Opera on the Natures of Drugs* (Yaoxing bangziqiang and Yaoxing xi).[27] The variety of titles and numerous extant printed and transcribed editions attest to the popularity of these plays.[28] Those that survive all have either eight or ten scenes, but they were written in different regions and as such their content and language vary somewhat. Rural theater plays contributed mostly to public entertainment, but these seem to have been written in response to a perceived need for public education and for this reason have been

termed "pharmaceutical didactic operas."[29] As the final rhyme in a
1932 manuscript copy of the play *Illustrated Study of Numerous Drugs* states,

> Although all diseases are different, and each has its own cause,
> A good physician will do his best
> Everywhere to raise the dead and bring them back to life,
> He also writes a play to be performed in the streets.
>
> Tree and leaves, herbs and roots become fantastic figures.
> Secret recipes assist to help everybody to be in perfect health.
> If, in the future, the actors have performed this play,
> There should be no patients any more.[30]

The didactic and charitable impulse here is quite explicit.[31] The lines
claim that a doctor wrote the play but that it transmits secret recipes
so that everyone who hears the play can treat themselves.

A late Qing manuscript edition of the *Caomu chunqiu* play has an
identical table of contents to that of *Illustration of Numerous Drugs*,
and the plots are very similar. One difference is that the former has
two prefaces. The first records the story of an official, who in 1894
"followed the Eastern campaign of the Xiang army under General
Xiong, and met an old priest on the way in Henan in the big temple
of Zhangdefuku," and who gave the official a medical book. The second preface is a sequel to the first. It tells how this official, from 1894
on, taught himself medicine: "Now, [I] gathered comments from all
authors on a broad scale, excerpted their essence, corrected their
errors, eliminated heterogeneity, supplemented omissions, explained
what had not been explained before, and selected what should be
the most important. And yet, I preferred not to be too concise in my
words. Rather, my presentation should be fun. Hence, I compiled the
piece *Caomu chunqiu*." One version of the *Caomu* play with similar
but not identical content dates from the Kangxi period, though it is
possible that this record refers to the novel of the same title.[32] Some
of the late-Qing versions of these plays copied in medical manuscripts
have a style of writing that indicates that they were copied from a
printed book.[33] It is difficult to say which was written first, the novel
or the play version of *Caomu chunqiu*,[34] but both became popular at
the same time, and claimed to have been written for the purposes of
charity, education, and entertainment.

There are some interesting differences between these pharmaceutical dramas. Plays with the title *Caomu chunqiu* are much

clearer and more detailed than the *Illustration of Numerous Drugs*. When characters come onstage, for instance, the *Caomu* does not introduce them with traditional designations, such as "girl speaks" (*danbai*) or "clown sings" (*chouchang*), but with abbreviated versions of their actual names. This is of definite advantage for understanding the plot if someone were reading the play, and it is a constant reminder that these are drugs speaking and singing. Both plays give dosages of the drugs to be used in pharmaceutical recipes, but they are more consistently given in the *Caomu*. This suggests that some versions were intended to serve more as practical textbooks, and others more as general guidelines. That these pharmaceutical plays were actually used in medical practice, at least by some, is borne out by a manuscript in the Berlin collection titled "Annals of Herbs and Trees, Rhymed Verses Used by Itinerant Physicians" (Caomu chunqiu lingyi zhudiao), which combines the play with the handwritten records of an itinerant healer. Another manuscript shows physical signs of use, with damaged margins and extensive marginal notes. The differences between these plays also suggests that they evolved over time. In the course of their transmission, either as texts or as performances, plots were revised and amended, and changed in accordance to medical theory and contemporary materia medica, just as other medical texts were amended, their errors corrected, heterogeneity eliminated, and omissions provided.

Household notebooks in the Berlin medical manuscript collection, such as the "General Notebook" (Zongjilu), which has entries from 1936 to 1951 in Ye County, Shandong, record both pharmaceutical treatments and various sacrifices. Sacrifices were made on many occasions, such as the seventh day after child was born, on children's birthdays, when a child was ill, when a child was cured from illness, when a child suffered from pain in the eyes, when there was an insect plague, and when a horse was sick. The "General Notebook" records that to make or redeem a vow to a sprit, rather than making a physical offering or animal sacrifice on the altar of the spirit, one should sponsor a dramatic performance.[35] It may have been on such occasions that the plays centering on medical-pharmaceutical issues were performed. Other plays with medical themes, such as the legendary stories of the physician Sun Simiao, *King of Medicine* (Yao wang) and *The Story of Medicine and Tea* (Yaochaji—a case of poisoning and the medicinal tea that saves the day), may also have been performed

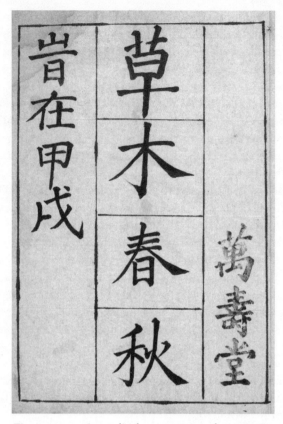

Figure 3.4. A medical manuscript that consists
only of the complete play *Annals of Herbs and Trees*.
The title page here is written to imitate the appearance of printed title pages, and carries what seems to
be the studio/name of the copyist/owner, Wanshou
Tang. The cover carries stamps of the bookseller.
Staatsbibliothek zu Berlin—Preußischer Kulturbesitz, East Asia Department Slg. Unschuld 8095.

on these occasions, though neither of these plays seems intended
to educate.

In the plays whose titles are *Caomu chunqiu* and *Illustration of
Numerous Drugs*, the characters and plots are basically identical.[36]
If they were meant to educate, their variety of entertaining and at
times bawdy plots surely aided in keeping the audience's attention.
The protagonist of the medicine plays is Gan Cao (licorice root), an

old scholar. He has a daughter named Ju Hua (chrysanthemum) who is engaged to Jin Shihu (dendrobium).[37] In scene 1 of most of these plays, titled "Zhizi is glib" (Zhizi douzui), four robbers, Da Ji (boor's mustard), Yuan Hua (lilac daphne), Gan Sui (euphorbia root), and Hai Zao (seaweed), plan to abduct and rape Ju Hua. When she learns of this, she falls ill with fear. Gan Cao calls on his servant Zhizi (Cape jasmine) to search for a physician, but he is reluctant to go, and argues with Gan Cao. The second scene, "Monk Tuo flirts with a nun" (Tuoseng xi gu), cuts to Mituo (litharge), the priest of the Red Stove Temple, who flirts with the nun Ci Gu (arrowhead). Zhizi, searching for a physician, happens upon them in flagrante delicto. The priest and the nun drug Zhizi with monkshood root (*caowu*), rendering him unconscious, and they throw him on a heap of sweet wormwood (*qinghao*). After that, Mituo and Ci Gu return to secular life. When Zhizi regains consciousness in the next scene, "The bewitching snakes emerge" (Yaoshe chuxian), he sees two beautiful women who are really Black-striped snake (*wushaoshe*) and White-banded snake (*baihuashe*) in human form. Zhizi makes an obscene offer to them, after which they drag him into their snake hole. Jin Shihu, who happens to be looking for these snakes, arrives in time to rescue Zhizi in scene 4, "Shihu subdues the monsters" (Shihu xiangyao). He enters into a fight with the snakes and kills both of them. Zhizi says he is looking for a physician to treat Ju Hua, and Jin Shihu reveals that she is his fiancé. In scene 5, "Lingxian invades for the sake of peace" (Lingxian pingkou), Jin Shihu asks his friend Wei Lingxian (clematis root) to help him defeat the four robbers who intended to abduct and rape Ju Hua. After a violent fight, they defeat and burn the four robbers to death. Jin Shihu returns to Ju Hua in scene 6, "Seeking refuge with relatives at Gan Mansion" (Ganfu touqin), but the robber Mu (*muzei*, common scouring rush) plans to break in at night to rape Ju Hua and rob Gan Cao. His plot is foiled, and Jin Shihu and Ju Hua marry. In scene 7, "Hongniang sells medicine" (Hongniang mai yao), the story returns to Zhizi's search for a physician. He encounters a girl, Hong Niang, selling medicinal drugs, and propositions her. The story returns to Jin Shihu in scene 8, "Calamity of the lost hairpin" (Jinchai yihuo), in which Shihu is traveling to the capital to take the examinations. On his way he stays at an inn run by Mituo and Ci Gu, who plan to kill their guests. Assisted by Zhizi, Shihu kills the former monk and nun. In the next scene, "Fanbie revolts" (Fan Bie zaofan), a foreign king's son-in-law, Fan Biezi, starts an uprising and

(a)   (b)

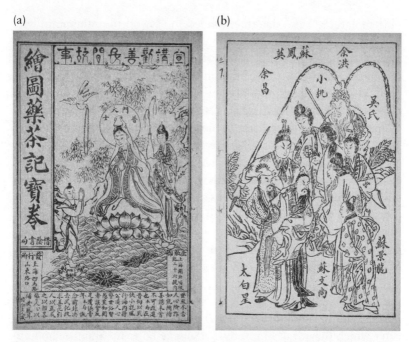

Figures 3.5a, 3.5b.   (a) The title page of the printed edition of *Medicinal Tea*
(Yaochaji), formatted like a scripture printed for distribution and merit accumulation (as were many *baojuan* published in the Republican period). (b) its
cast of (nonmedical) characters. University of Tokyo Library.

intends to invade China. Jin Shihu, who has passed his exam, and
been appointed to the position of military doctor, is ordered to repel
the invasion. A large battle ensues. In the course of the fight, Fan Biezi
uses the drug sal ammoniac (*naosha*) to blind thousands of Chinese
soldiers. In Act 10, "Gan Cao brings peace to the Country" (Gan Cao
heguo), Gan Cao comes to Jin Shihu's aid. He uses azuritum (*kongqing*) to cure the eyes of all soldiers. Fan Biezi surrenders, and Jin Shihu
returns in triumph.

So much action suggests that the intended audience was not very
sophisticated, and that the purpose of such a play was to employ
the structure as a comfortable rubric through which to disseminate
practical medical knowledge. There are few diseases featured in the
play—this was not the same kind of practical knowledge found in
encyclopedias and formularies (this disease, this prescription). Rather,
the knowledge transmitted depends on learning the hierarchy and
interactions of the characters to discern the natures and interactions

of drugs, the sort of information usually found in materia medica. Perhaps this is why the play was copied out in medical manuscripts, given that much of the knowledge it transmitted was foundational for elite medical practice rather than for quick home remedies. These pharmaceutical plays seem aimed at helping the uninitiated to begin the study of medicine, to disseminate knowledge that could be used by laymen to detect the false prescriptions of quacks by understanding drug interactions. It is also possible that the unsophisticated playgoer may have had enough medical knowledge gleaned from word of mouth or life experience that they were able to use that medical knowledge to better understand the play—the interactions between characters, the alternate hierarchies into which their pharmaceutical namesakes place them, the attribution of gender or office to one or another drug, and the humor of base drugs brought into submission by powerful ones.

There are a few different ways in which medical knowledge is woven into the librettos of these plays. The most common and obvious are the drugs with leading roles. For example, when Gan Cao enters the stage for the first time, he introduces himself, "This old man's family name is Gan; his personal name is Cao. His home is in the province of Shanxi in the district Fu [Fenzhou] in the hamlet of Pinghe." Fenzhou in Shanxi is the primary place of origin of the drug *gancao*. The village of Pinghe ("peace and harmony") is fictitious, but the name points to the mild effects of the drug and the ability of both character and drug to bring peace to the body politic.[38] Gan Cao then begins to sing:

> Who is my equal? My nature is sweet and balanced.
> I am good at balancing all drugs.
> I am also good at bringing them together and at dissolving all sorts of
>   poisons.
> My name has been famous for thousands of years.
> Simply apply me, and I will warm the center and eliminate cold.
> If roasted, I can be of help, too.[39]

Gan Cao subverts the conceit by explicitly describing the natures and interactions of his pharmaceutical namesake, though they are reminiscent of an old man's tolerant, honest nature. Gan Cao subdues the revolt initiated by Fan at the end of the play, which is an allusion to the drug *gancao*'s function of dissolving poison like the toxic drug *fanmubie* (nux vomica), the namesake of the rebel leader Fan Mubie. Gan Cao is awarded the honorary title of *guolao*, "elder of the state," which is one of the vernacular, alternate names of the drug *gancao*.[40]

According to the concept of "eighteen oppositions" (*shiba fan*), a famous list of dangerous drug interactions which Gan Cao also recites,[41] the drug *gancao* is "opposed" to the four substances *daji*, *yuanhua*, *gansui*, and *haizao*, the namesakes of the bandits out to rape his daughter. If drugs known to be "mutually opposed" (*xiangfan*) are consumed together, they will be toxic and evoke severe reactions in the patient. The play invokes this pharmacological conflict by portraying enmity between characters. It also illustrates drug affinities. For instance, the purgative rhubarb (*dahuang*) is often combined in medical formularies with the two substances hedge thorn (*zhishi*) and mirabilite (*mangxiao*), and correspondingly, the character Gan Cao, working with Da Huang, has two assistants named Zhi Shi and Mang Xiao.[42]

Toxic drugs tend to be cast in villainous roles.[43] A leading role in the play is the monk Mituo (Mituo seng). His name is a homophone of the pharmaceutical drug *mituoseng* (litharge), which is (mostly) lead monoxide, a toxic residue remaining in a furnace used to refine silver in Ming times and earlier.[44] It was also used to remove putrid flesh. The name includes the character "monk" (*seng*), leading the drug to be personified as an evil monk. Mituo introduces himself entering the stage:

> Prepared as an ointment, the loitering monk Mituo cures sores and
>   malignant boils.
> With liquor and meat he connects with his friends and is on good terms
>   with all sorts of physicians.
> I am the monk Mituo from the Red Furnace Temple
> In the temple, the old teacher Silver was not willing to keep me any
>   longer because my natural disposition is simply too poisonous.
> Many Mongolian physicians make use of me when they boil their
>   ointments; they resort to me to cure sores and malignant boils.
> Every day I go out to many places to meet my best friends, and all we do
>   is eat meat.[45]

This statement refers to the preparation of *mituoseng*, a leftover of the alchemical processes used to refine silver, hence "the old teacher Silver was not willing to keep" it any longer. It is frequently used in Chinese external medicine to cure various types of abscesses and to remove rotten flesh, hence "it goes out to many places" and "eats meat." Not only is the image of eating rotten meat off-putting, but since monks are not supposed to eat meat, it also implies taboo violation, adding to the overall villainy of the character. When Jin Shihu kills Mituo, he boasts of having "smashed him and thrown him into an oil cauldron to boil an ointment," a reference to the processing of *mituoseng*.

The opera structure allows for the easy insertion of poetry and rhymed instructions that were commonly found in pharmaceutical and recipe texts. In the *Caomu chunqiu*, characters also frequently quote verses verbatim from medical literature. For example, Mituo, Zhizi, and Ci Gu sing a verse often printed in pharmaceutical texts, the "nineteen fears" (*shijiu wei*), in which one drug's toxicity or action is counteracted or reduced by another. Similarly, the Black-striped snake sings to her sister a rhymed list of drugs pregnant women must avoid that is found in many medical texts.

The play is interspersed with brief statements of proverbial medical knowledge, such as "whether it is sore or not, immediately drink a decoction with dandelion [*diding*]" and "for pacifying a fetus, mugwort leaf [*aiye*] may be fine, but one must add donkey-hide glue [*ejiao*] to see a wondrous [effect]."[46] Generally speaking, the author takes pains to work the medical knowledge into the story in a logical way—the libretto is not just a hodgepodge of rhymed instructions sewn together. For example, Mituo's carnivorous inclination (taboo for a monk) is taken as an opportunity to discuss the medical properties of various kinds of meat:

> Today I ate donkey meat; it excites wind and stimulates lust. I ate dog meat. Dog meat is warm; it strengthens the yang and benefits the kidneys. I ate mutton. Mutton is hot. It causes massive sores. I ate pork. Although it nourishes the spleen, it also has the disadvantage of generating phlegm. I ate beef. It supplements spleen depletion and is very beneficial to people. I ate soft turtle meat. It has a turtle shell that nourishes the yin and pushes back heat. I ate chicken meat. It has a chicken gizzard. It is in great demand to rub away amassments.[47]

The plays repeatedly list groups of related substances, but the styles of such listings vary considerably. At times, drugs are mentioned together simply because their names all begin or end with the same character (such as *sha*, *zi*, *ren*, or *huang*), or because they contain homophones. For example, Mituo sings,

> Bat's dung [*yemingsha*] is able to cure sparrow eyes [i.e., night blindness].
> Climbing Japanese fern [*haijinsha*] cools heat and opens the passage of water.
> To harmonize the stomach and pacify the fetus, resort to amomum seed [*suosha*].

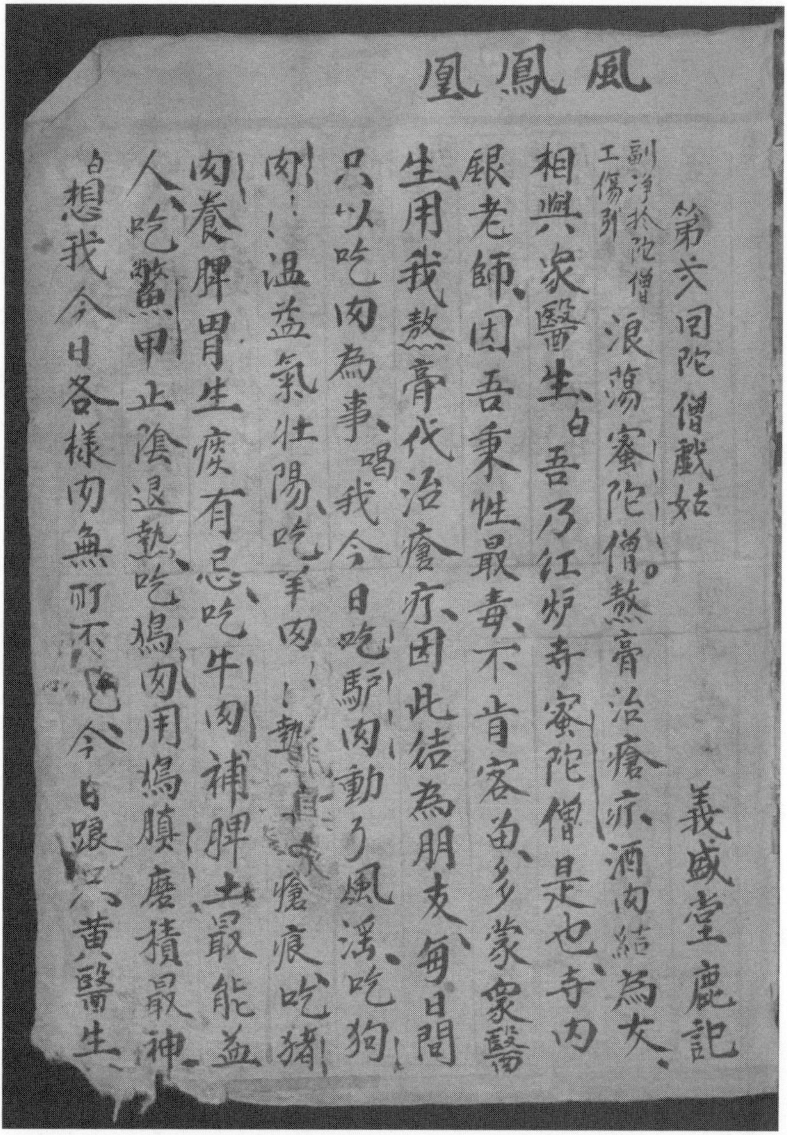

Figure 3.6. A Republican-era manuscript of *Annals of Herbs and Trees*, showing many writing errors (and calligraphy practice?), but with additional plot points and material added to the play. The scribe identifies himself at the bottom of the first line (Yisheng Tang, Lu ji). The scene is labeled as a "chapter" (*hui*), a usage more common in prose fiction and oral literature but which also appears, along with similar terms, in Pu Songling's songs. Staatsbibliothek zu Berlin—Preußischer Kulturbesitz, East Asia Department Slg. Unschuld 8801.

(a)   (b)

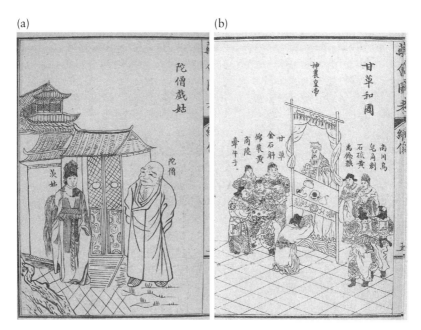

Figures 3.7a, 3.7b. "The monk Tuo flirts with a nun" (a) and "Gancao restores peace to the kingdom" (b). From a 1935 lithographic edition of *Illustrated Congregation of Drugs* (*Yaohui tukao*), Wellcome Library, London.

> To dissolve a swelling of the throat, there is borax [*pengsha*].
> To eliminate wind dampness, there is silkworm dung [*cansha*].
> To ease one's heart and calm the spirit, use cinnabar [*zhusha*].[48]

Printed pharmaceutical literature lacks these kinds of groupings, but they are certainly reminiscent of the many medical poems featured in practical medical texts such as the "Song on Natures of Medicines" (Yaoxing ge) that were designed to aid learning. Dai Baoyuan (1828–1888?), a doctor who compiled a set of medical verses, confessed that his reason for doing so

> was really due to the fact that I was slow and not gifted, and I put myself in the shoes of [other beginners]. I was ashamed that I had not been successful in [Confucian] study. That was the reason why I took up medical studies with my late father. I was then already over thirty, and had lost the sharpness of the youthful mind. . . . Things in [medical] classics were forgotten almost as soon as they were learned, and it was not because I did not concentrate, but because of my age.[49]

There was a perceived need for medical mnemonics, for practitioners or for the readers and audiences of plays. The presumption is that medical knowledge is difficult to learn, which is why it was put in verse, but these medical didactic plays also presume that medical knowledge was not interesting, and so had to place the mnemonics in the context of an opera.

Elsewhere in *Illustrated Numerous Drugs* and *Caomu chunqiu*, pharmaceutical substances of a similar nature or action are grouped together. For example, when Zhizi goes out to seek the help of a physician named Huang Qi (astragalus root), he partly speaks, partly sings, "I think that Dr. Huang lives in the village of the Warmth family. So there should be many [family members] with a warm nature." He then enumerates the male and female members of the family, all warming drugs, and the illnesses they treat. This speech is clearly a mnemonic device, personifying drugs with a warm nature as members of the same household, all of the "female" drugs being fragrant substances (i.e., having *xiang* in their names). This grouping relies on the medicine of systematic correspondence, but is also consistent with the taxonomy of practical medical texts that order drugs according to use.

Another approach to grouping substances is based on shared origins. In one scene of the play, Zhizi wants the medicine Hong Niangzi (red ladybug) is selling, but does not want to pay for it:

Female Clown [*choudan*]: You don't look like someone who can afford to buy drugs!

    Clown [*chou*]: How I look is none of your business. There's a saying: The poor consume drugs, the rich pay for them.

Female Clown: If you think you can consume drugs without paying for them, you are wrong!

    Clown: I don't want anything for free. I just happen to have no money!

Female Clown: If you have no money, then why don't you take drugs you can get for free?

    Clown: Drugs you can get for free? Which ones are they?

Female Clown: Listen to me. (Sings:)

You could take "the yellow in man" [*renzhonghuang*, a drug prepared from feces]. It is good to dissolve heat poison.

You could take "the white in man" [*renzhongbai*,

a drug prepared in urine]. It is capable of curing noma.[50]

There is also sparrow droppings [*baidingxiang*], which can break up accumulations of poison.

There is also rat droppings [*liangtoujian*]. It relieves head-wind.

Then there is boys' urine [*tongzibian*], which nourishes one's yin and brings down fire;

as well as flying squirrel droppings [*wulingzhi*], which regulates the blood and stops pain.

There is also hare droppings [*wangyuesha*]. It pushes back cataracts and clears the eyes.

Finally, there are maggots in feces [*fenzhongchong*]. If the intestines are blocked, they can penetrate the blockage.

Clown: Are you saying you want me to eat shit and drink piss?

Female Clown: If you won't eat shit or drink piss, why should I give you other drugs for free?[51]

This aria is similar to Crimson's (and this Hong Niangzi might be referencing that Hongniang) in *Story of the Western Wing*, in which a prescription suggests that Student Zhang is suffering from a condition brought on by lust. But the medicine plays are not consistent in their pedagogical strategy. These plays employ the names of drugs as homophones or puns simply for the sake of wordplay, similar to the verses in *Journey to the West* and *Plum in the Golden Vase*.

Drugs grouped into prescriptions further illustrate the didactic impulse of these plays. For instance, when Wei Lingxian falls ill, he says, "Today cold evil has directed itself against my stomach, with the result of vomiting and pain. In my heart I experience turmoil; my intestines have diarrhea."[52] His two wives, Zi Shiying (amethyst) and Bai Shiying (quartz), suggest the following:

> Master is ill today; he must get some medications to cure his vomiting, disperse the cold, strengthen the spleen, and eliminate wind, and then he will be fine. (*Singing:*)
> Take some beefsteak leaves [*zisuye*] to disperse the cold and bring down qi.

Take some esholtzia herb [*xiangru'er*] to discard summer heat and wind.

Take some Sichuan magnolia bark [*chuanhoupu*] to regulate the pain and dissolve the swelling.

Take some hyacinth bean [*baibiandou*] to benefit the spleen and harmonize the center.

. . . Zi Shiying says: "Ah! Now, I too have developed a chill on my body. I assume I have been affected by something adverse—wind and cold. But I am not willing to spend money to purchase medication. What should I do? I have it!" (*Singing:*)

"I will consume some radish [*luobo'er*]; this will remove any distension.

I will drink a bowl of onion and ginger soup [*congjiang tang*]; this will disperse wind and cold."[53]

This scene teaches the audience how to treat a very common illness using the most basic, cheapest drugs and household food. The didactic impulse or charitable impulse to spread knowledge is clearer here than in the clever displays of knowledge found in the poems randomly interspersed in Ming novels, but these prescriptions are not common in the plays. What is common in these plays, however, is a great deal of information about aphrodisiacs, which is in keeping with tendencies found in practical medical texts. Mituo, for instance, recites such a recipe for men to enhance their potency:

Seven grains of clove [*dingxiang*] and eight grains of pepper [*jiao*], Manchurian wild ginger [*xixin*], dragon bones [*longgu*], and cuttlebone [*haipiaoxiao*], as well as a little calcined alum [*kufan*] mixed with honey, will let a girl of eighteen years sway her hips.[54]

Providing the audience with such a prescription might seem to contradict or subvert the charitable impulse of these plays, but medical manuscripts, materia medica, and medical recipe books contain so much information about sexual dysfunction and aphrodisiacs that there must have been great demand for such information. The authors of these plays were at least sparing audience members from having to purchase such drugs from medicine peddlers, quacks, or charlatans. Moreover, Mituo's interest in aphrodisiacs serves the story in that it enhances his lechery and, as a presumably celibate monk, his villainy. These medical plays were popular in that they were printed and copied repeatedly, and were performed in different regions of the empire, but they were also popular in that they reflected the contents of popular, practical medical texts.[55] They gave the audience what they wanted, and helped them to remember it, too.

Anthropomorphism is the most unique mnemonic device sustained throughout the play. Pharmaceutical drugs become people, and not only do they interrelate in a way that reflects the natures of drug interactions, but the characters are described in ways that reflect notable features of the drugs. In addition to the self introductions that included their primary functions and place of origin, a character's appearance, armor, horse, weapons, and fighting style could reflect the drug's characteristics. Cape Jasmine describes the foreign villain (*fanzei*):

> (Sings:) When he was born, his complexion was that of green copper and he was able to cure festering eyes.
> As an adult, he had red lotus hair and he was able to supplement involuntary seminal emission.
> On his head he wore a white cockscomb and was able to administer a white girdle.
> He wore pig-hoof armor and was effective in the management of anal fistula.
> He availed himself of a horse the color of orange peel and converted phlegm and ended cough.[56]

This character's description explicates the effects of the drugs copper rust (*tongqing* / *tonglü*), red lotus (*honglian*), white cockscomb (*jiguan*), pig trotters (*zhuti*), and orange peel (*juhong*), as well as their appearance. In this play, the evil monk, the irascible servant, and the cheeky medicine peddler all have similarly striking features that elaborate on the appearance and functions of the drugs for which they are named.

None of these medical plays is known to have existed prior to the Qing dynasty.[57] Still, personifying drug names and associating drugs with social roles have a long history in Chinese literature. Possibly beginning with the Han dynasty, drugs were categorized as "ruler" (*jun*), "ministers" (*chen*), or "assistants" (*zuoshi*), to show their role in a recipe that was believed to function like a social body: with one ruler at the top, several ministers below the ruler, and even more assistants at the bottom of the hierarchy. In subsequent dynasties, literati wrote poems in which the names of drugs were used to imply certain emotions.[58] When composing medical plays, authors had a variety of models upon which to draw, such as *Story of the Western Wing*, *Journey to the West*, and *The Story of Mr. Sangji*. However, the primary aim of conveying pharmaceutical and medical knowledge to audiences by means of a folk opera appears to have been a completely new development in the Qing. The plays must have been the work of highly educated authors with a thorough knowledge of contemporary medicine, since they reflect contemporary concerns and discuss drugs that are not included in earlier works such as *Systematic Materia Medica*. These plays may have had an underlying purpose—to educate—but they did not lose sight of the crucial role entertainment played in the pedagogical project. A purely didactic play featuring the names of 550 drugs would likely have been as tedious then as it seems now, but the crafting of comic scenes, variety of word games, breaking of taboos, sexual innuendo, and regular use of low or vernacular speech were clearly employed to make these medical plays entertaining.

There is no way to know if these librettos were intended for performance. It may well be that the subtle allusions to certain pharmacological functions, as well as the passages with sexual themes, simply appealed to men of higher education and were written for their private reading pleasure. What we can be certain of is that these plays were written by authors with a great deal of medical knowledge, some literary and linguistic sophistication, and a charitable impulse to increase or standardize medical knowledge among those who could read—and perhaps those who could not. We also know from extant manuscripts and printed editions that they were used, annotated, supplemented, and commented upon.

ANNALS OF GRASSES AND TREES: A NOVEL

If the medical-didactic plays came first, the novel version of *Caomu chunqiu*, did not learn much from them. If the novel was first, the plays did not seem to garner much attention from subsequent literary critics. If the plays were meant to teach, or at least to entertain, the reason for the existence of the novel that shares their title is less clear. The sex, bawdy innuendo, taboo violation, witty repartee, and demons that entertain the reader or audience in medical plays are almost completely absent in the novel *Caomu chunqiu yanyi*. Its plot is completely different from that of the plays, and although almost all of the same characters reappear, they are often cast in different roles. The plot of the novel essentially has two parts. It opens with an introductory chapter in which Liu Jinu (wormwood) sits on the throne during the (fabricated) Zhongxuan years of the Han dynasty (there is no discoverable dynastic period in the plays). He is a benevolent king, and the people are happy. The "old man of the country," Gan Cao, along with two prime ministers, has helped to establish this long-lasting era of peace. The main characters are then introduced. The regional commander of Chang'an, Jin Shihu, has a large, loving family with two sons, Jin Yingzi (Cherokee rose) and Jin Lingzi (chinaberry), and a daughter, Jin Yinhua (honeysuckle). Jin Shihu, his sons, and his uncles are all skilled in martial arts. Jin Shihu was good friends from childhood with Huang Lian (Chinese goldthread), now the regional commander of the military in Yazhou, with three sons, Huang Qi (radix astragali), Huang Qin (scutellaria), and Huang Dan (lead oxide /minium). They, too, are well versed in the arts of warfare. The first chapter then moves to Buddha Cave on Mount Wudang, where Immortal Weiling (Chinese clematis) has four apprentices, but only one of them, Jue Mingzi (cassia seed), is unable to learn the secrets of the Dao.[59] Weiling predicts that the Kingdom of Hujiao (pepper), which is ruled by King Badou Dahuang (croton seeds and rhubarb), will invade the Han Empire, and he sends Mingzi down the mountain to assist Han.[60] Three years later, when Mingzi has quelled the invasion and restored peace, he may return to the mountain. Huang Lian visits Jin Shihu in the capital, and the two old friends agree to wed Jin Yinhua to Huang Qi. Yinhua had just recovered from an illness, and plans to travel to Temple Hai Jinsha (Japanese climbing fern) in Xuanzhou to redeem the vow she made to Guanyin when ill. Jin Shihu sends Jin Lingzi to escort and protect her. The first part of the novel (chapters 2 through 5) sees Lingzi and Yingzi set upon by bandits, but each is rescued by an immortal who brings them back to their abode and instructs them in medical and martial arts. They are told that they will see each other, and their parents, again in one year. Jin Shihu hears of his missing children and goes to wipe out the bandits. Shihu is joined by his brother-in-law, the regional commander of Xuanzhou, Mu Tong (*mutong* stem). With their combined troops, they defeat the bandits, and their leader, Tianzhu Huang (tabasheer), flees.

The second part of *Caomu chunqiu yanyi* makes up the bulk of the story. Chapters 6 through 32 follow the invasion of Han by Badou Dahuang and his army. The many characters from the first part of the novel are the primary heroes, particularly Jin Shihu, Huang Lian, and their children (Liangzi and Yingzi join the fight with new

powers), although the novel introduces over two hundred more characters, all of whom have the names of drugs. The great majority of
characters are mentioned only once or twice, and many are the disciples of some more important figure. Disciples are to their masters
as supplementing drugs are to a core drug. Each side has numerous victories and defeats, and each comes up with increasingly complex battle formations and increasingly severe weapons. Each side
begins to draw on the talents of various immortals and demons that
are loyal to their side, and employ their magic to inflict great losses
on the enemy. Hujiao is joined by two other foreign kingdoms, but
all are eventually defeated by a heavenly army of immortals called
down by Weiling Xian and deployed in the unbreakable "heavenly
web" (tianluo; luffa) formation; a deus ex machina that goes without explanation. Li Shizhen explains that when the fruit of tianluo
(aka tiansigua) gets old, its fibers are exposed. These resemble the
Channels and the Collaterals, which makes tianluo good for dredg-
ing them and for dispersing invading pathogenic wind, detoxifying
toxin, eliminating swelling, dissolving phlegm, relieving pain, and
killing worms. Hence, the name is useful in describing a weblike formation designed to purge invaders.[61]

The plot is thin, with little character development. Nor does it contain much in the way of direct speech, let alone banter. The complexity
of Caomu chunqiu yanyi lies almost entirely in the descriptions and
interactions of the many drugs introduced. The novel format allows
for certain groupings that would be difficult in a play. For instance,
Jin Shihu and his children all have names that are from the categories
of herbs or woods, even though they share the common surname Jin
("gold"), and the novel takes pains in the first chapter to describe how
Jin Shihu named each of his children, Jin Lingzi, Jin Yingzi, and Jin
Yinhua. The author was drawing on materials more contemporary
or popular than Systematic Materia Medica to make this grouping.[62]
The utility of these taxonomies is limited, though, because the drugs
have nothing in common—their flavors, natures, origins, and treatments all differ markedly, they do not occur in prescriptions together
very often, and it is only their names that have some overlap. The
immortal Weiling, for instance, who in the novel is the originator of
Daoism, has four disciples—Jue Mingzi (cassia sophera), Tian Xianzi
(henbane seeds), Yi Zhizi (alpinia oxyphylla), and Yu Zhizi (akebia
fruit—the names of which, aside from being medicinal drugs, sound
like higher states that have been honed through spiritual devotion

("clear decision," "immortal," "growing wisdom," and "anticipation," respectively). Classification based on these sorts of homophonic puns might suggest that the author was appealing to a readership with a bit more literary sophistication than the audience of the bawdy medical plays.

Some characters fight alongside others to indicate that those drugs are often used together in prescriptions, but providing the reader with useful recipes is clearly not a primary concern of the author. One common grouping, and perhaps the most significant for aiding memorization, is that of a character with its weapon and mount. For instance, Mituo is one of the primary villains in the novel. He is a powerful warrior and sorcerer and is put in charge of the invading army. He is cast as a villain, as he is in the plays, because it was a common role for strange monks in novels, who seemed particularly evil when transgressing their oaths of poverty, vegetarianism, abstinence, or nonviolence. The drug *mituoseng* is not particularly toxic or dangerous, though its uses enhance the monk's evil image because it "eats" necrotic flesh and treats diseases of the nether regions—dysentery, hemorrhoids and anal fistula, sores and itching of the genitals, and bone infection due to having intercourse with a blood relation in the first month of pregnancy.[63] In battle formation, Mituo rides a tiger cihu (litharge) carrying a halberd huzhang (knotweed) in his hand.[64] He is associated with the tiger (*hu*) and the huzhang because the drug *mituoseng* was said to come from the Hu region.[65] But the drugs homophonous with Mituo, his tiger, and his weapon do not have much in common in terms of geographical provenance, effects, natures, or treatments, or as ingredients in the same prescription. *Mituoseng* also does not occur with or have much in common with his sister drug, pale butterfly bush (*mimenghua*), his master pumice stone (*haishi*), or king (*badou dahuang*). The rebus seems to mark a particular kind of allegorical thinking—it is blatantly literalistic, draws on homophones to signal basic information about a drug, and brings that knowledge to life.

The wordplay in the *Caomu* novel relies on information that is more like materia medica literature—giving natures, origins, or alternate names of a drug—than popular recipe books that pair drugs according to a taxonomic aim of practical remedy. For instance, the king of the invading country has the mandate of heaven in his own country, and is a good ruler. The drugs from which he takes his name, *badou* (croton) and *dahuang* (rhubarb), are two of the most

common drugs in Chinese medicine. *Badou* is toxic and a strong purgative, and it was used to treat stagnation in the viscera and bowels,
as well as to facilitate urination, eliminate malignant flesh, and purge
vicious agents such as invading ghosts or worms. *Dahuang* is nontoxic and is sometimes referred to by the name "military general"
because "the drug pushes away the old and brings in the new, like a
military general putting down a riot and bringing peace."[66] Most of
the prescriptions in which it is the primary ingredient are for treating
accumulation and stagnation. "Attack" (*gong*) is one of the standard
verbs used to describe the action of drugs that purge and break up
stagnation, and it is likely for this reason that the author cast these
useful drugs as benevolent invaders. One early Ming account criticizes doctors for thinking that it was always necessary to "attack
and lead away" (*gongli*) stagnations of blood when treating traumatic
injuries. It describes how, to treat the injuries of soldiers defending
a besieged city, doctors used rhubarb (*dahuang*), switching to croton seed (*badou*) when they ran out.[67] Presumably these two drugs
were thought to be pharmacological "doubles," thus justifying the
only such pairing of names in the novel. However, many of the most
useful drugs in the physician's arsenal were not cast in starring roles.
Ginseng (*renshen*), to cite just one example, is a minor character in
the invading army. Obviously (as we have seen with *hongniangzi*,
mituoseng, and *weilingxian*), some drugs lend themselves to anthropomorphism simply because their names sound like those of a young
woman, a monk, and an immortal, respectively. Other primary characters, such as *badou dahuang* and *huangqi*, were commonly used
drugs in prescriptions, though just as often major characters, such as
Fupen Zi and Mu Lan, are drawn from drugs that occur infrequently
in pharmacopeia.[68] The *Caomu yanyi* employs vernacular knowledge
of pharmaceutical drugs drawn from works of materia medica but
rewrites it, not according to utility but according to literary logic. In
this regard, it is like a "literati" novel in the respect that it relies on the
reader having enough familiarity with the textual tradition to make
sense of its rubric. But the texts it draws on were themselves compendia of all kinds of information, much of it popular and practical, and
much of it reliant upon linguistic correlation, figurative language, and
literary devices.

It is possible that the author of the *Caomu* novel had little practical medical knowledge or that he was just arranging the contents of
some pharmaceutical text into taxonomic categories according to the

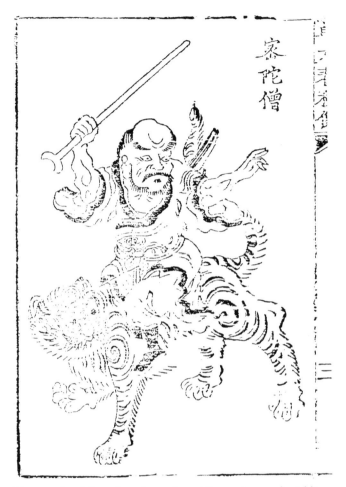

Figure 3.8.   Mituo Seng frowning, riding a tiger and wielding a sword that creates a medical rebus. University of Tokyo Library.

demands of conventional military romance plots. He may have been criticizing the same sort of doctor lampooned by the author of *Journey to the West*, or perhaps he was even satirizing those who aped Sun Wukong in reality. In chapter 69 of *Journey to the West*, Wukong ("Monkey") plays the doctor to the ruler of the scarlet-purple kingdom. He palpates the king's pulses and prepares a prescription for the king's illness. Wukong first asks for three pounds of each of the 808 different kinds of medicines to disguise the ingredients and quantities of his marvelous prescription recipe (*shenmiao zhi fang*),[69] evoking the language of generational doctors rather than medically trained ones.[70] Wukong tells Bajie, "Bring me an ounce of *dahuang* and grind that into powder." Sha Monk speaks up, "Dahuang is bitter in flavor; its disposition is cold and nontoxic. Its nature is sinking and not rising, and its function concerns movement and not fortification. It can take away various kinds of pent-up feelings and unclog congestion; it can conquer chaos and bring about peace. Hence its name is 'General,' for it is a laxative. I fear, however, that prolonged illness has weakened the person and perhaps you shouldn't use it." Smiling, Wukong says, "Worthy Brother, you don't realize that this medicine will loosen phlegm and facilitate respiration; it will also sweep out the chill and heat congealed in one's stomach. Don't mind me. You go also and fetch me an ounce of *badou*. Shell it and strip away the membranes. Pound away the oil, and then grind it to powder." Bajie speaks up, saying, "The flavor of *badou* is slightly acrid; its nature is hot and toxic. Able to pare down the hard and the accumulated, it will therefore sweep out the submerged chills of one's internal cavities. Able to bore through clots and impediments, it will therefore facilitate the paths of water and grain. This is a warrior who can break down doors and passes, and it should be used lightly." Monkey responds, repeating the sentiment, "Worthy Brother, you too don't realize that this medicine can break up congestion and drain the intestines. It can also take care of swellings at the heart and edema in the abdomen. Prepare it quickly, for I still must use an auxiliary flavor to lend the medicines further assistance." To this passage one commentator adds, "Bajie and Sha monk both have read some materia medica literature."[71] Another commentator finds Monkey's prescription esoteric: "I fear that the ten famous Ming physicians also have not heard of this [prescription]."[72]

Monkey also puts soot from the bottom of a frying pan into the prescription. "The proper name for this kind of soot is Hundred-Grass Frost [*baicao shuang*]," he says, "and you have no idea that it can soothe a hundred aliments."[73] This soot, not unlike *mituoseng* (the ash residue left from refining silver), is good medicine, but the idea of feeding it to a king is a carnivalesque image that might elicit laughter in the reader. The humorous nature of this prescription is pushed further when Monkey requires half a flask of urine from their horse.[74] Laughing, Sha Monk responds, "Elder Brother, this is no joking matter! Horse urine is both pungent and stinky. How could you put that into the medicine? I have seen pills made from vinegar, aged rice soups, clarified honey, or pure water, but never from horse urine. That stuff is so foul and pungent, the moment a person with a weakened stomach smells it he will vomit. If you feed him further with *badou* and *dahuang*, he'll be throwing up above and purging down below. You think that's funny?" It is doubly disconcerting that Bajie, who is himself the novel's clown, is worried that Monkey's medicine is a bad joke. Perhaps most interestingly, a chapter-end comment reads, "These days, there is no short supply of this sort of '*badou dahuang* doctor.' As for those who use *dahuang*, *badou*, pot soot, and horse urine to make a secret prescription, they know nothing . . . "[75] There is no doubt that this scene is meant to be comical. Bajie has a difficult time getting the urine from the horse, and Monkey says he also needs as an adjuvant "the fart of an old crow flying in the air, the piss of a carp in swift flowing streams, the elixir ashes in Lao Tzu's brazier," and other similarly difficult-to-obtain ingredients.[76] If these are unavailable, Monkey says, they can take the medicine with sourceless water,[77] but in the end he substitutes dragon spittle. The humor of this passage is multivalent—all readers can understand that the king is going to be given strong and disgusting medicines, but for those readers who understand the natures of these medicines, and their practical effects, the scene is even more ribald, while showing how Monkey apes common practitioners.

Bajie and Sha Monk laugh when Monkey explains the name of his secret prescription to the king: "This is called the Elixir of Black Gold." Smiling, Bajie and Sha Monk say to themselves, "There's soot mixed in it, it has to be black gold!" One commentator had never heard of this medicine, saying that it had a strange name, but this only reveals his own highbrow background (or general ignorance), since "black gold" was the name of various prescriptions common among hereditary doctors. In fact, it was mentioned in the *Systematic Materia Medica* repeatedly, and Xu Dachun recommends it in *Medical Cases of Huixi*, so it was not exclusively the purview of nonelite healers.

"Black gold pills" (*wujin wan*) was a name and a concoction similar to "elixir surpassing [the value of] gold" (*shengjin dan*) and "black spirit pills" (*heishen wan*).[78] All of them were core formulas that could be modified in their effects by ingesting them with different liquids. These "black gold" medicines, along with the likes of "the prescription offering Guanyin's all-encompassing help" (*Guanyin puji fang*) and "pills prepared with old ink" (*gumo wan*), treated a wide variety of ailments (in one medical manuscript, twenty-nine, forty, and seventy-one ailments, respectively), and were extremely common formula in the Qing. The "black gold" formulas had at their core the drugs *dahuang* and *badou*. One medical manuscript from the Republican period states in its introduction, "Black gold powder [*wujin san*] cures all ailments, just as the wind bends the grasses. Other names [of this prescription] are 'pine smoke elixir' [*songyan dan*] and 'black spirit pills' [*heishen wan*]. It cures thousands of illnesses, just as the sun melts the frost."[79]

Black gold pills (*wan*), powder (*san*), paste (*gao*), and elixir (*dan*) were commonly employed to cure gynecological issues. A prescription named "black gold powder" was first recorded in the Song work *A Spring of Recipes in the Magic Park* (Lingyuan fangquan)[80] and was followed by references in the Southern Song prescription collection "Complete Collection of Effective Prescriptions for Women" (Furen daquan liangfang, 1237), *Formulas for Universal Benefit* (Puji fang, 1390), and other works. Over the centuries, numerous formulas, each with different ingredients, became known under the names "black gold powder," "black gold pills," and "black gold elixir." The three designations of this formula result from the use of pitch (*mo*), a vernacular name for which is the "black gold" of these prescriptions.[81]

Monkey's prescription reflects a historical reality, namely that the advent of the imperial pharmacy (*huimin yaoju*) in the Song required doctors who had previously relied on simple medicines with one or two ingredients to employ formulas with numerous substances whose composition followed theories of systematic correspondences.[82] From this conflict between empirical and theory-based recipes arose a new type of prescription eventually consisting of a nuclear formula that could be adapted to the requirements of a given patient's disease by omitting or adding individual constituents in accordance with his pathological condition. Monkey is preparing simple, trusted medicine at the core, namely *badou* and *dahuang*, and adding to it many exotic, unobtainable ingredients.

Badou features prominently, and usually with gynecological implications, in a few short stories of the late Ming and early Qing. Perhaps the most notorious is the alternately macabre and ribald comedy "The Female Chen Ping Saved Her Life with Seven Ruses" (Nü Chenping jisheng qichu, 1654), the fifth story in Li Yu's *Silent Operas*.[83] In it, Geng the Second's Wife, Geng Erniang seeks to protect herself from being attacked by bandits who have overrun her village during the Ming-Qing transition. One bandit in particular tries to force himself on her. Erniang uses a rag soaked in her menstrual discharge to pretend that her period is not yet over to ward him off. On the second night, she applies *badou* around her forbidden area, so that its "jade skin became swollen, haloed with a purple hue. The deep slit rose to a shallow fold. There was no entrance door, because two halves became one. Though it still had a seam, it was very difficult to pry open. It looked like a steamed bun laid out for five nights, or rather, a mussel soaked in water for ten days."[84] Erniang, an illiterate peasant woman, is compared to the resourceful Han tactician Chen Ping, who was famous for his stratagems, duplicity, and ruthlessness, hence the term "female Chen Ping."[85] *Badou* here is medicine to repel men, and the description of its effects is both gruesome and coarsely comical.

The Geng Erniang story has a parallel in *Journey to the West*. It is funny, raunchy, and seems to critique the authority of kings, physicians, or both. This is particularly the case considering that Wukong diagnoses the heartsick king as having a "cessation of the menses" and then prescribes for him a common recipe to treat gynecological disorders. To understand this aspect of the carnivalesque comedy, or to realize that it was a mistake in the incorporation of medical materials into the novel, readers would have had to be quite familiar with medicine, at least enough to know that the medicine Monkey is preparing is consistent with his diagnosis.[86] Casting *badou* and *dahuang* as the invading king in *Caomu yanyi* likely does not reflect a negative attitude toward those drugs' properties of purgation. It also does not seem to be the case that the author is critiquing *badou dahuang* physicians, since the invading drugs were all part of elite medicine too. If anything, the author is just as guilty of their overuse. Nor is the author of the *Chunqiu yanyi* making a clear distinction between domestic and foreign drugs. Some that are foreign in origin do seem to have been cast on the side of the invading country, but the author is not consistent in that regard. He does not regularly refer to the invaders as coming from the Black Pepper (Hujiao) kingdom. Most often they are said simply to be "Fan," which could mean that the author was drawing on the medical plays or on some other source that discusses the foreign rebellion as coming from Fan, and being led by Fan Biezi, or it could simply mean "fan" in the generic sense of the term—"foreign."

The *Caomu chunqiu yanyi* is thus not a cohesive or consistent allegory. There is no medical lens that adds meaning to the overall point of the novel.

Good, domestic heroes and immortals best evil, invading ones, but such situations do not correlate to the drug interactions. The overall story, the battle between Han and Fan, is not enhanced by the strange fact that all of the characters involved—and their weapons, mounts, formations, and many places—all have the names of medicines. If the author of the preface is to be believed, though, the benefit of this novel (other than simply naming medicines, which seems like a useless project given the availability of pharmaceutical literature at the time), was in the various groupings of medicine names that might facilitate memorization. While obviously sharing many of the categorical groups that we can find in similarly titled plays, the *Caomu yanyi* does take advantage of the novel form to group some medicines according to linguistic, homophonic, and symbolic relationships. The only other justification that the author gives for writing such a novel—that the *Caomu Chunqiu yanyi* was a useful method to disseminate medical information—is borne out in reality given its multiple printings and its fame as a literary display of knowledge.

Despite the claims of the author, the novel does not seem to be terribly useful, especially compared to the play versions of these stories.[87] So, if it is not useful, what is its entertainment value? One answer to this question was that it drew on the narratives and metaphors found in pharmaceutical literature. For instance, Liu Jinu is cast as the Han Emperor, likely because, as the *Systematic Materia Medica* recalls, the drug is named after an emperor:

> Li Yanshou in his work *History of Southern Dynasties* [Nan Shi, 420–589] recorded: Liu Yu, with the nickname Jinu, Emperor Gaozu of the Song, was once leading his troops to conquer rebels in Dixin prefecture before he was crowned. He saw a big snake and shot at it with his bow and arrow. The next day, returning there, he heard a sound of husking. He saw a group of young lads husking herbs under a brush. When Liu asked them what they were doing, the youths replied, "Our master was shot by Liu Jinu and we are preparing drugs for him." Knowing that the lads were preparing drugs for the wounded serpent, he realized these were not ordinary people. So, Liu asked again, "Why not kill Liu Jinu since he wounded your master?" The boys answered, "No, Liu will be a king and cannot be killed." Liu shouted at them, and the boys disappeared. So, Liu took back the drug and used it to treat those suffering from battle wounds. It was very effective. Later the drug was called Liujinucao [herb of Liu Jinu].[88]

Badou, as Monkey reminds us, is a warrior who can break down doors and passes, a statement echoing that of Zhang Yuansu, who is quoted in the *Systematic Materia Medica* as saying, "*Badou* is a warrior that fights fiercely and bravely."[89] The same text calls *dahuang* "the general who pushes out the old to make way for the new."[90] The metaphors and stories found in pharmaceutical literature are the guiding logic for casting Liu Jinu and Badou Dahuang as leaders, since they are all drugs placed in a metaphorical military hierarchy, and all were used to treat injuries sustained by soldiers. The entertainment value in this regard is to highlight or develop the literary aspects already extant in materia medica literature. There are wars and alliances between drugs metaphorically scattered about and hidden in the classificatory structures of pharmaceutical literature. In other words, the *Caomu chunqiu yanyi* is not a medical allegory, it is a hodgepodge of collected medical metaphors, based on their descriptions, origins, and actions. *The Caomu Chunqiu yanyi* is pharmaceutical literature as entertainment; it highlights the literariness latent in materia medica literature and at the same time strips materia medica literature of its usefulness.

The *Systematic Materia Medica*, with the exception of some early chapters devoted to particular diseases and their remedies (*baibing zhuzhi yao*), gives a historical survey of each drug, along with first-hand accounts of its uses. Entries typically begin with an explanation of names (*shiming*) that discusses the drug category, followed by definitions and variant names as found in a wide variety of texts. Li often refers to the early dictionary *Explaining the Graphs and Analyzing the Characters* (Shuowen jiezi) in this section and gives his own opinion as to which name is most fitting, and which are not. Collected notes on origins, harvesting, and production (*jijie*) follow, with lengthy quotations from previous medical, historical, and literary works. Li provides his comments on each throughout. A section that expresses doubts and corrects errors (*bianyi* or *zhengwu*) follows, as do sections for adapting and preserving the medicine (*xiuzhi*), the smell and toxicity of the drug (*qiwei*), and indications and curing efficacy of the drug (*zhuzhi*). The last two sections of each entry for a drug consist of Li Shizhen's and his predecessors' experience with the medicine (*faming*), and prescriptions (*fufang*), including methods of preparation, quantities, and evaluations of effectiveness. In the narrative of one drug army invading the kingdom of another there no explicit discussion of any given drug's properties, and when alternate names, drug affinities, origins, properties, or uses are mentioned, they are done so obliquely (though not necessarily subtly) through the historical romance paradigm.

If its compass and utility were far inferior to materia medica literature, at least the *Caomu yanyi* shared a similar general project: to classify and reclassify the potent natural world.[91] The *Systematic Materia Medica*, according to some, was innovative in its reclassification of the entire materia medica according to a new logic that was to a greater or lesser extent motivated by the "investigation of things" (*gewu zhi xue*).[92] The *Caomu yanyi*, clearly not beholden to the *Systematic Materia Medica*, reclassified materia medica according to a literary logic—that of linguistic correspondence and metaphors drawn from stories of derring-do. In this regard it could be said that the *Caomu yanyi*, rather than being a materia medica stripped of its usefulness, was rather an attempt to reveal the literary logic that tied these drugs together in a web of relationships.

Some were still reading and writing about this novel in 1926, such as Liu Dabai (1880–1932), who, for instance, suggested that the eighteenth-century comic novel *Which Source?* (He dian), a collage of standard sayings and clichés, was descended from "reductionist" literary ancestors, in which only a single aspect of reality, or single register of the language is used, such as *Annals of Herbs and Trees*, *History of Roaches* (Zhang shi, late Qing), and poems composed entirely of names of things from a certain category, such as stars (*xingming shi*) or medicines (*yaoming shi*).[93] Others in this genre would include *Story of Various Fruits* (Baiguo zhuan, late Qing), in which all characters have the names of fruits (which is apparently a late imitation of the *Caomu chunqiu*), and *The Story of Beheading Ghosts* (Zhangui zhuan, 1688), in which the world is described as being inhabited only by various kinds of ghosts. In some cases this limitation seems to have been chosen as a means of attracting special attention to a given area of literary virtuosity, but often the one-sidedness is clearly a device for satire and caricature.[94] Based on the number of late Qing and early modern editions, *Annals* was popular among readers, but it was also notorious for its peculiarity, and often mentioned in essays on literature. The twentieth-century writers Lu Xun and Mao Dun both mentioned it, although both recognized it only as a curiosity.[95]

The *Caomu yanyi* does not feature any explicit prescriptions, as do the medicine plays, and very few characters receive medical treatment.[96] Since the novel warranted so many editions and at least one imitation, it must have been the delight in uncovering these drug names that made the conceit worthy of preservation.[97]

Why, in light of so much Western medicine being transmitted to China, and of the decline of traditional literati novels, was *Caomu yanyi* reprinted so many times in the first decades of the twentieth century?[98] The preface to a 1923 edition recommends the novel despite its many demons and spirits, and its violence. It claims that the novel is worth notice for its "amusing" (*huaji*) use of medicines, and is nonetheless helpful and interesting (*zhuqi*). The modern preface places the value of the *Caomu yanyi* on its timely reminder of the threat of foreigners and its notable military strategies. Du Ji, the author of the modern preface, writes,

> Thus, this book, the *Caomu chunqiu*, although it uses strange names, and features spirits and mad demons, yet its principles and results are deep indeed. Precisely because it is a book that startles [the reader] and reveals the fearful and unreasonable that it will enlighten the reader. For instance, take the simple narration and detailed language of the book. Its worth is deepened because it alleviates the melancholy of even those who peruse it.[99]

It may seem odd to deemphasize the medicine in a novel that is so conspicuously titled (in this edition) *Searching for Hidden Pharmaceuticals: Annals of Grasses and Trees* (Yaowu suoyin caomu chunqiu, 1923), clearly indicating its function as a teaching text or medical word-search.[100] Yet, the value in reading the *Caomu yanyi*, at least to some, lay in the ability of its method to shock the reader into enlightenment—or at least alleviate his melancholy.[101]

NOVELS AS RECIPE BOOKS

In premodern novels, when characters discuss diseases or when a doctor makes a pronouncement, often included is the name of a prescription (without details on the recipe for it) or a discussion of the primary drugs to be used to cure the patient. But some popular and well-esteemed works of narrative fiction did transmit practical medical prescriptions. Two early novels (possibly the earliest) to include full medical prescriptions in their texts, complete with weights of ingredients and preparations, were *Sequel to Plum in the Golden Vase* and *Marriage Destinies to Awaken the World*. Both of these two novels seem to have had a didactic intent. The authors defend their use of the vernacular, saying that they were following the precedent of the great Ming novels,[102] or that they used "plain" (*fuqian*) and "unrefined" (*li*) language so that peasants and women would be able to understand.[103] Although these claims were not uncommon apologies for writing in the vernacular, the degree to which these novels borrow from daily-use encyclopedias and similar helpful sources is extensive.[104] The impulse to bring knowledge to readers may have been inspired by *Plum in the Golden Vase*, to which both novels are heavily indebted.

In chapter 49 of *Marriage Destinies*, the Chao family celebrates the birth of Chao Liang's son with a banquet, at which a Daoist guest thanks the Chao family with a prescription for smallpox (*douzhen*). His prescription gives the exact amount of each ingredient and the steps for making the medicine. In chapter 57, Madame Jiang sends a servant to fetch a pill (*lanji wan*) from her father, and the narration inserts a detailed formula for the prescription, ostensibly because it is a "marvelous prescription" (*shenfang*). Unlike the prescription in chapter 49, this one is set off from the text, as if it were a poem or some other quoted text. It likely was drawn from another source, since there are many pills with this name in contemporary medical literature.[105] It is also consistent with the impulse to propagate good prescriptions for merit, but why bury one in the text and make another so pronounced?

Marriage Destinies presents two other prescriptions that are set off from the rest of the narrative, both aphrodisiacs.[106] Prescriptions, it might be needless to say, are a jarring break from the narrative in the same way that novels written as vehicles for poetry often do not transition well between prose and verse. Like publishing poetry, transmitting these prescriptions was important, though perhaps not important enough to justify writing an entire novel. There are not many prescriptions in these two novels: *Sequel to Plum in the Golden Vase* gives two prescriptions in full, for stomachache and for cold (*hanzheng*), quoted in chapter 17.[107] Many other prescriptions are named but not detailed. In chapter two of *Marriage Destinies*, for instance, Grand Physician Yang is described as "a notorious charlatan. He was the type of doctor who would prescribe the 'Decoction of Four Ingredients' [*siwutang*, a medicine for blood disorders] for toothache and the 'Powder of Three Yellows' [*sanhuangsan*, a laxative] for diarrhea." Yang usually prescribes "the ten [ingredient] completely and greatly supplementing decoction [*shiquan dabutang*],"[108] a common recipe in early modern China, regardless of the ailment, sometimes with healing effects, other times with fatal results. Clearly, readers were expected to be familiar with these prescriptions, since the comedy would be lost if they were not. But it seems just as clear that the

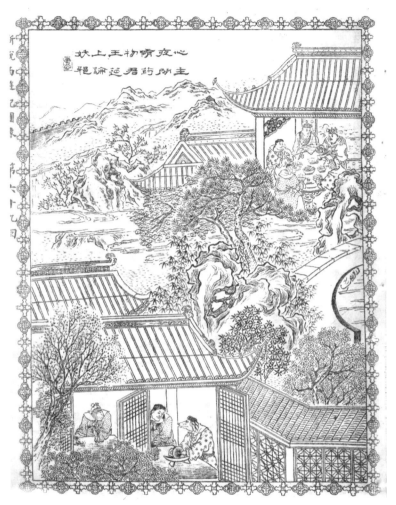

Figure 3.9.   Wukong and Bajie prepare medicine for the king in *Journey to the West* (chapter 69). Cornell University Library.

prescriptions that are detailed in these novels, while they account for a tiny portion of those texts, must have been there because the author assumed his readers were not familiar with them and should be.

It is difficult to say if any of these medical recipes were original. Some were available in daily-use encyclopedias such as *Seeking No Help from Others for Myriad Things* (Jianqin Chongwenge huizuan shimin wanyong zhengzong bu qiu ren quanbian), which is even mentioned in chapter 2 of *Marriage Destinies* as a book that Chao Yuan's household owns. The prescription for stomachache in *Sequel to Plum in the Golden Vase*, "decoction for reversed cold of limbs" (*sini tang*), is reprinted in many daily-use encyclopedias of the time and likely borrowed from such a source.[109] Aphrodisiacs are often included in late-Ming daily-use encyclopedias, in which sexual cultivation (*fengyue*) was an essential category.[110] Almost all such books also discuss the prevention and treatment of smallpox and related illnesses, and many devote a chapter to it. It is possible that these novelists were trying to enter into dialogue with encyclopedias and to correct or supplement what they found there. The inclusion of these particular prescriptions in the novel text suggests that the author had firsthand experience with them and knew them to be particularly useful, efficacious, and in need of propagation.

The Qing dynasty saw an increased interest in local charity work of all kinds, and some harnessed the charitable impulse to justify becoming a professional physician.[111] Some notable literary men pushed the well-documented defense of medicine as a charitable (or humane, benevolent, or *ren*) practice further.[112] Chen Hongmou (1696–1771), a well-known Qing scholar-official, wrote that even more than practicing medicine, "if kind-hearted gentlemen could share what they know [about efficacious herbal formulas] and post it wherever people gather together, then they will have accumulated more merit than giving away herbal medicines."[113] Printing effective prescriptions in novels may have been the penance authors needed to pay for writing them in the first place.

Some of the medical manuscripts in the Berlin collection include passages from novels copied by doctors who seem to have copied them simply for their own enjoyment.[114] Other medical practitioners, though, read novels differently—making careful notes on the prescriptions they copied from novels such as *Flowers in the Mirror*, *Biography of Jigong* (Jigong zhuan, 1744), and *Record of Wiping Out Bandits* (Dangkou zhi, 1831).[115] *Wiping Out Bandits* by Yu Wanchun was published shortly after *Flowers in the Mirror*), with at least twenty-two Qing editions, most of them in the Tongzhi (1861–1875) and Guangxu periods.[116] *Flowers in the Mirror* was similarly popular in those periods, when nineteen of at least thirty-five Qing editions were published.[117] Although *Biography of Jigong* was published in 1744, there were at least twenty editions in the late Qing and Republican period in Shanghai alone, with particular interest in the Guangxu period.[118] All three manuscripts that copy the medical information from these novels attest to their popularity, though none of them shows any interest in the novels themselves.

The practical prescriptions contained in novels do not bear any relationship to the narrative either.[119] They are dropped into the novel, seemingly without any literary value other than heightening the realism of a quotidian scene. Setting prescriptions off from the narrative would have made practical bits of information easier to find and use. A variety of records attest to various people using the prescriptions from *Flowers in the Mirror*.[120] There was plentiful and real medical information in that novel, according to readers.[121] A late Qing account remarks, "[*Flowers in the Mirror*] is filled with medical prescriptions, and they have never failed to have effect for those who employ them. Mr. Shen of Zhejiang has collected them in a book called *Tried and True Prescriptions* [Jingyan fang]."[122] The recipe for a salve to treat burns taken from chapter 26 of *Flowers in the Mirror* differs slightly from the prescription found in *Systematic Materia Medica* (which in turn quotes *The Materia Medica of Food* [Shiwu bencao]). The *Systematic Materia Medica* recommends grinding okra (*kuicai*) and applying it directly to burns or scalds. The prescription in the novel says to mix fresh flowers from the okra known as *qiukui* or *jizhuakui* with sesame oil, and if they are not in bloom, to substitute rhubarb (*dahuang*).[123] The Wu Taichong preface to a Shunzhi (1644–1662) edition of the *Systematic Materia Medica* (originally published in 1596) laments that it "has already been in circulation for a long time, and yet most doctors do not use it for guidance, let alone the rest of the population."[124] Presumably the *Systematic Materia Medica* and some other medical works were simply too large or expensive or contained too much information to sift through if someone was looking for prescriptions for particular problems. Or, if it had fallen out of use, it was perhaps because there were more people who had taken the practice of medicine into their own hands, and found the *Systematic Materia Medica* too difficult to use because of its organizational scheme, which starts with medicinal drugs and then explains what they are good for, rather than starting, as novels did, with symptom sets, then naming the illness and listing prescriptions to cure it.

Different materia medica books were written for different reasons, but their main use was to deepen practitioners' understanding of drugs and their usefulness. The *Systematic Materia Medica* is enormous, comprised of over two million characters, and the length alone must have been daunting for anyone seeking to look up specific information. Moreover, the *Systematic Materia Medica* was just one of roughly ten thousand extant medical books written before 1911, a quantity of literature that would have been overwhelming to a filial son who wanted to find a good prescription for an ailing parent, or for a local doctor who did not have extensive education. These were likely the people who found prescriptions in novels. In any case, whoever these users of novels were, it was partly because novels shared their content and, to some extent, format with daily-use encyclopedias and guidebooks to daily life that they could be so construed. The pharmaceutical knowledge they contained was more like the practical, middlebrow, and vernacular medical texts that collected good prescriptions, more like formularies that listed diseases and recipes, than they were like elite medical texts that discussed whole-body imbalances and debated warm or cold pathogenic influences.

The belief in the practical applicability of *Flowers in the Mirror* was widely held throughout the Republican period, with some even referring to it as a "scientific novel" on the basis of the prescriptions given out by the protagonist, Tang Ao.[125] Yet, despite the fact that Tang Ao is presented in the novel as being interested in the collection of a variety of kinds of knowledge and specimens, among which materia medica figures prominently, much of his materia medica knowledge does not seem to be exactly canonical. In one scene, he eats "walk-on-air plant" (*niekong cao*) that allows him to jump to superhuman heights, and during that leap, he finds and eats "jade paste" (*yujiang*), which turns him into an immortal.[126] But this did not seem to confuse readers about which prescriptions were useful, or about the fundamental utility or purpose of the novel. In chapter 27, Tang Ao's sidekick, Duojiu Gong, uses "man and horse, safe and sound powder" (*renma pingan san*) to cure Tang Ao's dysentery (*liji*). Xu Xiangling's marginal commentary says, "This prescription is truly effective, not simply idle theorizing."[127] He claims that this is a tried-and-true prescription from the mid-Qing, saying that the earliest reference to it is Xu Dachun's *Standard Criteria of the Orchid Dais* (Lantai guifan, 1764), and that it is also called "elixir worth a thousand gold" (*qianjin dan*).[128] Xu Dachun does indeed discuss this recipe, and clearly indicates that it is a "secret prescription" (*mifang*).[129] Xu Xiangling, familiar with this passage, must have believed that Li Ruzhen, like Li Shizhen, was popularizing secret prescriptions for charity and to combat quacks.[130] But Xu's comment about the prescription being effective (*youxiao*) and not just idle theorizing (*zhishang tanbing*) is also interesting because he does not consider that the prescription might be fictional, only that such medical recipes may be based on theory and not experience. The majority of prescriptions in *Flowers in the Mirror* do not seem to exist in previous printed literature, leading many to believe that they were the invention of Li Ruzhen himself—drawn from his experience (*yanfang mifang*).[131] This is at least the case for those prescriptions that were put into practice. Whether or not Li Ruzhen authored the prescriptions in his novel, it was their perceived originality that made them important. That they were thought to be secret prescriptions (and therefore potent) made available through the widest possible method of dissemination, the novel, seems to have been proof enough that they were helpful. These may have been folk prescriptions, but, unlike many culled from that tradition, the prescriptions found in *Flowers in the Mirror* were deemed trustworthy because they had modest claims and treated everyday ailments.

Just as some in the mid- and late Qing claimed that novels such as *Warning Lights at the Crossroads* (Qilu deng, mid-eighteenth century) were fictionalized household instruction manuals (*jiaxun*), so they also believed certain novels to be instructive compendia of medical knowledge.[132] *Flowers in the Mirror* explicitly claimed this role. Tang Ao expresses his goal of making effective medical prescriptions available to wide audiences. Duo Jiugong helps to heal Tang Ao's dysentery, and Tang Ao says to him, "Since [your prescription] is so efficacious, why don't you publish it and make it accessible to the public? In that way, everyone would be able to avoid this malady and they can extend their lives. Isn't that a great benefit?" Jiugong refused at first: "Our family depends for its livelihood on secret medical prescriptions. If I publish them, everyone will have the access to the prescriptions. In that case, who will still buy medicine from me? I know that it is meritorious to make secret prescriptions known to the public, but aren't I just adding to our troubles if I do that?"[133] In the conversation that follows, Tang Ao elucidates the benefits of making all hereditary secret prescriptions known to the public and eventually manages to persuade Duo Jiugong to publish his prescriptions. Duo says, "I will surely publish all of the secret prescriptions I've inherited from my ancestors, and give them out. In this way I will benefit the world *yiwei jishi zhi dao*]."[134] This is the very prescription the medical manuscript (likely written in the early Republican period) copies into its margins.[135]

Xu Xiangling said about the three prescriptions in chapter 29—"protecting pregnancy no worries powder" (*baochan wuyou san*) "iron fan powder" (*tieshan san*), and "seven *li* powder" (*qili san*)— "these three prescriptions were all hand-picked by [Li Ruzhen], and put out into the world for the public. It was his desire that this book would transmit them, echoing and validating the claim of the chapter title 'transmitting wonderful prescriptions / an old man helps the world.'"[136] Xu Xiangling mentions only three prescriptions in chapter 27, but there are five. The other two are very simple prescriptions, juice from onions, wine, malt, shrimp, and urine, so perhaps they were not remarkable for that reason. But this omission suggests that Xu does not particularly agree with Tang Ao, who says, "The world is filled with wondrous prescriptions, but from antiquity these are rarely transmitted, and become lost. Perhaps it is because the ingredients are not particularly precious that people ignore them, and so many become buried. Now, knowing medicines that are of little value, [I] am able to cure disease . . . if you take the value of the drug in order to determine its worth, that is truly harming the common people in the extreme!"[137] In chapter 55, Tang Ao laments, "People nowadays have forsaken the old ways and esteem only luxury. Among the transmitted prescriptions that contain expensive and precious drugs, the common people see them regardless of their efficacy, and there are none that do not look like silver bullets [gods]. If the transmitted prescription does not contain valuable and precious drugs, even if it is effective, people look at it and ignore it, saying that buying it is of no use."[138] Yet some readers thought these prescriptions of particular use, and *Flowers in the Mirror* intentionally charitable because its prescriptions were comprised of widely available and cheap medicines.[139] If readers of *Flowers in the Mirror* trusted these prescriptions, they were at odds with the Qing dynasty doctor Zhao Xuemin in *Listing the Elegant Practice* (Chuanya), who claimed that mendicant doctors always use terms like "honest," "cheap," and "ordinary" (*lian, jian,* and *bian*) to describe their prescriptions.[140] Since many mendicant doctors were recorded by the likes of Xu Dachun as being quacks, readers could just have easily associated cheap medicines with medical charlatans.[141] Li Ruzhen must have been responding to this ambivalence when he cast characters as humane mendicants and proponents of simple, inexpensive (and unprofitable) drugs.

Some of the medical manuscripts in the Berlin collection similarly encourage readers to distribute one or another medical recipe to gain

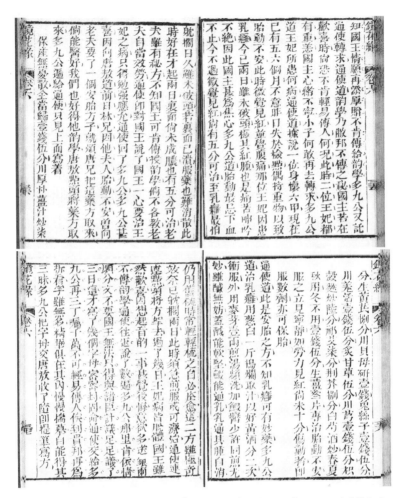

Figure 3.10. Prescriptions in *Flowers in the Mirror* for easy childbirth (*top, indented*) and for abscessed breast (*bottom, within the text*). From chapter 29 of the 1832 edition, Waseda University Library, Japan.

merit. In some cases, a message is attached to these "retributive recipes" informing users that they "must not be kept secret" (just as in others there are directions to keep it secret).[142] Once a person has obtained such a prescription, he is obliged to pass it on and make it known to as many other people as possible. Disseminating such a retributive recipe results in reward, and keeping the formula for one's own use invites disaster. In manuscripts that contain lists of

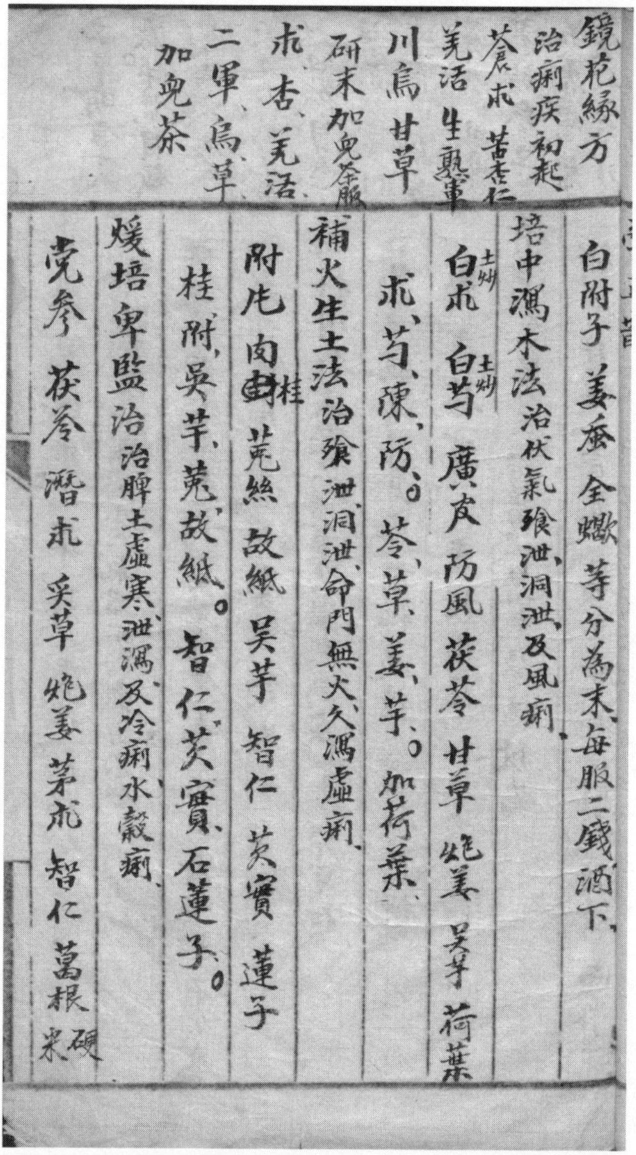

鏡花緣方

治痢疾初起

蒼朮 苦杏仁

羌活 生熟軍

川烏 甘草

研末加兜茶服

朮、杏、羌活、

二軍、烏草、

加兜茶

白附子 姜蚕 全蠍 等分為末、每服二錢酒下、

培中瀉木法治伏氣飧泄洞泄及風痢

白朮土炒 白芍土炒 廣皮 防風 茯苓 甘草 炮姜 吳芋 荷葉

朮、芍、陳、防。苓、草、姜、芋。加荷葉。

補火生土法治飧泄洞泄命門無火久瀉虛痢

附片 肉果桂 蔻然 故紙 吳芋 智仁 芡實 蓮子

桂、附、吳芋、蔻、故紙。智仁、芡實、石蓮子。

煖培卑監治脾土虛寒泄瀉及冷痢水穀痢

黨參 茯苓 潛朮 炙草 炮姜 茅朮 智仁 蒿根 米硯

Figure 3.11. Medical manuscript quoting *Flowers in the Mirror* prescription for dysentery (*liji*). Staatsbibliothek zu Berlin—Preußischer Kulturbesitz, East Asia Department Slg. Unschuld 8315

prescriptions, authors frequently identify one as needing printing and distribution. Some manuscripts also contain a "secret merit text" (*yingongshu*), which discloses single-ingredient prescriptions recommended for treating often-seen ailments. Retributive recipes banked credit that would later be spent by asking a sprit for help with another medical cause, such as an illness or a birth. Some manuscripts record prescriptions that were given out by a pharmacy.[143] Tang Ao's predilection for simple, cheap medicines led some of his readers to think of his novel as just such a book of merit.

Some readers wanted to see the authors doing this work themselves, and so cast them as characters in a similar plot to disseminate medical knowledge to the masses. For instance, there are some stories (*chuanqi*) that feature the miraculous healing powers of *The Story of the Stone*'s author, Cao Xueqin.[144] In one story, "A Tried and True Prescription Saves the Villagers" (Minjian yanfang qiu xianglin), the reader is told that Cao "understood the ways of medicine, he knew efficacious prescriptions, and every day he gathered effective prescriptions from among the people in order to propagate them and thereby cure commoners of illnesses. Stories concerning his medical prowess spread far and wide." Cao cures three cases of "yellow sickness" (jaundice, *huangbing*) by getting patients to eat live mudfish (loach). The first, a young scholar named Liu Xianglian, courageously perseveres in coming every day for three months and swallowing whole, large mudfish to cure his illness—this after Cao saved him from his attempt to drown himself in the lake. The narrative tells us that his faithfulness in following Cao's prescription and their subsequent mutual respect led Cao to cast Liu in *Story of the Stone*. Cao modifies his prescription in elaborate ways for an old woman and a pregnant woman, demonstrating that he has real medical knowledge, and effects cures in all three cases.

Similarly, Cao cures patients with simple medicines after many preceding doctors have failed to do so. Specifically, he often employs Chinese celery, the *qin* (*yeqin, shuiqin*) of his name. In one story he cures a poor, elderly man of liver disease with it, and in another, cures a young woman of consumption (*lao*).[145] These stories, like the tale of eating loaches, emphasize the local origins, simplicity, and cheapness of the drugs, but also the ingenuity of Cao in thinking to use them, both tailoring the medicine to the disease and to the person who cannot otherwise afford medicine. Cao, like the typical good doctor in literati fiction, always turns down payment: "All of the medicine I use I have collected with my own hands. I don't need a penny. I see patients and practice medicine in order to help the sick and relieve suffering, not so I can profit. It is proper for village and farm [i.e., ordinary] doctors to have this medical virtue."[146]

Cao finds celery so effective for his poor patients that he buys a small tract of land and cultivates the celery that grew wild in the Western Hills.[147] He calls this plot Celery Garden (*qinpu*). That Cao had cured the young woman's consumption spread throughout the white banner, and many came from far and wide seeking his treatment.[148] These people did not call Cao by his given name, Zhan, nor did they use his courtesy name, Mengruan; they called him only Master Celery Garden (Qinpu Xiansheng), which pleased him. Thereupon he took Qinpu as his nickname. Another story similarly remarks that this is why he is known today as Cao Xueqin.[149] Cao, like Tang Ao, is made into a charitable doctor, though, according to the novels that feature them, both are poor. It is somewhat curious that Cao is chosen for this role, since the medicines in his novel are either very complex or clearly fictional, as in the case of Xue Baochai's "cold fragrance pills."[150]

Authors, commentators, and critics of the late Ming through Qing periods continually emphasized the didactic value of traditional fiction. *Marriage Destinies to Awaken the World* and *Sequel to Plum in the Golden Vase* both focus on retribution; so it seems sensible that prescriptions might be included as an example of the sort of merit characters and readers need to accrue.[151] If there is a relationship between the story and the prescriptions that they transmit, it might have to do with charity, and with helping others even if they seem foreign or alien. The mundane medicines Li Ruzhen and Cao Xueqin supposedly employed reflected the practical sensibility of literati medical practitioners who also read novels. To apply these fictional prescriptions and propagate them as effective cures, acts of merit, and ultimately evidence that *Flowers in the Mirror* was a "scientific" novel was to be completely unfazed by the fact that the story in which the prescriptions are found is brazen fantasy, even if that fantasy is satire. The authors of *caomu* literature took advantage of literary devices and formulaic plots to convey relationships between drugs, but the authors of novels such as *Marriage Destinies* and *Flowers in the Mirror*, at least to those who used their prescriptions, seem to have believed that they used narrative as a delivery mechanism for medicine, like a sweet coating or delectable adjuvant. For them, reading fiction was reading everything but fiction. If becoming obsessed with fiction caused depletion and harm, ignoring the fictionality of fiction altogether and blithely appropriating bits and pieces of it for real, practical use was cost-effective, meritorious, and healing.

CHAPTER 4

Diseases of Sex

*Medical and Literary Views of Contagion
and Retribution*

Ximen Qing drunkenly stumbles into the room of his most lascivious wife, Pan Jinlian. It is late and he has been complaining of fatigue the past few days. No wonder, since he has been disporting himself with Laijue's wife, Ben the fourth's wife, Wang Liu'er, and three of his own wives in recent days, and in all of those sexual encounters, Ximen has employed a powerful aphrodisiac obtained from a mysterious foreign monk. Now in his wife's room, he falls asleep immediately. Unable to produce an erection from her husband in his drunken slumber, Pan Jinlian gives him an overdose of the monk's medicine and makes love to him. He ejaculates all of his semen, followed by blood and cold air. He slips in and out of consciousness. The following day he is dizzy. It becomes difficult for him to urinate, and his scrotum swells. Pan Jinlian continues to make love to him since the effects of the aphrodisiac have not yet abated. Finally, his scrotum bursts, and days later he dies.

This notorious scene from chapter 79 of *Plum in the Golden Vase* is invariably interpreted as a case of the unwise overexpenditure of limited bodily resources. However gruesome, it is a prime example of the dangers of sex and, by extension, all kinds of excessive behavior. The reader is told that Ximen "sought only his own sexual gratification but did not realize that 'when its oil is used up the lamp goes out.'"[1] Title couplets and illustration captions imply similar diagnoses: "Ximen Qing in His Licentiousness Incurs Illness" (Tanyu de bing). These kinds of excesses were a major concern of doctors and scholars in the late Ming, a period often thought to be the height of sensuality in premodern China.[2] Death by excess is read as a metaphor for the entire novel, the age, and the dynasty.[3]

Yet, Ximen's case is not so cut-and-dried. The narrative of *Plum in the Golden Vase* subverts and supplements a straightforward reading of his illness and death as one brought on by simple cause and effect. Death from excess is a kind of worldly retribution, a simple result of unwise behavior,[4] but Ximen also dies from haunting by the ghosts of people he has driven to death. Ximen's illness is identified by a variety of characters knowledgeable about medicine as "poison in the region of relief" (*bian du*) and "yin cold" (*yinhan*), diseases found in the medical texts with a range of symptoms and causes.[5] The novel also occasionally refers to Ximen's disease as something *contracted* through sex. The lesions on his groin that emit a yellow fluid, lower back pain, and painful urination are symptoms of diseases known at the time to be transmitted by sexual intercourse—namely gonorrhea (*baizhuo*) and syphilis (*yangmei*).[6]

Given the interest in syphilis among medical and other authors during the period in which *Plum in the Golden Vase* was written, it is not surprising that it finds mention in the novel. It is surprising, however, that it does not play a more prominent role. Prescriptions for *bian* poisoning in the *Systematic Materia Medica*, for instance, were said to also treat numerous diseases caused by or related to sex and resulting in skin lesions.[7] Most often we see *bian* poisoning occurring alongside "evil chancre" (*echuang*), "carbuncle and chancre (*dingchuang*) and "fish mouth" (*yukou*).[8] Some drugs for *bian du* also cure syphilis sores and bug or worm bites (*chongyao*). Most often, *bian du* "breaks out" (*chufa*)—it is latent on the inside and becomes manifest.[9] The *Systematic Materia Medica* also discusses *bian du* as being caused by the following pathoconditions: sexual overexertion, restraint of ejaculation, or failure in love affairs, which cause stagnation of vital essence and blood or retention of sperm. *Bian du* can also be caused by "excessive anger that has damaged the liver, bringing with it stagnation of vital energy and blood in the channels and veins. A hard mass may appear in the groin area, which may develop into ulceration."[10] References to *bian du* in fiction and medical texts drop off after the Ming and disappear almost entirely by the eighteenth century.[11] This malady seems to have been a precursor to contagious venereal diseases, such as *yangmei* in its many symptoms and often sex-related causes, but it also evokes emotional disorders such as consumption, since it can be caused by anger and disappointment in love affairs. *Bian du* was a malady caused by a broadly defined desire that encompassed both excessive carnality and extreme feelings.

A story contemporary with *Plum in the Golden Vase*, "A Husband Leaves His Wife in Xi'an Fu and in Heyang County a Man Becomes a Woman" (Xian fu fu bie qi, Heyang xian nan hua nü, 1632) features a man, Li Liangyu, who contracts *bian du* syphilis (*bian du guang-chuang*) from visiting a prostitute.[12] His penis ulcerates and "festers to the root," and he loses all of his facial hair, which makes him look like a "stunning lady-in-waiting." He is taken to see King Yama, from whom he learns that a clerical error caused him to be reborn a man rather than a woman. Yama thus has him changed into Lady Li. The story makes clear at the outset that "if one can uphold one's morality, then one is most likely a man; if one cannot keep one's virtues, then one is most likely a woman," and Li, having violated his morality as a man, is turned into a woman both by syphilis and by Yama. His disease punishes men with mundane and karmic retribution for immoral acts.

Medical case histories that included treatment of *yangmei* patients invariably identified those patients as men. All of the maladies recorded in Wang Ji's *Stone Mountain Medical Cases* (Shishan yi'an, 1531) related to sex are attributed to men.[13] Although this does not reflect the reality of his day (perhaps Wang did not treat prostitutes, or perhaps women with diseases related to sex would not ask to be seen by him), that his records show men suffering primarily from sex and exhaustion (and drink) contributed to a public perception that these are diseases of men.

Ximen Qing's illness and death are most often and most simply read as stemming from sexual depletion. While he develops *bian du* from excessive sex and from being morally corrupt, it is interesting that his female doppelgänger develops consumption. Pang Chunmei is the most licentious character in the novel after Ximen Qing and Pan Jinlian die. Chunmei indulges in a variety of sexual affairs, living for nothing but pleasure. She gives herself over to her passions for her new lover, Zhou Yi. They enjoy themselves in bed without the slightest restraint. Chunmei,

> because of immoderate lust, developed consumptive bone steam-ing. Although she took medicine, she lost her appetite. Her spirits were depressed and her body became very thin, but she never gave up indulging in lust. . . . She stayed in bed with Zhou Yi all day. They were having intercourse when suddenly she exhaled cold breath and

her lusty juices emanated from her vagina. She died right there upon Zhou Yi's body. She was twenty-nine *sui* [twenty-eight years old].[14]

Later in that last chapter of *Plum in the Golden Vase* (admittedly a point of crisis in the text), when the ghosts of the dead are assigned their lot in the next life, they appear before the monk who will assign them described only by their bodily descriptions upon their deaths. Chunmei, whose face is pale and thin, says that she died of "sexual consumption" (*selao zhi si*).[15] Hers is a reenactment of Ximen Qing's death from overindulgence in sex, only this time it is gendered female. Not only is Chunmei's depletion disorder related to lust and sex, it is the female equivalent of *yin* coldness and *bian* poison.

Ximen Qing's disease, whatever its name, is complicated and tied to his sexual activities. But the vector of his illness is not well defined. It is caused by both retribution and contagion. The concept of interpersonal contagion was, if not completely new, undergoing redefinition in the medical texts of the late Ming, largely in response to syphilis epidemics. Contagion became tied up with retribution and gender. It was a cause of illness that incorporated new knowledge into old beliefs. Contagion implicated border crossings of all kinds, but, as with Ximen's case, also moral transgressions, supernormal vengeance, and mundane accumulations in the body. Because contagion is a concept foundational to medicine and rich in metaphorical possibilities for literature, and since it forced somewhat of a paradigm shift at the moment domestic fiction was becoming so popular, it is worth investigating how the concept was used in medicine and fiction.

A BRIEF HISTORY OF *CHUANRAN*

In early twentieth century China, the term *chuanran* quickly became the standard translation of the biomedical concept of contagion. In traditional Chinese medicine, illness was usually perceived as being the result not of microorganisms but rather of blockages or the improper flow of qi within the body. Before the nineteenth century no one in China suffered from plague, cholera, typhoid fever, or malaria. Millions, though, died from yin deficiency (*yinxu*) and foot qi (*jiaoqi*) and cold damage (*shanghan*),[16] not to mention bone-steaming (*guzheng*), flying corpse (*feishi*), and ghost infection (*guizhu*). Before the biomedical revolution of the late nineteenth century, neither physicians in China nor Europe had any notion of syphilis's spirochete or of the mycobacteria that cause tuberculosis. *Chuanran* was a new concept with modern, Western, and scientific implications.

But *chuanran* is an old word, used as early as the tenth century to express complex concepts about the spread of disease from person to person. In premodern Chinese medicine, several different kinds of transmission fall under the conceptual umbrella of *chuanran*. *Chuan*, "to pass on," for instance, referred to the transmission of a pathogen from a corpse, place, or other nonliving source to a living body, while *ran*, literally meaning "to dye," described the movement of a disorder between living things, including processes of "mutual dyeing" (*xiangran*), "exchange by dyeing" or "dye and exchange" (*ranyi*), and "affect by dyeing"(*ganran*).[17] Thus, the binome *chuanran* literally meant "transmission by dyeing" or "dye by transmission."

The word *chuanran* appears in many medical texts from the premodern period. In the tenth century, *chuanran* began to replace *ranyi* as the preferred term for describing the flow of qi between people.[18] In medical texts of the Ming and Qing, there are essentially three ways in which something could *chuanran*: by direct or indirect physical contact with the sick, by hereditary transmission, and by transmission through sexual intercourse.[19] Gong Tingxian, a sixteenth-century palace doctor, uses *chuanran* to describe modes of transmission from a sick body to a healthy one when he observes, "If one is careless while traveling, *mafeng* [probably leprosy] could be transmitted [*chuanran*] in toilets, in living quarters, or by bedding and clothes."[20] Family and members of the community often worried that the qi or physical corpse of a *laozhai* (consumption) victim could contaminate objects, which in turn could contaminate those who come into contact with them. People could be infected by a residence (*wuchuan*), by clothes or bedding (*yichuan*), or by food or medicine belonging to the deceased (*shichuan*). If a patient died of "corpse pouring" (*shizhu*) or depletion-consumption (*laozhai*), his clothes, utensils, and residence were all likely to retain harmful qi, which could then infect his relatives and neighbors if they could not afford to dispose of them.

The second type of *chuanran* was hereditary transmission, particularly within a household. Although some Daoist texts as early as the Southern Song recognized *gu* poison contagion "irrespective of family relationship," it was common to think of disease transmission as something that happened primarily among family members.[21] The concept of *gu* contagion reveals a conflation of spatial proximity with lineal proximity—families transmit disease to members through shared sin and through shared space and objects. Gong Tingxian presents family ties as another potential vector for the transmission of *mafeng*: "[The disorder could be] transmitted to others from ancestors or parents [to descendants], from husbands and wives, or other members of the family."[22] Hereditary transmission could mean the passing of some irregularity or contaminant from mother to child, through breast milk or blood, but it also included illnesses inherited from the father as well as from ancestors, both living and dead.

The third type of *chuanran* was by sexual intercourse. An early concept related to this was "*yinyang* exchange" (*yinyang yi*), an ailment transmitted by sexual intercourse when one partner had not yet fully recovered after being cured from "harm by cold" (*yinhan*).[23] In the case of a man's illness transmitted to his female partner, Li Shizhen prescribes the ashes from the burnt crotch of the man's trousers. In the case of a woman's illness transmitted to her male partner, physicians should treat him with the ashes from the woman's burnt pubic hair. Both of these cures obviously relied on sympathetic medicine and carried the symbolic stain of sexual intercourse. "*Yinyang* exchange" referred to the pouring out of essence, which enabled noxious influences to enter the body during a period of depletion. Sexual transmission was primarily discussed in the late imperial period in the context of a new disease called *yangmei chuang* ("plum-blossom sores")—also called *Guangdong chuang* ("Guangdong sores"), as the disease was believed to have originated in Guangdong province—which modern historians of medicine often identify as syphilis and which was first recorded in southern China during the first decade of the sixteenth century. The section "Essentials of Authentic Methods in External Medicine" (Waike xinfa yaojue) in the *Golden Mirror of the Medical Lineage* (fig. 4.1) makes it clear that "there are two types of *yangmei chuang*: those that have at their essence a change in *jing* [essence] and those that have a change in qi. The change in *jing* is the result of licentiousness and desire, [while] the change in qi is the result of contagious [*chuanran*] qi."[24] This disease was caused by evil or heteropathic qi entering the body, and also by (or aided by) a depletion of "original essence" (*yuanqi*) as a result of (excessive) sexual activity and, more specifically, illicit sexual contact outside the family.

Most doctors throughout China's long literary and medical history did not define *chuanran* clearly as three modes of transmission. The term meant contamination not only by contact with the sick but also

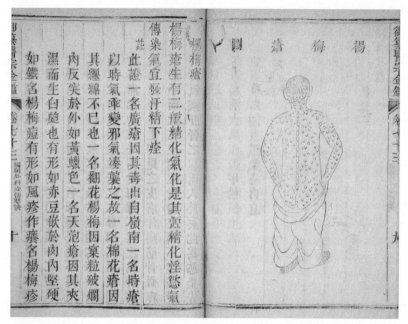

Figure 4.1. Entry on syphilis in the "Essentials of Authentic Methods in External Medicine" section of *Golden Mirror of the Medical Lineage*, 1742, *juan* 73. Waseda University Library, Japan.

by contact with a pathogenic qi that could be epidemic or individual, an old idea originally expressed by "mutual dyeing" (*xiangran*). From the late Ming onwards, many southern doctors distinguished between the noncontagious qi that provoked "cold damage" disorders and contagious, local, impure, epidemic qi.[25] *Chuanran* also meant that members of the same household or people related by blood were believed to be more vulnerable to contamination by the patient, a notion already described in seventh-century texts. *Chuanran* was a nebulous, plastic concept, and it was not an important topic in medical discourse until the late Ming. Up to the modern period, *chuanran* was never the only cause of a disorder.[26] A polluted location, unseasonal weather, the weak physical constitution of the victim, extremes of emotion, bad geomancy of a residence, or moral flaws or wrongdoings were equally valid or more important causes. However, disorders considered more prone to *chuanran* tended to be particularly deadly, such as severe epidemics caused by impure qi, chronic disorders with conspicuous poisonous sores such as *yangmei* sores and *mafeng*, or

those ending in a slow, painful death such as *laozhai*. Some of these
disorders were closely associated with sexual transmission, and all of
them provoked fear or disgust in Late Imperial society.[27]

SEXUAL TRANSMISSION, SEXUAL HEALING

It might seem logical to investigate sexual contact as the origin of
the notion of interpersonal contagion. Sexual transmission of disease
seems like an obvious vector given that the symptoms of venereal disease appear at the locus of contact and affect the parts of the body
used to transmit blood, essence, and qi from one body to another.
Diseases of this type did indeed receive more attention in medical
texts in the late imperial period, considering the increased concern for
women's reproductive health in the Ming and Qing periods, marked
by a proliferation of medical publications that specialized in female
disorders, and noted by many scholars.[28] The importance attached to
conception and reproductive health is apparent in the large volume
of books published on obstetrics, childbirth, and pediatrics. Medical discourse attempted to restrict sexuality to a marital context by
drawing on the pathological consequences of sexual excess for the
health of future progeny. Sexual disorders were also approached in
the context of reproduction, and a number of publications referred
to diseases enabled, caused by, or transmitted by sexual intercourse.
Yangmei chuang ("red bayberry sores" or syphilis) in particular was
the object of medical attention starting in the late sixteenth century.
The symptoms of this condition were described in a number of medical texts with detail and consistency, but the root cause of it was given
as sexual excess rather than contagion.[29] Li Shizhen quotes Wang Ji as
saying, "Recently, among those who are fond of licentiousness, many
have become ill with sores of *yangmei* poison [*yangmei du chuang*],"
but Wang Ji did not suggest that they had contracted this ailment
through sex, and explains the etiology of this disease according to
normal pathogenic models: "Humidity accumulates together with
heat in the muscle and the interstices, resulting in the emergence of
carbuncle and swelling with contractions and spasms."[30] Li Shizhen
underlined how this disease had spread (*chuan*) from the Lingbiao
region in south China to the four corners of the empire. He pointed to
the humid climate, the spicy food, and the sexual intemperance of the
locals, all thought to contribute to an accumulation of wetness-heat
and to the appearance of *yangmei*. But the nature of the transmission

seemed to have two vectors—either *yangmei* is contracted directly by heat, humidity and spiciness, or indirectly by sex with someone who has the lesions that form from those conditions. Li writes, "Dampness and heat accumulate thickly to form a pathogen [*e*, lit., "evil"] that causes the development of malignant sores that are mutually contagious among people [*huxiang chuanran*]."[31] The climate of the south is brought north in the bodies of those with excessive dampness and heat.

Although the infection may have been caused by the climate, as in *yangmei feng* ("red bayberry wind"), once the *yangmei* sores form, they are transmitted through intercourse, since Li writes explicitly, "All those who become sick with it are lascivious people."[32] This term, literally "people of lascivious evil" (*yinxie zhi ren*), suggests that sex invites disease through depletion, and invasion by pathogenic wind or demons. But there did not necessarily need to be invasion by malicious forces for an illness to develop. Excess itself was a cause of disease, whether it was excessive emotion, excessive food or drink, or excessive sex. Other maladies were caused by excess, too, as is evident in the Ming discussions of obsession in which a *pi* (hobby, habit, or mania) can literally form a *pi* (hardness or stone), and block the flow of qi and food.[33] One Yuan dynasty encyclopedia, for instance, has a prescription for "pathogenic desire that turns into chancre" (*e zhi yu cheng chuang*).[34] This particular malady is an instance of a sexual disease, though one grown rather than contracted.

A detailed account of syphilis was published in 1632 by Chen Sicheng, titled *Secret Account of the Rotting Sores Disorder* (Meichuang milu), a work based on an epidemic that had occurred at the beginning of the 1630s.[35] Chen similarly wrote that *yangmei* has its origins in the Lingnan climate, where "it is humid and hot, snow never falls, snakes and *chong* [worms, bugs] never hibernate, and all manner of nastiness and filth are stored up. When the first *yang* [transition from spring to summer] arrives, damp poison and miasma [*zhangqi*] steam [under the sun]. Things in contact with it easily rot and perish. Human beings in contact with it are easily infected with rotting sores."[36] *Yangmei*, according to Chen, can be transmitted sexually and lineally: "This ailment is not transmitted only through sexual intercourse. When people with weak constitutions go to use toilets in town, or talk with patients that have the disorder, they are sometimes infected with toxic qi. . . . The disease can also be transmitted [by a husband] to members of the inner chamber. Even if the wife or concubine does not fall ill, the disease can be transferred [*yi*] to sons and daughters, nephews, or grandchildren."[37] That the disease can be passed directly to nephews or grandchildren is clearly not the simple sort of transmission of modern biomedicine, and suggests that once it has contaminated one member of the household, even if originally contracted through sex, it can contaminate relatives through other means. Chen blames not just sex but lasciviousness as the mode of contagion. In response to the question "How is it that these sores are transmitted and contagious [*chuanran*] without end?" he replies,

> In the past *ran* worked like this: relatives did not live together [with the patient], when eating and drinking, they did not share utensils [with the patient], they would place themselves quietly in their rooms, and thus wait until they recovered, and hence *chuanran* was infrequent. Recently, [the current generation] has become weak [*shibo*], and men rashly submerge themselves and hide in brothels. Many neglect to shun taboo. They repeatedly visit poisonous prostitutes, the fire of lasciviousness burns in them, and this is the true origin of their weakness. The poisonous qi takes advantage of this weakness, and attacks. Before they realize [that they are infected], they have already transmitted [the disease] to their wives and concubines or to their pretty boy servants. In previous generations, there were few medical books to correct this, which explains the endless transmission and contamination [*chuanran buyi*].[38]

For Chen, *yangmei*, among other modes of transmission, was a disease of moral weakness, of taboo violation, excess, carelessness, and recklessness. It was moral weakness that allowed evil qi to invade the body, and once inside, it could be passed to innocent sexual partners or nearby relatives.[39]

Chen Sicheng and Li Shizhen, in discussing the ostensible transmission of climate (miasmas, evil qi) through sex, were aligning themselves with Confucian moralists of a century or two earlier. The concept of miasma (*zhang*), usually a feature of environment, that was now being applied to lascivious southerners in Lingnan had previously been used to characterize Burmese women, who were seen as promiscuous. Zhang Hong, who visited Burma in 1407, recorded, "The Mian people [Burmese] often cultivate promiscuous women to seduce our soldiers. Anyone who has sex with these women will die. Hence, these women are called human miasma [*renzhang*]." He lectured his soldiers: "When you left for here, your parents, wives, and children cried farewell, knelt and prayed to heaven, and longed for your return. If you die of human miasma, and your wives then marry other men, how will your parents be able to bear it?" Zhang Hong claims that his men were touched by his words, and they did not dare to contract human miasma.[40] The discourse on *yangmei* now cast lascivious people as the carriers of a poisonous southern miasma that was circulating around the empire. Bodily invasion by bad local qi was not the only geospatial concern related to *chuanran*. Ultimately, deceased ancestors also caused diseases of place. The return of vengeful ancestors required people to leave a certain place to "avoid the killing" (*guisha* or *bisha*). Victims of disease are often victims of places. Dirt is matter out of place, but in many instances, in China, illness was a matter of people out of place. *Chuanran* meant that the infected had brought climates out of their regions. The infected were the embodiment of an unhealthy climate: they had become bottled wind.

In the eighteenth century, the "poison of the plum" (*meidu*) was thought to be transmitted in three different ways: by semen (*jing*) during sexual intercourse, by vitiated air (qi) emanating from a contaminated person, and from the mother to the fetus. Wu Qian published the most systematic account, in which he claimed that "absorption of air through the nose in encounters with people who suffer from these chancres, eating unclean substances in error, or using toilets infected with the vitiated air of *meidu* could lead to infection."[41] Prostitutes in particular were said to harbor the poison in their vaginas. Diseases caused by unhealthy emanations were considered to affect the surface of the body only, while syphilis transmitted by intercourse would infect the bones and marrow of victims.

Despite growing interest in sexually transmitted diseases, epidemics, and the concept of *chuanran* as person-to-person transmission of disease in the late imperial period, many physicians still had reservations about the concept of interpersonal contagion.[42] Most accepted the possibility of mutual contamination within the same household because members shared similar physical traits, habits, air, food, and living space, but it was not yet commonplace to think of these as facilitating person-to-person transmission of an agent of disease. Xiao Xiaoting (d. 1801), for instance, wrote, "[Since] the qi and blood of a person each follows its own vessels, how could [a contagion] be transmitted from one [person] to another?"[43] For many who were not physicians, it was difficult to understand *chuanran* contagion as the primary reason that someone was sick, when the vital blood and qi of a person were believed to circulate in a closed system corresponding to and interacting only with the cosmos. It is difficult and often anachronistic to draw sharp distinctions between interpersonal contagion and shared miasmas (*zhangqi*). The primary concern was that people became sick through "mutual dyeing" (*xiangran*) or "communicated dyeing" *chuanran*. The source of the evil qi with which one became dyed, whether endemic to the area or emanating from a particular individual, was secondary.[44]

Descriptions of *yangmei* in medical literature, though they emphasized sexual excess and sexual transgression as foundational reasons for the spread of disease outside of its natural habitat, were also beholden to traditional frameworks for explaining illness. In premodern China, "people fell ill, in short, for many different reasons, but two factors mattered most: emotions and the weather. Weather was *the* external threat. . . . Demons, heavenly displeasure, the attacks of wind and cold, and the emotional exhaustion that makes one susceptible to attack—these are, by far, the dominant themes."[45] *Yangmei*, though at times described as something almost subversive of dominant medical paradigms and always discussed in the Ming as a new disease, upon greater scrutiny borrows from traditional metaphors of invasion by wind, unseasonal climate change, and borderland "barbarian" people who are themselves the embodiment of miasma.

Although vectors of transmission were a topic for debate, the meanings of *yangmei* and its association with sex and prostitutes were part of its earliest descriptions. It was a disease to be embarrassed about, and as such was often the purview of itinerant doctors, who could treat the illness in the patient's home and then move along out of town, enabling the patient to more easily keep his condition a secret from neighbors and community members. Itinerant physicians were most often asked to treat abscesses and other such ailments associated with the specialty of external medicine. One medical manuscript, for instance, lists numerous therapies recommended for treating ailments such as "chancres and sores" (*ganchuang*) and "lower chancre" (*xiagan*), both terms referring to syphilis or similar ailments, and "vaginal-itch" (*yinyang*).[46] Stories in other manuscripts, such as the one attached to the prescription "Guanyin's recipe to save one from suffering" (Guanyin jiuku fang), make clear that these are afflictions about which patients were embarrassed, and people avoided seeking physicians for treatment of them. There is a story of a pious widow who suffered from vaginal itch and was too embarrassed to seek help from a physician. Guanyin assumed the form of a beggar and gave her an effective remedy.[47] Treating these ailments was obviously an important source of revenue for itinerant doctors, given examples from manuscripts like that written by a physician named Yang Xiu-wan, in which he records following the recipe for a "scent causing the red bayberries [i.e., syphilis] to immediately disperse [*yangmei lixiao xiang*]" and about which he admonishes, "This is a secret treasure that must not be divulged to outsiders. Watch it, treasure it!"[48] Syphilis was also frequently discussed in daily-use encyclopedias, presumably meaning that patients could relatively easily self-diagnose and treat themselves to spare themselves the embarrassment or shame of sharing their condition with a doctor.

At first glance, *yangmei* and other venereal diseases seem not to be represented often in fictional literature. If it was understood as a disease simply contracted during sex, it might have limited use as metaphor, but that clearly was not the case. Syphilis came to China at approximately the same time that the domestic novel gained popularity—with its focus on relationships within the household and quotidian details such as medicine and sex—it might seem particularly odd that venereal disease did not enter more largely into novelistic discourse or even gain more than passing mention in fiction.[49] Given that *yangmei* and related maladies were discussed in vernacular texts such as daily encyclopedias, almanacs, practical medical texts, and medical manuscripts, as well as by scholar-doctors such as Wang Kentang and Xue Ji, and official works such as the *Golden Mirror of the Medical Lineage* (Yizong jinjian, 1742), we might expect that novels particularly known for depictions of sex would be eager to portray maladies such as *yangmei*. These novels do exhibit traces of these diseases, and such traces infect the depictions of illnesses related to desire (*yu*) and to sentiment or passion (*qing*).

In the late Ming and certainly in the Qing sex is often presented as something that is dangerous—in excess, in taboo violation, in careless disregard for procreation. But sex is also something that can be used, usually sympathetically, to cure certain unhealthy conditions. The tension between a disease transmitted by sex and one that is cured by sex is illustrated in discussions of the practices of "passing *lai*" (*guolai*)[50] and "selling the sickness" (*maibing*). An example found in an 1850 account by Chen Jiongzhai (d. 1857) titled "Transmission of Lesions" (Liyang chuanran) records, "In the southeast the land is low and the climate is humid. The inhabitants are plagued with sores [*liyang*], which beyond the mountains are called *damafeng* [leprosy or syphilis]. This disease is contagious [*chuanran*] and cripples entire families. Those who get it are abominated by others and ostracized from their own kind."[51] Here we find a traditional notion of *chuanran*: namely the belief that transmission is facilitated by weather, climate, and geography, wherein the qi of an environment provides the medium for transmission. Chen explains that the treatment is a combination of quarantine and rigidly controlled marriage: "In Guangzhou and Chaozhou there were formerly *mafeng* colonies where [the infected] came together, like with like, and lived as a community. They were led by a *feng*-chief. In their ranks were *fengren* [persons with *mafeng*] of the second and third generations. The chief arranged their marriages in strict order, ensuring no mixing of generations. By the third generation the disease had run its course, and the children were allowed to leave the colony—hence the saying "*Mafeng* lasts only three generations."[52] In this interpretation of the disease, it becomes less powerful over time, the infected must be quarantined from the healthy, and "generations" of infected must be quarantined from those whose parents or grandparents had it. While in the colony, contagion passes along vectors of heredity and sexual contact. Unless subjects are reinfected, the disease diminishes over time, such that by the third generation children are born free of the disease and are therefore permitted to leave the colony. The disease affects families and at the same time is *cured* by a series of carefully monitored marriages. A disease that can be transmitted by sex is cured by the maintenance of proper marriage traditions.[53]

There are some accounts of "selling the sickness" in fiction, but they tend to be very late. Wu Jianren (1866–1910), in his novel *Bizarre Happenings Eye-witnessed over Two Decades* (Ershi nian mudu zhi guai xianzhuang, 1905–1910), for instance, writes,

It really isn't funny, but it is hard not to laugh. In fact, as far as this disease *mafeng* is concerned, it's not that other provinces don't have it. In fact, I've even seen one case in Shanghai; it's just that other provinces don't fear [such cases]. In Guangdong, people dread those with it [*fengren*]. Now, why they would or would not fear them is inscrutable. Perhaps because it is so hot in Guangdong, that it makes the disease fester, and in other provinces it doesn't fester, and so you have some that fear it and some that don't. In Guangdong, people are so offended by those that have this disease that their fathers and sons act as though they don't recognize them. Moreover, they have even created a *mafeng* colony, to adopt this group of people and to prevent their *chuanran*. Not only can this disease *chuanran*, it has no visible symptoms after being transmitted through heredity [*chuanzhong*] for

three generations, yet the root of the disease remains in the bones.
This kind of person will have to try to pass it to others [by sex]. It is
easy for men to do that, but women can only seduce passersby in the
countryside [where they will not encounter people they know]. They
only need to do it once or twice, and it will be passed [to others], and
the man that has been deceived will have to move into the *mafeng*
colony. This is called "selling the *feng*." The burdened have to do this
outside the home under the cover of darkness. No one does this publicly or in the light of day in their homes. It doesn't take even a month
to get rid of [the disease] completely.[54]

This might be related to the concept of transmission by "pouring,"
but just as likely draws on the notion of a rudimentary bodily economy of spending or saving essential essences, fluids, and qi. More
importantly, one contracts and cures oneself of these diseases by the
same method, and in this regard the transmission of illness via sex
or down a lineage obeys a similar logic: taboo sex cures taboo sex,
and passing disease to one's children eventually cures descendants of
diseases originally contracted from one's parents. Wu Jianren seems
to suggest that these two modes of transmission are also interchange-
able. The passing of generations cures diseases contracted through
sex, just as sex rids patients of the latent root of the disease.

Sex was not something universally to be feared—at least not by
women. The late-Ming scholar-official Wang Linheng (1548–1601)
noted that "when women are afflicted with *feng* they pretend to run
away from their families or get lost on the road in order to seduce
men. Once they have had sexual intercourse, the ailment passes to
the men. The custom is called 'passing on *feng*' [*guofeng*]."[55] It is due
to this custom, Wang claims, that most of those who suffer from the
ailment in Guangdong were men. According to Xiao Xiaoting, "It is
rare for a man to transmit [*mafeng*] to a woman, and common for a
woman to transmit it to a man."[56] Moreover, the disease itself affects
men and women differently. According to Chen Jiongzhai,

> The face of a [male] *fengren* is swollen, his hands and feet ulcer-
> ated; the sight is nauseating. Female *fengren*, on the other hand, are
> transfigured: their complexion takes on a rosy bloom, and they have
> no other visible symptoms of infection. They often deck themselves
> in finery to tempt men to fornication. When some stupid young rake
> falls into the trap, he contracts the disease. It attacks his vitals, and in
> no time his limbs begin to itch unbearably. As the man takes over the
> woman's disease, her own chronic condition immediately improves
> and she is restored to normal.[57]

These medical theories that women were much more likely to infect others and cure themselves through sexual contact must have played on the fears of Confucian moralists that men were too often frequenting brothels or having extramarital encounters while traveling. They also reveal an attitude that remained quite consistent between late Ming and the Republican period that men, much more so than women, were likely to contract (or less able to rid themselves of) sexually transmitted diseases.[58] Despite the cult of female chastity that prevailed throughout the Qing, in medical discourse, sex was an activity that was particularly dangerous to men.[59]

CHAOS AND THE STONE WOMAN

Another form of "sexual healing" in fiction concerns the curious case of the stone woman or stone maiden (*shinü*). Ming and Qing medical writers showed a great and systematic interest in biological variation.[60] Doctors, especially scholar-doctors, naturally showed a great interest in fertility, and the variety of medical practitioners did a brisk business in enhancing reproductive power.[61] Li Shizhen, to take just one example, discusses at least thirty drugs that can be used to treat female infertility or enhance fertility in women. In a social milieu concerned with creating male heirs, the figure of the stone maiden, who suffered from a condition in which her vagina was impenetrable, or even closed entirely, stands out among anomalies.[62] Li Shizhen includes them in a description of those who are desexed in the last chapter of the *Systematic Materia Medica* on "human anomalies" (*rengui*):

> Qian [man] becomes the father and Kun [woman] becomes the mother. This is a normal condition. But there are five types of men who cannot act as fathers and five types of women who cannot act as mothers. Why is this? Isn't it that [these] men have a deficiency of yang qi, and [these] women have a blockage of yin qi? The false females are the corkscrew [spiral stria of the vulva?], the striped [stricture of the vagina], the drum [imperforate hymen], the horned [elongated clitoris?], and the pulse [amenorrhea or menoxenia]. The false males are the natural eunuch [impotence], the bullock [castrated], the leaky [seminal emission], the coward [inability to ejaculate when having sex], and the changeling [genitals have forms of both sexes].[63]

Li and other medical writers who repeated these classifications explain that four of these five terms applied to women refer to genital abnormalities of the sort that would make sexual penetration impossible.[64]

Those referred to in medical texts as the "drum" (or, in other versions, "small door"), well-known in popular lore as a "stone maiden," one who has an impenetrable vagina (vaginal atresia).[65] Medical writers addressed the issue of biological variation in physical sex characteristics most systematically in the late Ming and Qing periods, but many stopped at observing and cataloging this syndrome and did not venture a "cure" for it.[66] Stone maidenhood was a wonder of the universe in medical texts. Since sexual determination was women's work to be done at birth by midwives or the like, variation in female sex organs was doubly mysterious to men.[67] Stone maidenhood was also a malady happily assigned meaning and treatment by writers of fiction.

The stone maiden was an object of humor, a female clown, in much fiction from the Northern Song compendium of story, lore, and anecdote *Broad Gleanings of the Era of Great Peace* (Taiping Guangji), through works by late-Ming and Qing authors such as Li Yu and Yuan Mei.[68] Perhaps the best-known stone maiden comes from the late Ming play *Peony Pavilion*, in which Sister Stone (Shidao Gu, nicknamed for her malady) of Purple Light Convent is a bawdy nun, born a *shinü*, failed in marriage, and fit only for the "shaman's robe." In her self-introduction, one of the funniest passages in all of *Peony Pavilion*, she misapplies many quotations from the *Thousand Character Classic*, a primer for writing known to virtually all literate people. She tells her own story as a stone maiden:

> My shit was like "twigs of the chaste tree"
> My piss was like "drips from the lotus leaves"
> At the delta where there should have been "a vast lake or swamp"
> There was only a stretch of land, which is "a dried pond with an arid
>   rock"
> Although the pebbled path could "clutch the scholar-trees,"
> How could the barren land "grow corn and millet"?
> Who would marry me for "unproductive echoes in the empty valley"?[69]

As the burlesque speech of Sister Stone suggests, in popular idiom the stone maiden could be a figure of fun, an old crone, or a termagant wife, for what is more useless in the Confucian milieu than a woman who cannot reproduce, much less even have sex? But the nature of her malady, however humorous, is consistent with previous descriptions in nonfictional texts. This is a congenital problem, and one that Li Shizhen would agree stems from the mysteries, even the chaos, of the universe. Sister Stone refers (hilariously) to her young husband trying to penetrate her closed vagina as "trying to drill a hole into fleshy chaos of 'black sky and yellow earth,'" a description made doubly poignant, since it misappropriates the first line of the *Thousand Character Classic* that in turn references a famous parable in *The Zhuangzi* about the interdependence of regularity and irregularity.[70] Li Yu's story "The Hall of the Ten Weddings" (Shijinlou, 1658) features a protagonist who is a *shinü*.[71] Eventually, after she suffers from an infection, her vagina proves penetrable. Her condition is also referred to as "primal chaos" (*hundun*), and her recovery is the restoration of order.[72]

If Miao women had previously been represented as elemental anomalies, human miasmas, a threat to the family because they can infect through sex and have rapacious sexual drives, they are brought under control in the novel *Humble Words of an Old Rustic*. Wen Suchen heals a Miao stone maiden's deviant body and sexuality through his yang embodiment of moral force. This stone maiden has a body of pure yin, which makes her pallid and prevents the proper development of her sexual anatomy, resulting in an impenetrable vagina. Although she is nineteen years old, the girl has received no marriage proposals. Compelled to sleep in the same bed as the stone maiden during his travels to the Miao frontier, Wen, with his body of pure yang energy, warms the stone maiden's cold body.[73] In fact, Suchen is said to "steam" (*zheng*) her. "As he slept . . . she gently took his hand and first massaged her breasts, then her abdomen, and then her vagina. She felt even more stimulated and excited, all over her body. She was numb in every spot and couldn't stop moaning and cooing."[74] Eventually, her menses begin to flow. Suchen's cure is described as an act of "boring open chaos and destroying heaven's neglect" (*zao hundun er po tianhuang*).[75] The chapter-end commentary also characterizes Wen Suchen's massaging of the stone maiden's vagina to affect the cure as the "boring open of chaos" (*zaokai hundun*).[76] When massaging Shinü's body, Suchen instructs her to curb her chaotic sexual drive and enlightens her about Confucian sexual norms. Domesticating these chaotic creatures is all the more important because Shinü (the name by which she is called) was conceived when her mother dreamed that she was being raped by a horse. Suchen achieves his civilizing project by marrying Shinü to the descendent of a wronged Han Chinese general who had been exiled to the Miao frontier in a ceremony strictly conducted according to Confucian rituals. Cured and civilized, Shinü (no longer a *shinü*) is now endowed with extraordinary fertility and rejuvenates the decimated family line of the displaced

Han general by giving birth to twenty-eight sons. The chapter-end commentary calls this outcome "chaos transformed into civility" (*hundun bian wei wenming*).[77] If disease contracted through sex or in conjunction with sex happens because of carelessness, the maladies of sexual impossibility are forms of natural chaos. Sexing the desexed was a project that required the transgressive use of sexual proximity to cure something fundamentally in need of sex (or yang), and also a way to bring order to the chaos of nature.

COMEDY

Stories such as "The Fan Tower Restaurant as Witness to the Love of Zhou Shengxian" (Nao Fanlou duoqing Zhou Shengxian), published around 1627 in Feng Menglong's *Constant Words to Awaken the World* (Xingshi hengyan), in which a grave robber violates the corpse of a beautiful maiden and surprisingly thus brings her back to life, also display the curative properties of sexual intercourse. Bringing ghosts back to life with an infusion of yang relied on a literary logic more than a strictly medical one. In this story, the maiden falls ill from longing, but her wealthy father categorically refuses a match when her mother broaches the subject. Upon overhearing their exchange, the girl is so shocked and upset she dies on the spot. The narration describes her surprising return to life with the words "it turned out that the young lady, with all her heart set on Second Brother Fan, had died a few days ago from a fit of rage against her father when he was lashing out at her mother. Now, however, upon the infusion of yang qi, so soon after her death, her soul revived and she came back to life."[78] A dominant medical explanation of anger during the Qing was that it caused an upsurge of liver fire, and it is not logical that yang qi would have addressed this medical imbalance, nor would the semen to which "yang qi" likely refers. Rather, ghosts and fox demons are yin qi by definition, therefore they benefit from taking the yang of living beings. The robber is curing death itself, not the cause of death. The yinyang ideology in this story seems to owe less to medicine than to stories of female fox fairies who nourish themselves by seducing human men and acquiring their semen during intercourse.

Despite this recurrent motif in vernacular literature, it was also a shocking, and even humorous, proposition, as evidenced by the surprise that characters in such stories always display at the revival of the dead or the revival of the ghost.[79] *Peony Pavilion* (subtitled *The Soul's*

Return [Huanhun ji]) was phenomenally successful, and its popularity was due in no small part to the widespread fascination with the death and resurrection to love of the beautiful, talented heroine, Du Liniang. The play was the culmination of the late Ming glorification of *qing* (sentiment, love, passion, desire) and also a primary vehicle for the promotion and dissemination of *qing* as a cardinal virtue for the next two hundred years. As Tang Xianzu defined it in his manifesto-like preface to the play, "The origins of *qing* are unknown, but it runs deep. The living can die of it, and with it the dead can come back to life."[80] For all of its claims to sentiment, and its obvious effect on literature written on that theme, *Peony Pavilion* is also a bawdy work of entertainment that was clearly meant to appeal to those with less refined tastes as well. The humor was ribald, and the play's attitude toward sexual malfunction and disease irreverent. Sister Stone is obviously a hilarious clown, and her physical deformity a source of comedy, but even the sentimental death of Du Liniang, the archetypal lovesick, talented beauty, is also about sex. Tang Xianzu uses the phrase "to perish because of longing for beauty and sex" (*muse er wang*) to describe Du Liniang's death by amorous longing for the handsome young scholar in her dream.[81] A "longing for beauty and sex" (*muse*), updates traditional romances, which disguise the heroine's love for the hero as "appreciation for literary talents" (*liancai*).[82] In addition to the "longing for sex"–based nature of her illness, Du Liniang's maid Fragrance (Chunxiang) cheekily drops references to venereal disease (though Du Liniang, the reader must assume, remains innocent of these references), and one commentary edition notoriously reads virtually every symbol in the play as a reference to sex.[83] Even if some argue against these readings, Du Liniang's illness is still explicitly a "shameful sickness" (*aza zheng*), and the maid is beaten for speaking flippantly about it. Her mother asks what illness it is, and Fragrance replies that it is "spring fever" (i.e., lovesickness, *chunqian bing*), though the possibility of having run afoul of a flower spirit who sapped her strength is also a possibility. All of these potential causes of Liniang's "shameful sickness" are tied to longing—for sex or for passion.[84]

Tang Xianzu was familiar with the very real effects of syphilis, and made light of it in his personal life as well. In 1605, Tang wrote a series of ten poems for his friend, the writer Tu Long (1543–1605). The long title of the poem is "Changqing [Tu Long] My Friend, Suffering from the 'Sores of *Qing*' [*qingji zhiyang*], That Have Devastated

Your Muscles and Bones, You Cry Out in Insufferable Pain, but You Will Get Some Relief with Your Whole Family Praying to Guanyin for You. Here I Compose Ten Long *Jueju* in Jest."[85] A couplet in one of the poems reads, "What are the causes for this strange disease? / You should regret having allowed your heart to float in clouds and rain [i.e., overindulgence in sex]," and another, "Your flesh and eyes played with rakshasa women / your lusty body has become old visiting whore boats.[86] Despite the fact that Tu Long was certainly very ill when Tang composed these poems (he died shortly after), that did not stop him from writing about the consequences of his promiscuity in such an admittedly playful manner. Although Tang insists that these poems were composed playfully, their content is quite serious and returns again and again to his friend's culpability for his own suffering. We might infer from these poems that the reader or viewer of *Peony Pavilion* did not necessarily ascribe venereal disease to the lower classes but to those with enough leisure to frequent brothels. If anything, syphilis in men was a literal and metaphorical marker of corruption, of corrupt officials. Tu Long was secretary in the Ministry of Rites in Beijing but was impeached after only one year due to his sexual misconduct. Tang mentions on the one hand that "the only medicine is to give up prostitutes," and on the other that "the only effort you can make is to comply with Guanyin's power." If there is levity in these poems at all, it is pointed toward the heavenly and earthly repercussions for licentiousness, the poetry of karmic justice, since the syphilis that caused his friend pain unto death could not have been much of a laughing matter.[87]

SEX AND RETRIBUTION

While romantic literati may have played with the poetic justice of *yangmei*, others were more sober in discussing the disease. Li Shizhen, for instance, was critical of the social mores of his day. He claimed that in remote antiquity people had medicine but did not need it because they rarely got ill. As morality declined, people needed more and stronger medicine, down to the present day, when excess and wantonness has made illnesses more intractable and many toxic drugs are needed to treat a case.[88] In premodern fiction, when sex enters into the discourse of medicine, it is usually in the form not of disease contracted through sex but disease brought on by indulgence in sex. Illness derived from sex is emphasized not as contagion but as

retribution. Retribution usually concerns excess and the poor man-
agement of bodily resources, but also carelessness, transgression, and
the logical outcomes of those actions. The most notorious examples
come from *Plum in the Golden Vase*, in which retribution (*bao*) is one
of the most important structuring themes and the agent of cosmic and
earthly morality.[89] Ximen Qing and two of his wives (though notably
not his most notoriously lascivious wife, Pan Jinlian), Li Ping'er, and
Pang Chunmei, all die from sexual transgressions, either of excess or
breaking taboo, or both. Critical terms in fiction commentary often
use the language of retribution, and Zhang Zhupo employs it frequently in his commentary on *Plum in the Golden Vase*.[90]

Despite the clear cause-and-effect nature of Ximen's illness, it is
conflated with vengeful spirits (retribution) and with venereal disease
(contagion). The opening lines of chapter 79 warn the reader against
excess, saying that "a surfeit of tasty foods will end up making you
sick / Pleasurable events, once over, are sure to result in disaster."
While this message that excess leads to illness seems straightforward,
the narrative further explains the meaning of these lines of poetry by
Shao Yong: "The way of Heaven ensures fortune for the good / Both
ghosts and spirits are hostile to excess." Under this interpretation,
sexual disease is not so much an issue of quotidian retribution as of
heavenly retribution for evil deeds. A poem from chapter 62 of the
novel relates excess, venereal disease, and retribution:

> Lust does not delude people, they delude themselves.
> But if they become deluded they will suffer the consequences.
> Their vitality will be dissipated; their countenances grow pale;
> The marrow in their bones will dry up, and their strength will wane.
> Those who engage in fornication find that their families will break up;
> Once venereal disease is contracted, it is difficult to cure.[91]
> As always, "A full stomach and warm body give rise to disorder";
> Those for whom disaster is imminent never seem to realize it.[92]

Venereal disease (*sebing*) is contracted (*rancheng*), but it is still
related, in a traditional way, to excessive sex and intemperate food
and drink. In a comment at the beginning of chapter 79, when Ximen
Qing begins to falls ill, Zhang Zhupo writes, "Behold the precision
of retribution [*baoying*],"[93] and, after describing Ximen's symptoms,
"This is clearly the working of retribution."[94]

Ghosts have always been considered pathogenic factors in the medical tradition. Doctors at least as late as Xu Dachun argued that the
"ghosts and spirits" of classical medical theory were not supernatural

beings but heteropathic forces such as wind, cold, damp, and heat that invaded a body with weakened defenses. He nonetheless admitted that in true cases of illness induced by wronged and vengeful ghosts, medicinal drugs were powerless, since such afflictions were the wages of sin or destiny.[95] Sexual excess was punished both by quotidian retribution and vengeful ghosts—sometimes in the form of *yangmei*. Syphilis demanded a paradigm shift of medical theory but not of fiction, since, in the words of a character from the 1905 novel *A Flower in the Sea of Sin* (Niehai hua, 1903), "Contagion is just retribution" (*chuanran jiushi baoying*).[96]

XIMEN QING'S (TAINTED) LEGACY

Sequel to Plum in the Golden Vase (Xu Jinping mei) presents three characters who suffer from *yangmei* (none of whom feature in the original novel), but their retribution is quotidian rather than karmic. One is a corrupt official, one a womanizer, and one the madam of a brothel. Perhaps syphilis began to be seen as a disease that was naturally retributory, indicative of an inner rottenness, a punishment fit for transgressions in this life rather than those graver sins for which it was not severe enough. Or perhaps the etiology of sexually transmitted diseases was understood widely enough by 1660 to make syphilis an ill-fitting karmic punishment, in which the transgressor would have to be born with it (and his immediate biological parents then must also suffer the disease), or at least susceptible to contracting it. If characters had syphilis, it was because they dallied with prostitutes, or they metaphorically received a rotting disease because they were morally rotten.

Marriage Destinies to Awaken the World is a novel about mundane rather than karmic retribution, and in many instances retribution for excessive or illicit sex. Likely published after the 1695 Zhang Zhupo Edition of *Plum in the Golden Vase* and its sequel, it indicates remarkable plateaus in the punctuated evolution of venereal disease, retribution, and gender in Chinese fictional literature. According to some scholars, the novel depicts a world divided in two. One realm is a utopian paradise of temperate climate, morality, and peace, in a rural setting, while the other is a dystopian place of expanding market towns and commercial centers that foster decadence, extravagance, and decrepitude, and threatens to engulf the entire Chinese empire.[97] It is the story of the town Mingshui as it transforms from a rural village into a booming market town, and its consequent moral fall. The narrator portrays this with voyeuristic glee, and portrays the decline of the town with an exaggerated realism, detailing the grotesque and profane in a mode surpassed by few of its predecessors.[98]

Although a large part of the population regarded syphilis simply as one of many diseases that plagued the empire at regular intervals, the fact that *Marriage Destinies* repeatedly refers to syphilis as "sores of heavenly retribution" (*tian bao chuang*) implies that readers were familiar enough with the etiology of this particular disease to attach it to certain immoral or excessive actions.[99] The patients who suffer these retributory sores contract them as the logical outcome of transgressive behavior, not as some karmic debt that still needs to be paid from some former lifetime. The evil scholar and teacher Wang Weilu is repaid for his misconduct with syphilis, and his sores are used as a symbol for moral corruption.[100] He gives up the pursuit of Confucian scholarship and goes into business, and his name puns on this fall: "the perversion of Confucianism" (*wang wei ru*). He becomes a money broker, who, like Ximen Qing, cheats and maltreats his clients and greedily covets the property and wealth of others. In fact, it is because he loses all of his facial hair to syphilis that officials are able to identify him as a criminal.[101] The description of *yangmei* is detailed and graphic to highlight the depravity of a character that would contract such a disease.[102] Wang Weilu's deathbed scene is also reminiscent of Ximen Qing's end in *Plum in the Golden Vase*, yet *Marriage Destinies* takes its grotesque effect even further.

Marriage Destinies depicts other syphilitics as well. The first, Shan Bao (whose name puns on "good retribution," *shanbao*), falls from his position as a good Confucian son to one who beats his wife and abuses his parents. He tries to prevent his father's proper burial and to destroy the corpse. Shan Bao indulges in drunkenness and lechery, and he dies of syphilis (*tian bao chuang*) as the consequence of his lascivious lifestyle. The retributory nature of the disease might have been interpreted as "karmic sores" by some readers, at least in part a punishment for his father's way of life, the punishing teacher who competes with his students even to the point of killing some of them. Yet it is also a retributory illness for frequenting brothels in the immediate and being unfilial in the long term. It is clear that the other characters who suffer from syphilis in the novel do so as a fairly speedy result of a particular kind of action.

Two Buddhist monks, Wu Bian and Cheng An, suffer from venereal disease. Wu Bian is promiscuous and frequently visits brothels, having slept with every girl in the forty or fifty houses of ill repute along the riverbank.[103] Because of his excessive fornication, his originally strong physical constitution is depleted, and he dies of a venereal condition identified by desiccation of bone marrow.[104] His death, like Wang Weilu's, is depicted in gruesome and bawdy detail. The other monk, Cheng An, explicitly suffers from syphilis (*yangmei*) by the time he succeeds Wu Bian.[105] Because he fears doctors he tries to hide his disease and engages in self-medication, employing *qingfen* calomel, a treatment for syphilis including primarily mercury found in *Systematic Materia Medica* and other medical texts of the late Ming and early Qing.[106] Treatment is of no avail; as "syphilis and insanity broke out together ... following the heart sutra, first he lost his eyes, and then he lost his nose, then his tongue, and finally his entire body."[107] The retributive morality, and the ironic appropriation of scripture for medical case, cannot be missed. Cheng An suffers a disease that results directly from visiting brothels, and because that practice is morally questionable, especially for a monk, he is punished with the particular disease whose symptoms parallel those depicted in the heart sutra.

The detailed and carnivalesque depictions of syphilis in *Marriage Destinies* are reserved for its corrupt, lascivious, selfish, and minor male characters. These sufferers were all engaging in the same practices and trades as their counterparts in *Sequel to Plum in the Golden Vase*, and they all contract the same illness. Consistent with contemporary medical case histories, there is a conspicuous absence of female syphilis, with prostitutes constituting the major exception, though they usually function as human miasma—unnamed and unvoiced contaminants. This is not to say that women escape the workings of retribution, they merely contract other maladies.

Syphilis was not sufficient punishment for rapacious main characters. It had limited use as metaphor, at least as it was represented in fiction, where sexual exhaustion followed by haunting or sexual dreams was much more significant and longer in coming for those such as Ximen Qing than was a simple diagnosis of sexually transmitted disease. Representing a disease as something contracted through or a result of sexual intercourse belies fears that boundaries, particularly boundaries between high and low, civilized and uncivilized, domestic and foreign, were being crossed—or worse, blurred. Fiction and medicine agreed that it was men who were most likely to transgress these boundaries, particularly in looking for sex in brothels and "prostitute boats." But sexual intercourse was not the primary mode by which disease was contracted—it is just one aspect of the increasingly complex understanding of disease transmission. When it came to diseases contracted through sex, late-Ming and early Qing fiction diverged quite a bit from contemporary medical sources that saw maladies such as *bian du* and even *yangmei* as having multiple causes, particularly geography (south) and boundary crossing (foreigners and ethnic minorities). Fiction represented venereal disease as a disease of immoral men, particularly un-Confucian scholars, corrupt officials, monks, wastrels, and merchants.

Fiction cast *yangmei* as a disease of those engaging in excessive or illicit sex, and therefore it often seems to be a malady to which men, often marginal and symbolic characters, were subject. But *yangmei* was also a symptom of being punished by avenging ghosts and by heaven itself. A similar malady, not of passionate expression but of repression, came to be frequently and prominently portrayed in late-Ming and Qing fiction and often discussed in medical texts. These depletion disorders, consumption-like illnesses, are the subject of the next chapter.

CHAPTER 5

Diseases of *Qing*

Medical and Literary Views of Depletion

Some doctors traced the ultimate cause of Li Ping'er's illness to blood loss, beginning as it had with the birth of her son. Ping'er had always had a delicate constitution, however, and had a history of falling ill from worry and longing (*youchou silü*) over her lover and fiancée's neglect of her. At the time, a doctor diagnosed her with a "melancholic congestion in her chest which cannot be resolved" (*yujie yu zhong er busui*). By reading her pulses, he further asserted that her ailment derived from her "six desires and seven emotions" (*liuyu qiqing*),[1] and said that if she were not treated in time, "it may develop into a "bone steaming disease" (*guzheng zhi ji*), which is of the family of [fatal] melancholic disorders."[2] These maladies are also related to Li Ping'er, in her longing, being visited by a fox spirit (*huli*) in her dreams. Every night he slept with her, sapping her vitality until she grew wan and emaciated.[3] The doctor was incredulous as to why a healthy young woman of twenty-three, born and bred in respectable circumstances, with ample means to supply all of her needs, would have been suffering from a melancholic congestion and deficient condition (*yujie buzu zhi bing*).[4] The doctor cured her easily enough, but whether it was his prescription or his marrying her that did it is not clear.

Now, years later, Li Ping'er had again lost her appetite, become lethargic and feverish, and suffered from bouts of delusion and derangement. Dr. Jiang had not able to fulfill her sexual desires and satisfy her longing well enough, and she had returned to Ximen Qing, for whom she had left her first husband. She became one of his wives and gave birth to a son. Her rival sister-wife, Pan Jinlian, endeavored to kill

Li Ping'er by haranguing her to death. Li Ping'er weakened, suffering
from significant vaginal blood loss. Jinlian's ferocious cat attacked the
baby; he had convulsions and died. Li Ping'er despaired and dreamt
of a visitation by her former husband, Hua Zixu, who accosted her
for her unfaithfulness and her role in his ruin. A nun explained to Li
Ping'er that the baby actually came into this life to trouble her for some
past sins (*yuanjia*).[5] Ping'er, tormented by Jinlian, mourning and losing
blood, grew weaker and died. The cause of her death, according to her
ghost, and the cause many scholars thus assume to be the ultimate one,
is "a case of acute metrorrhagia."[6] But her case is overdetermined, her
death the result of a different cause, depending on who is speaking. Yet
a full description her illness and death is not ambiguous; it integrates
mundane bodily, emotional, and demonological causes—a multivalent
condition that was more in line with an inclusive, robust medical diagnosis than with a metaphor or simple literary device.[7]

SEX, LONGING, AND DEPLETION

Most clearly, Ping'er's illness has to do with blood, grief, and resentment. Ximen and Old woman Feng both suggest this, and try to employ
emotional counter-therapy by shocking her out of her disposition by
showing her the coffin that has been made for her.[8] Ximen tells Second Sister Shen that Li Ping'er is so preoccupied by her child's death
that it has given rise to this ailment. "She's just a woman after all, and
doesn't know how to put [the grief] behind her," and "it is this excess
of grief that has brought on her illness."[9] Further, Dr. Hu said that
anger has disrupted her blood, and the nursemaid makes it clear that
her ailment began as a result of suppressed anger, and then she wore
herself out with worry over her sick baby that was then compounded
by grief at his death. The nursemaid says, "When someone is suffering
from suppressed anger, it helps to discuss it with someone else, but the
mistress won't let anything out."[10] There are two emotional causes of
Li Ping'er's illness—excessive emotions and repressed emotions. Those
emotions result in physical symptoms: her anger disrupts her blood,
and the taxation results in depletion from continual blood loss.

An example of the interrelatedness of these various illnesses
comes from the *Materia Dietetica* (Shiwu bencao, early 16th century), an herbal in four volumes.[11] In *juan* 27 there is an illustration of black bean sauce (*douchi*) and a description of its properties
and uses that reads, "Black bean sauce is bitter in flavor, cold in

thermostatic character, and nonpoisonous. It is efficacious against conditions such as cold damage [*shanghan*] and headache [*touteng*], miasmas [*zhang qi*], malign poisons [*edu*], impatience-melancholy [*zaomen*], depletion exhaustion [*xulao*], difficulty breathing [*chuanxi*], ague/malaria [*nüeji*], and bone steaming [*guzheng*]."[12] Dr. Jiang Zhushan says of Li Ping'er's condition, "It is like *nüe*, but it is not *nüe*, it is like [*shang*] *han*, but it is not [*shang*] *han*.[13] In eliminating these two, Jiang is, at least according to the *Materia Dietetica*, delimiting Li Ping'er's disease to one of depletion, emotion, and bone steaming.

Emotions (anger, grief, and melancholy), taboo violation (Ximen insisted that they have sex while Ping'er was menstruating) that allowed semen into her blood, and the conflict of blood and anger results in hemorrhaging, according to the aged physician in *Plum in the Golden Vase*, Old Man He.[14] If blood was seen as the root of the most serious female maladies, and that which characterized an illness as female, it seems to have been a fact widely known by educated people. Doctors, healers, shamans, and acquaintances draw on their own knowledge of medicine to diagnose her. Ximen says that he knows Li Ping'er is in possession of some *sanqi* ginseng, which "is certain to cure all those troubles from which women suffer."[15] He may have relied on pharmacological literature when he mentioned that it came from Guangnan, a fact also recorded in the *Systematic Materia Medica*. Li Shizhen says that this drug was discovered only recently, and that it is also known as "[drug] that cannot be traded for gold [*jinbuhuan*]."[16] It stops bleeding, removes blood stasis, and relieves pain. It treats profuse menstrual and uterine bleeding, disperses remaining blood stasis after childbirth, and reduces pain due to blood disorder.[17] The local prefect recommends that Ping'er take ash of the palm leaf and white cockscomb flower, both recommended by *Systematic Materia Medica* for uterine bleeding.[18] If readers were savvy enough to recognize these drugs, they would know that the characters who recommend them see Li Ping'er's illness as one common to women postpartum. Whether because of excessive emotions, the blood-based nature of the illness, the violation of sex taboos symbolized by semen in blood, or the confluence of all three, Li Ping'er's illness is the emblem of women's illnesses in the late Ming.

These earthly, logical, cause-and-effect kinds of explanations for her illness are supplemented by a variety of shamans and diviners who make it clear that Li Ping'er is paying for sins committed in this life

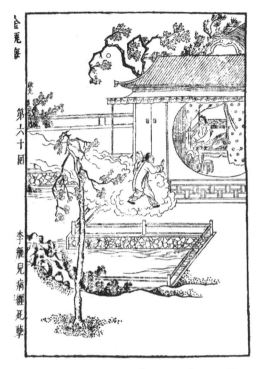

Figure 5.1. Li Ping'er dreams of Hua Zixu
demanding her life in *Plum in the Golden Vase*.
Xiaoxiaosheng, *Jinping mei cihua*.

or a previous one. Immortal Wu predicted in her twenty-seventh year
she would face a catastrophe, and that is the year she dies.[19] Master
Huang, after being given the dates and times of Li Ping'er's birth,
says, "If it is the horoscope of a female, it is very unpropitious. The
judgment reads: given over to sorrow without respite / if you want to
know why this woman is so afflicted, / and as unlikely to endure as a
tangle of threads: / Ponder the events before conception and postpartum."[20] Which is to say that she is fated to suffer postpartum blood
loss exacerbated by sorrow as retribution for past misdeeds. Li Ping'er
herself "fears that there are evil influences at work," and Ximen asks
Abbot Wu for "a couple of written spells which can be pasted up in
her room with a view to suppressing them."[21]

But more than generic evil influences, Ping'er knows that her former husband is the cause of her suffering; he says as much to her in

a dream. Daoist Master Pan (who is able to perform exorcisms and write effective prescriptions, reads incantations) performs rituals and confirms that it is a court case against her in the underworld that is the cause of her suffering.[22] Finally, Yinyang Master Xu reads from his little black book (*heishu*)[23]:

> In her former life, she was the son of a family named Wang in Pinzhou and was guilty of killing a pregnant ewe. Consequently, in this life she was reborn as a female in the year of the sheep, her nature was gentle and compliant, and she was given to artifice from her earliest years . . . her fate was crossed by the three penalties and six banes.[24] Although she acquired a distinguished husband in her years of maturity, she suffered from continual ailments and the 'matched shoulders' in her horoscope. She gave birth to a son, but he died prematurely, and her suppressed anger brought on hemorrhaging from her lower body that resulted in her death.[25]

The *yinyang* master diagnoses everything at once—proximal, distal, and ultimate causes.

How was a reader to understand the meaning of such a polygenetic illness? The various editions and recensions of *Plum in the Golden Vase* are themselves conflicted about the primary cause of Li Ping'er's death. The chapter 60 title couplet in the earliest edition reduces Ping'er's issue to one of emotion: "Li Ping'er becomes ill because of grief and anger."[26] The later *chongzhen* and Zhang Zhupo commentary editions have "Li Ping'er's illness invokes death and retribution." It is tempting to say that ultimate, karmic causes are the most important, most meaningful, in understanding illness, but then why include such detailed diagnoses, prescriptions, and medical information? Obviously the nature of the illness reveals something about a character, but if a character is fated to die, that removes the agency for contracting a disease either through contagion, infection, or moral transgression.

Li Ping'er is clearly the victim of Pan Jinlian's machinations, but the narrative; the shamans, Daoists, and Buddhists; the chapter titles; and, not least, the depiction and diagnosis of her illness and death make it clear that she is also being punished for sins in her previous life, for her role in the death of her previous husband, and for her role in bringing disharmony and ritual violation to her own house. If readers were conflicted about judging Ping'er as harshly as her fate seems to demand, it may be because her major sins come early in the novel and she is basically kind and generous, because she is overshadowed in lasciviousness and deceit by Pan Jinlian, or because there is a crisis in the text when the most authoritative doctor is giving his diagnosis of Ping'er. At the end of chapter 54, Dr. Ren feels her pulses and proclaims:

> Her liver conduit is hyperactive. People do not understand her. The element of wood [in her liver] has overcome the element earth [in her stomach], so that her stomach qi has been weakened. As a result there is no way for her vital energy to be replenished, or for her blood to be regenerated. . . . Because her blood is depleted, her two kidneys and the joints through her body all ache, and she has lost her appetite for food and drink. . . . Do not assume that this is an ailment of exogenous origin. It is not that at all. The symptoms are all those of deficiency. Her original store of vital energy was weak, and her postpartum conditions have not been stabilized, with the result that her blood has become depleted. It is not a case of blockage that would require purgative medications. Only if she is treated gradually with a regimen of pills can she be induced to come round and make a recovery. . . . It is only necessary to know that these are the symptoms of deficiency. The pain in her chest beneath the diaphragm is caused by an inflammation and is not of exogenous origin. The unusual pains afflicting her waist and the area of her ribs are due to depletion of her blood, and not to stagnation of the blood. Once she has taken the prescribed medications, these conditions should naturally be alleviated, one by one. There is no cause for alarm.[27]

The language of this passage is oddly and significantly repetitive, as if the author were repeatedly copying out of a medical text so as to get it right and to make it clear that this is a disease of a beautiful, delicate, and refined woman that concerns her personality, her predisposition to depletion, her weak qi, and her blood depletion from sex and resentment. The reader of *Plum in the Golden Vase* turns the page and in the first passage of chapter 55 goes back in time and reads all over again the diagnosis Dr. Ren gives Li Ping'er, in slightly altered version:

> The story goes that after Doctor Ren had palpated Li Ping'er's pulses, he returned to the reception hall and sat down. . . . "This illness of your wife's," said Doctor Ren, "is the result of inadequate care in the treatment of her postpartum conditions. . . . Right now, the pulses on your wife's two wrists are feeble rather than replete. When palpated, they are both scattered and large, as well as flaccid, and unable to recuperate themselves. These symptoms are all indications of inflammation, resulting from the fact that in the liver the element earth is deficient, and the element wood is in the ascendant, causing an abnormal circulation of the depleted blood. If these conditions are not treated at once, they will only grow worse in the future."[28]

The discontinuity and redundancy of the opening of this chapter are two of several indications that this chapter was probably not by the same hand as the two preceding chapters, or perhaps not edited by the same person.[29] If this is the case, and this passage was written by another hand without reference to the preceding chapter, it shows remarkable consistency in the diagnosis of depleted blood with liver fire and wood (liver) encroaching on earth (spleen).

Disregarding the textual issues surrounding Li Ping'er's diagnosis, there is little doubt that Dr. Ren views her condition as one of yin depletion, and consequent yang heat. Yet there are so many possible causes of her illness: anger, grief, postpartum issues, being an orphan, being highborn, having bad luck, being beautiful but neglected, having an excess of sexual activity, having semen in the blood, having a vengeful, dead husband, and having a karmically meager fate. Women were not soldiers. For them, simple blood loss did not cause death. Blood loss caused haunting, dreams, and fantastical and phantasmagoric sex. For Li Ping'er, contagion is retribution, but there are multiple kinds of retribution at work all at once, karmic (killing a ewe in her past life), vengeful ghosts (Hua Zixu), chronic (repressed emotion), and immediate (sex during menstruation). All of these are medical conditions, though only the karmic explanation is not found in the *Systematic Materia Medica*. None may be characterized as venereal disease, as could *bian du*, since the contagion (namely the causes of Li Ping'er's disease that stem directly from another person) are from ghosts. On a more quotidian level, Ping'er's blood loss and depletion fatigue occur when she is wracked with longing, when she suffers from anger and resentment, and when she engages in excessive and taboo sexual activity. The paradox of her illness symbolizes how women were always in medical jeopardy, regardless of their sexual situation.

DEPLETION AND THE PROBLEM OF SEMINAL EMISSION

Among the many diseases Li Shizhen lists in the *Systematic Materia Medica* under the category of depletion and decrease (*xusun*) are those caused by the five overstrains and seven impairments (*wulao qishang*), and those marked by depletion with much dreaming (*xu er duomeng*), depletion and taxation with fever (*xulao fare*), excessive sexual intercourse with spitting blood (*fanglao tuxue*), and "cold and hot feeling in the penis with pain" (*jingzhong hanre tong*).[30] Li mentions parenthetically that diseases of depletion and decrease can be caused by qi deficiency (*qixu*), blood deficiency (*xuexu*), essence deficiency (*jingxu*), deficiency of the five viscera (*wuzang xu*), deficiency of heat (*xure*), and deficiency of cold (*xuhan*), but he details only those deficiencies of qi, blood, and essence.[31] This category of disease, depletion and decrease, or depletion and exhaustion (*xulao*), was one of the most discussed in late-Ming medical texts, and one from which both men and women suffered.[32] Xu Dachun, for instance, wrote frequently about depletion in his medical cases and other texts.[33] Strengthening yin and bolstering vital essence (*qiangyin yi jingsui*) was a common approach for doctors to overcome these diseases, because although there were clearly a number of things that could be depleted in the body, the most often discussed seem to be qi, blood, and essence, and particularly blood and essence.

Blood was often associated with women's maladies, and, correspondingly, essence often came to mean "semen" in medical cases of the Song and later periods and to be associated with illnesses of men.[34] Although on a basic level essence and (menstrual) blood would seem to be paired opposites yang and yin, given their complimentary roles in procreation, from the Yellow Emperor's *Basic Questions of the Inner Canon* on, in medical literature both seminal essence and menstrual blood are grouped together as "yin blood" (*yin xue*), and "in this sense, male seminal essence [*jing*] is also yin, a specific form of a more general and primary yin, blood."[35] Depletion from sexual excess was, medically speaking, a disease related to loss of yin. Like prescriptions that treated *yangmei* and female blood loss, there was a great deal of overlap in the prescriptions recommended to reinforce the sexual ability of men and the ability of women to have babies. These drugs were also good for treating consumptive disease with exhaustion of the vital essence (*xulao jingjie*). Zhu Zhenheng, writing in the Yuan dynasty, warned, "Human beings' sexual desire can be boundless. How can yin qi, which is hard to develop but easy to deplete, provide supplies [to meet the demands] of such desire?"[36] He was not alone in his concern about the proliferation of depletion diseases.

Although emotional causes seemed to fade from descriptions of venereal diseases that featured sores and chancres, in both fiction and medical literature, emotions were very much a part of depletion disorders. Anxiety, physical labor, irregular regimen, sexual deprivation, losing oneself in art, obsession, mental overstimulation, aimless imaginings, pining away for a desired object, and disturbing dreams were all types of experience in addition to sexual overindulgence that resulted in depletion of semen. In fact, loss of semen for reasons other than sexual intercourse was considered particularly dire. This type of taxation, called "loss of essence taxation" (*yijing lao*), was a major illness discussed widely in medical texts.[37] There was a virtual epidemic of spontaneous seminal emission in the twentieth century, and it was a serious concern dating back at least to the fourteenth century.[38]

Seminal emission was inherently dangerous because it wasted precious bodily resources and because the depleted emptiness created by seminal loss left one vulnerable to attack by pathogenic factors such as ghosts and cold wind. From at least the Ming, to the end of empire and through the Republican period, spontaneous seminal emission was a key concern of elite and vernacular medicine. One of the Berlin manuscripts, for instance, contains a "discourse on involuntary/ spontaneous emission of semen" in which the (anonymous) author records the rhymed statement, "It is better to have sex ten times than to [involuntarily] lose one's essence even once."[39] Seminal emission was often grouped in the late Qing medical manuscripts with treatments and discussions of the venereal diseases *yangmei*, *bian du*, and others.[40] Late Qing and early twentieth-century clinical records suggest a disproportionate concentration on this malady.[41] Perhaps medical fear of the ailment was extreme because of the connotations of immaturity or impotence. One of the *Annals of Herbs and Trees* plays has the evil monk Mituo sing to the nun Cigu:

> I have produced my black curculigo root [*heixianmao*; popular term for penis]. It strengthens the yang and benefits the kidneys. / There is this little red bean [*chixiaodou*; popular term for clitoris]. It takes away the pain and dissolves ulcers. / Let us produce some mixed quiet and running water [*yinyang shui*; suggesting the mix of male ejaculate and female fluid]. It is effective against cholera. / Quickly, let your soft lotus stamen [*lianrui*] cure my involuntary seminal emission.[42]

The *Annals of Herbs and Trees* play, like many medical manuscripts, presents a number of treatments for this condition, some presented in mnemonic fashion.[43] Perhaps it was because this malady was so closely linked with those with postpartum bleeding or menorrhagia that it was felt to be particularly shameful and dangerous and thus so widely discussed.

Emotional excess was also a cause of yin depletion, and thereby linked to sexual excess. Zhu Zhenheng states the connection clearly, "Both the liver and the kidney depot harbor minister fire, and both have a link to the heart above. The heart is the ruler fire. When it is excited and brought in motion by desires, the minister fire willingly follows it. The chamber of semen is disturbed and, as a consequence, the semen flows off in the dark, discharged and drained even when not having intercourse. That is why the sages always instruct people to withdraw and nourish the mind."[44] An early Republican-era medical manuscript copies a 1730 text by the Shanghai physician Shen Fan (*zi* Luzhen). This work, the "Medical Case Histories of Mr. Shen Luzhen from Tiesha" (Tiesha Shen Luzhen xiansheng yi'an) copies the above quote from Zhu Zhenheng but adds, "the patient must calm down [his desires] to nourish his mind. This way, the original semen can be stabilized. Otherwise it is trying to put out a burning cartload of lumber with a cup of water."[45]

Wang Kentang names four sources of the disorder, cited for centuries, in his *Guidelines* for *Treating Illness* (Zhengzhi zhunsheng, comp. ca. 1597–1607).[46] These are "excessive mental exertion" (*yongxin guodu*), which causes seminal loss (*shijing*); "unsatisfied lascivious thought" (*si seyu busui*), which causes "semen to leak out" (*jing er chu*); "too much sex" (*yu taiguo*), which causes "the semen to flow uninterrupted" (*huaxie bu jin*); and "abstinence when in life's prime" (*niangao qisheng jiuwu seyu*), which causes "the *jingqi* to overflow" (*jingqi manxie*).[47] Zhu records a case history in which a man over twenty contracted this disease from overexerting himself studying for the official examinations. Another contracted it through an invasion of yin evil when caressing the statue of a maiden at a temple and subsequently obsessing over it.[48] Seminal emission was a chaste form of sexual excess. "The illness is in the heart," writes Zhu, "[seminal emission] arises from thoughts/lovesickness [*sixiang*]."[49] Seminal emission often accompanied erotic dreams, another form of sex without sex. Li Shizhen, in his chapter on seminal emission and emission with dreams (*yijing mengxie*), writes, "When excessive melancholy damages the heart, seminal emission occurs."[50] This was an illness brought on by excessive emotion, and longing resulting from erotic dreams or resulting in erotic dreams, a condition Li Shizhen calls "depletion and exhaustion with dreams and leaking" (*xulao mengxie*).

Though the medical literature rarely if ever discusses disease explicitly as being the result of retribution—either karmic retribution or worldly retribution—fiction was much clearer about these etiologies.[51] Medical literature tends not to pass judgment on victims of particular illnesses, but diseases linked to sex were clearly thought to be dirty in the popular imagination, and those who suffered from them were being punished for moral lapses.[52] Like sexual exhaustion, involuntary seminal emission is a disease of quotidian retribution in novels. As a result of lovesickness, it is also at times identified as stemming from a karmic debt, implied in terms such as *guobao* (retribution / karma), *yinguo* (cause and effect / karma), *yezhang* (retribution for sins in a previous incarnation), *yuannie*, and *yuanye* ("injustice curse"). But some of these, particularly *yuannie* and *yuanye*, become conflated with quotidian retribution for transgressions related to love.[53] For instance, in *Story of the Stone*, one of the claims that Baoyu's jade talisman makes is that it cures retributory illnesses, *yuanji*.[54] The word *yuan* is essentially a negative term referring to enemies, or, in the Buddhist view, sin, but it is also often used for love relations, especially in the words *yuanjia*, *yuanye*, and *yuannie*, all of which may refer either to enemies or, playfully, to lovers, the usage most common in *Story of the Stone* and *Plum in the Golden Vase*. Love and desire are seen as the results of karmic retribution for sins in earlier lives, and they are the cause of harm in this life. In this view, that which Baoyu's jade cures is a disease of retribution or lovesickness or both. This is the same malady from which Jia Rui, the obsessed masturbator, suffers (*yuanye zhi zheng*).[55] Jia Rui dies from misreading and from obsession, and from the expenditure of his bodily resources, but the real clue to explaining his death is the pool of semen in which he dies. Jia Rui masturbates while longing for Xifeng, which brings him to a dire strait, but once he is given the mirror for the romantic, the fantasies he encounters in its reflection result in involuntary seminal emission (*xiaji yile yi tanjing*).[56] Jia Rui dies from mistaking fantasy for reality, from misreading, but that misreading causes a fundamentally emotional taxation, a longing and frustration that result in a depletion disorder. Lovesickness and sexual exhaustion are thus fundamentally linked in fiction by their symptoms and retributory etiology.

Seminal emission was closely related to exhaustion from sexual activity on the one hand, and depletion with coughing blood on the other. Wang Ji's case histories record a patient debating with the doctor about his condition, and the patient shows his (presumably popular) understanding that "exhaustion from sexual activity, coughing blood, and nocturnal seminal emission are all disorders of the blood."[57] Xu Dachun has a treatise in which he discusses how, during depletion from sexual excess or seminal emission, "when the [blood and qi] are decrepit and exhausted [ghost] evils can consequently enter [the body]," resulting in raving, mumbling nonsense, and hallucination. But the primary cause of involuntary seminal emission, from the *Yellow Emperor's Classic* down to the twentieth century, were obsessive thought and feeling, particularly longing (*sixiang*).[58] Uncontrolled depletion came from uncontrolled emotion. Because of the link between *yijing* and emotion, it may seem strange that women fade from the medical discussions of these essence loss disorders early on.[59] Of the over two hundred drugs that Li Shizhen discusses that treat seminal emission, only a few of them also explicitly treat women's erotic dreams with discharge of secretion.[60] In the medical manuscripts there is also little mention of female emission, though one early Republican manuscript implies a difference between the sexes. In view of involuntary seminal emissions (*yijing*), "emissions come, and emissions go. The bone marrow is depleted." In view of vaginal discharge (*daixia*), "discharges come, and discharges go. The body is depleted."[61]

This paucity of cases detailing female involuntary emission of essence may well be because women were often depicted as having their own disease of depletion: consumption (*xulao, xusun*). This was one of three broad internal syndrome clusters defined by women's medical texts in the late Song. This category assembled afflictions marked by slow, chronic wasting, where the sufferer grew emaciated and debilitated, accumulating a host of secondary symptoms, from pallor, indigestion, and shortness of breath to hair loss, hot sensations on palms of hands and soles of feet, and palpitations, while also experiencing a destabilized psyche marked by disturbed dreams or insomnia and fits of melancholy or anger. Coughing with bloody sputum was an important but not definitive symptom in this syndrome.[62] Consumption in its many forms becomes in fiction of the Qing a disease almost exclusively of romantic heroines.

EMOTIONS, GHOSTS, WORMS, CORPSES, AND DREAMS

Li Ping'er's illness, in its multivalent iteration, presents a picture almost exactly as fully as did medical texts contemporary with *Plum in the Golden Vase*. There is an etymological link between *lao* 勞 exhaustion, and *lao* 癆 "exhaustion illness" with the sickness 疒 radical. Terms such as "exhaustion sickness" (*laobing*), "exhaustion disease" (*laozheng*), "taxation disease with cough" (*kesou laozheng*), "illness of exhaustion and depletion" (*lao sunxue zhi bing*), and "depletion exhaustion" (*xulao*) are all synonyms for *lao*. In some medical texts, *laozhai* 勞瘵 ("exhaustion consumption") is simply an alternate term for *laozhai* 癆瘵 ("exhaustion-illness with consumption"). In the case of taxation and depletion, most medical texts refer to depletion (of qi, blood, or essence) in one of the five viscera, though, as Dai Yuanli, a physician of the early Ming, wrote, "Although all five viscera can have taxation, that of the heart and kidney happen most commonly. The heart is ruled by blood, and the kidney is ruled by essence—when the essence is exhausted [*jie*], and blood is dried up [*zao*], this gives rise to *lao*."[63] Excessive emotion was thought to cause depletion, but was often accompanied by different kinds of taxation—from writing, thinking, worrying, and fatigue.[64] These strains were thought to take many shapes, particularly in women, in whom one could find thirty-six different maladies caused by the "five taxations, seven harms, and six extremes."[65]

Sun Simiao wrote in the Song, "Women's longings and desires are more intense than those of their husbands, and they are more frequently stimulated to become ill. Add to this that in women envy and dislike, compassion and love, grief and sorrow, attachments and aversions are all especially stubborn and deep-seated. They cannot themselves control these emotions [*qing*], and from this the roots of their illnesses are deep, and their cure is difficult."[66] According to the standard treatise *One Hundred Questions on Female Disorders* (Nüke baiwen, 1279), a major cause of female sickliness was women's "inability to control their emotions." The resulting excesses of "compassion and love, aversion and envy, melancholy and grief lead to bodily imbalance."[67] Although these emotions existed in a relationship to one another that implies equality, in that each can conquer or give rise to another emotion, certain emotions caused illnesses to which women were particularly prone. Anger caused liver fire (*ganhuo*), and melancholy engendered "static congestions" (*yujie*). The *New Book of Childbearing* (Taichan xinshu, 1793) classified menstrual and fertility disorders according to a woman's physical and emotional type. Thin and repressed women suffer from "static congestion," and hot-tempered and jealous types are afflicted with "liver fire," while lethargic and plump women can be expected to suffer from "phlegmatic stagnation."[68]

It seems that this paradigm was widely understood, given that the three most prominent female characters in *Story of the Stone* conform to it: the thin and repressed Daiyu, the hot-tempered and jealous

Xifeng, and the plump and reserved Baochai. These characters fit the types defined by the *New Book of Childbearing*, but the causes and significance of their illnesses are more complex than personality archetypes. Women were seen as being particularly prone to anger, which could cause miscarriage (as in the case of Wang Xifeng) or a variety of functional blood disorders. Anger was visualized as a kind of heat associated, when extreme, with the fire of the five phases that caused heat, the upward movement of qi in the body, and drying up of blood. However, women were also particularly subject to static congestion, a kind of melancholy syndrome of congealed blood associated with spleen system dysfunction. This syndrome was experienced as feelings of oppression and suffocation, pressure or tightness in the chest, languor, and loss of appetite, all linked to pent-up resentments and repressed desires. Physicians knew that static congestion and liver fire were related, and despite their differences in marital status and sexual experience, this link is quite clear through a medical analysis of Lin Daiyu and Wang Xifeng in *The Story of the Stone*. "Static congestion" and "static anger" (*yunu*) were often paired. Congestion that blocked yin could produce reactive heat, as excess yang surged in the vacancy left by underlying yin depletion, with manifest "wind and fire ascending" and overconsumption of blood.[69] Static congestion was seen primarily as a syndrome of women because of its metaphorical implications with blood and emotions. As the *Golden Mirror of the Medical Lineage* explained it, "Women must follow others and do not command their own persons; therefore they suffer from worry, resentment, and static qi."[70] Further, this disorder particularly afflicted young women whose circumstances did not allow them to "fulfill their desires." "Maids and concubines often suffer from stasis; their emotions are not outgoing and unimpeded."[71] "Static congestion" implies sexual frustration, just as loss of blood and essence points to sexual excess.

Medical practice associated static syndromes in women with grave, potentially life-threatening "depletion and wasting disorders" (*xulao*). "Bone steaming" (*guzheng*) was often presented as a final, fatal transformation of such disorders. Immediately following his chapter in the *Systematic Materia Medica* on depletion and decrease (*xusun*) in which these links are made, Li Shizhen details treatments for similar maladies that fall under the category of "malign influx" (*liaozhu*), and those in the category of "ghosts and demons" (*xiesui*). These are diseases that share symptoms and treatments with *laozhai* and *guzheng*, maladies caused by an accumulation of "worms" (*chong*) and corpse qi (*shiqi*), and those caused by malignant qi taking advantage of depletion resulting in congestion of phlegm, blood, and fire.[72] In these chapters (and throughout the *Systematic Materia Medica*), depletion illnesses (*xulao, guzheng*, and *laozhai*) are closely related to, share common treatments with, or are proximally caused by corpse transmission (*chuanshi*), corpse infusion (*shizhu*), ghost infusion (*guizhu*), flying corpse (*feishi*), demonic influence (or sex with demons; *guimei*), evil [heteropathic] qi (*xie'e qi*), attack of malignant forces (*zhong'e*), or worm infusion (*chongzhu*).[73] Li gestures at a complex matrix of syndromes that are ultimately caused by depletion and taxation but which are essentially contagious, resulting from more immediate causes. These disorders were messy metaphors in fiction—although emblematic of women's' problems, they were also overdetermined, suggesting personal responsibility for uncontrolled emotions or desires, retribution from worms or ghosts for immoral lapses, or simply an unfortunate encounter with a pesky demon or proximity to the corpse of someone who had died from such. The tendency of authors of fiction to deemphasize retributory aspects of consumption,[74] or its ghost and worm causes, might be explained by the general trend in Ming and Qing medicine to replace such older explanations with those that emphasized internal disharmony and unfulfilled desire as root causes.[75] The demon- or worm-centered explanation still persisted, but learned doctors displayed their superiority by recognizing and addressing the root internal disharmony that allowed the invasion to occur in the first place. Thus, the Ming-Qing authors who emphasize emotion and depletion are actually consistent with broader developments in learned medicine.[76]

Learned healers in the late imperial period increasingly attributed the root cause of disease to internally generated imbalances and pathologies rather than to invasions of external pathogens.[77] An important result of this was that doctors in the Ming and Qing increasingly attributed a variety of illnesses to internal damage caused by unregulated emotion.[78] Yet emotions themselves are contaminated by these exogenous, supernatural forces. Depletion disorders, caused by demons, ghosts, worms, or malevolent wind give way to *dreaming* of demons or spirits, a fictional, illusory version of invasion by pathogenic forces. The external pathogens that once caused consumption become internalized. Although in *Plum in the Golden Vase* consumption could be caused by sexual excess and transgression, as

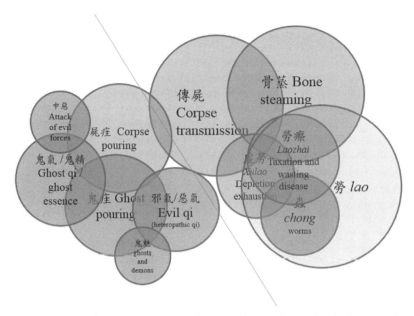

Figure 5.2. Relative occurrence of terms discussed together in Systematic Materia Medica, chapters 3.35 and 3.36.

it becomes an illness of emotions and repressed sexual desires in the hands of Qing authors, it also takes on the stain of ghosts, corpses, and worms. Increasingly, these female depletion disorders are associated with emotions and with dreams. Dreaming of sex with demons was both a symptom and a cause of excessive emotions, in the same way that reading fiction was both a symptom and a cause of excessive emotionality.

Anxieties about excessive emotion paralleled anxieties about the sexual activity of women. A useful example of the problem of female sexual activity and its metaphors is presented in *Sequel to Plum in the Golden Vase*. Jingui, the reincarnation of Pan Jinlian, repeatedly dreams of a rendezvous with her lover under a grape arbor (reminiscent of Jinlian's infamous scene in the original) and becomes physically drained. She soon becomes unable to function sexually, and becomes a stone woman (*shinü*):

> Like Pan Jinlian, [Jingui's] sensual tendencies made her fall easy prey to the demons of voluptuousness and concupiscence. It was all too easy for them to make their way into her soul through the gaping holes in her defenses and master her. But Jingui's unbridled license in

the realm of fantasy had been too much for her; even her strong passions had been drained and exhausted. She was now nothing but an
empty shell. And that was not all. . . . She could only stammer mean-
ingless and disconnected words; her legs were incapable of supporting
her body. She could not eat or drink. In short, she was seriously ill.
She lay on her bed for ten whole days, seemingly lifeless.[79]

Jingui (Jinlian) is punished by being desexed, which makes sense
according to literary logic, but not medical logic—the complete loss
of yin essence results in her becoming a stone woman, who is a creature of pure yin. One commentator writes in the margin that "these
symptoms are all those of Li Ping'er's illness," defining that malady,
too, as one that had sexual excess at its root.[80] Jingui *dreams* of sex,
which saps her essence. Traditionally, dreaming of sex was tantamount to dreaming of sex with ghosts or demons, and that was a
result of demonic invasion. Since the Han, "dreaming of intercourse"
(*meng jienei*) was interpreted as the function of deficient qi dwelling
in the "genital organs" (*yinqi*). The Eastern Han physician Zhang
Ji (ca. 150–219) categorized erotic dreams in terms of "fatigue disorder" or "depletion taxation" (*xulao*). He believed that such consumptive diseases resulted in women's "dreaming of intercourse," and
contrasted this with men's "loss of semen."[81]

According to *Prescriptions Worth a Thousand in Gold* (Qianjin yaofang, seventh-century), in men sexual desires exhaust human
thoughts and result in the illnesses of "depletion and damage"
(*xusun*), such as "losing semen," "turbid urine," and "having sex
with demons" (*guijiao*).[82] In women, it was not sex but dreaming of
sex, and particularly dreaming of sex with demons, that was tied to
an internal fatigue disorder resulting from external stimuli.[83] The
late-Ming physician Zhang Jiebin not only addressed the emotional
origin of cases of women "dreaming of sex with demons," he also
contributed to a new nosology of "stagnation disorders" (*yuzheng*)
in which unmarried women's love sickness and widows' sexual frustration were now included.[84] Repressed passions and unfulfilled
desire were seen to cause blockages such as "ghost fetus" (*guitai*)
and invited sexual dreams with demons, which either produced or
were caused by internal taxation vacuity. The imbalance of emotions owing to lovesickness and sexual frustration then became a
new perspective through which physicians interpreted the diagnosis of women "dreaming of sex with demons." The medical basis of
these dreams shifts from "mutual affection with demonic qi" (*xieqi*

jiaogan), "demonic influence" (*guisui*), and unsatisfied sexual appetite to increased emphasis on the seven emotions diminishing the
heart's blood.[85] The late Ming physician Zhang Jiebin, in particular,
discussed in depth the condition of women "dreaming of sex with
demons" in terms of both internal emotions and external demonic
influence. Excessive emotion led to fatigue and lethargy during the
day, and "dreaming of sex with demons" (*meng yu guijiao*) at night.
Zhang Jiebin writes that the emotions of pensiveness, anger, and sorrow often transformed themselves into disorders of static congestion
yu.[86] These concepts extended from elite to mundane medicine, with
one instance from an 1847 medical manuscript including a recipe for
"pills to end passions," (*duanyu wan*), which were recommended for
"virgins, widows, and nuns, whose longing for a man cannot be ful-
filled, in order to prevent these more severe consequences of longing.[87]
Diseases that were historically tied to sex increasingly became tied to
thoughts of sex, dreams of sex, and ultimately simply prolonged feelings of passion, longing, or resentment. This progression in medicine
and fiction coincided with (or happened just after) related trends, such
as the "cult of *qing* [passions]" and the "cult of female chastity."[88]

Xulao and *laozhai* were the quintessential disorders of female
blood, and had their counterpart in the spontaneous seminal emissions expected in men who came down with depletion and wasting
disorders.[89] In Ming fiction and vernacular literature prior to that
period, these female maladies, like seminal emission, were diseases
associated with sexual exhaustion, even though sufferers often were
loyal wives, chaste widows, or virgins. Sexual dreams, medical wisdom had it, were especially likely to trouble celibate women such as
widows, nuns, palace women, and those whose marriages were too
long delayed. Static congestion and depletion and wasting disorders,
as gender-linked syndromes, were associated both with sexual frustration and with the results of sexual fulfillment. They became disorders of anxious and longing virgins that manifested in menstrual
irregularity and bodily lassitude. But depletion and wasting disorders
were also endemic in worn-out mothers, who had expended their sexual vitality in childbearing or through rage and worry.

The gendering of *laozhai* and *guzheng* extended to the gendering
of their victims. That is, women who suffered from these conditions
were gendered as male or as hyperfeminine. If women engaged in
excessive sex, as men were wont to do, they suffered depletion of their
yin, allowing yang heat to increase, leading to bone steaming and

frequently to vaginal bleeding. They were depleted women, but they were also women who had depleted their femininity. However, depleted yin in virgins with repressed and excessive passion resulted in consumption and bone steaming, and those illnesses come to be represented in fiction as the malady of young women and virgins par excellence.

Although Li Ping'er's illness is represented as being the result of almost every one of these forces, many later authors of fiction took the gendering of depletion disorders to even greater lengths than did Ming medical writers. Seizing upon the notion that depletion disorders were really caused by emotions, and ignoring that they also were commonly thought to be caused by agents of retribution such as ghosts and consumption worms, suggesting sexual excess and transgression, we find statements about *xulao* stripped of retributory notions: the illness, with symptoms of consumption, was "brought on partly by melancholy [*yuzheng*], partly by lovesickness [*sizheng*], partly by cowardice [*qiezheng*] and partly by fright [*jingzheng*]."[90] Emotional disorders belied the sexual and retributory implications of this malady.

THE CONSUMPTIVE HEROINE IN THE QING

Given that the complex of symptoms and causes surrounding depletion and retributory agents became increasingly one of women and their emotions, it should not be surprising that *Story of the Stone*, which is perhaps the first long work of fiction in the Chinese tradition in which emotions are of primary importance, features these diseases so prominently. This focus on the novel's emotionality and language also ironically reinforces the traditional (and still widely prevalent) tendency to read the novel as "autobiography" and its characters as historical people. Not only was *Story of the Stone* read as autobiography, but more than that it was read, the novel claims, as "a true record of real events." The poetic status granted to the novel through its emphasis on emotions further bestowed upon it the veneer of truth, since, as we have seen, poetry, and particularly often-quoted poetry, served medical writers (as well as writers of encyclopedias, guides to daily life, and other such texts) as evidence, most often captured in the formulation "there is a poem as proof."[91]

If *Story of the Stone* was about emotions, it was equally about young women, and it acted as a medical case history of female emotionality.

Lin Daiyu, Qin Shi, Adamantina (Miaoyu), Skybright (Qingwen), and Wang Xifeng all suffer from a wasting disease brought on by abundant and unexpressed emotion (*qing*).[92] Their maladies are all are tied to blood. The nature of this illness was recast by *Story of the Stone* as one primarily of emotions, stripped (mostly) of sexual connotation, ghosts, demons, worms, and corpses. The different manifestations of these depletion disorders in the world of *Story of the Stone* all became related to one malady that had at its root extreme emotion. However, even in this novel of female emotion published at the height of the "cult of female chastity," the vestiges of transgressive behavior are still visible beneath the veneer of transgressive emotionality.[93]

Xifeng has persistent blood loss postpartum,[94] but she, like Daiyu, also has repeated bouts of coughing and vomiting blood.[95] Each manifests the symptom set of a consumptive who suffers from passion, grief, worry, or ambition. Qin Shi's diagnosis is notably almost exactly the same as Daiyu's (and very similar to that of Li Ping'er's in chapters 54 and 55 of *Plum in the Golden Vase*). Dr. Zhang says of her,

> A deep and agitated left distal pulse indicates a febrile condition arising from the weak action of the heart; the deep and faint median pulse is due to anemia caused by a sluggish liver. A faint and feeble distal pulse on the right wrist comes of debility of the lungs; a slight and listless median pulse indicates the wood element of the liver is too strong for the earth element of the spleen. The fire produced by the depletion of heart qi results in irregular menses and insomnia. A deficiency of blood and sluggish condition of the liver produce pain in the ribs, delayed menses, and heartburn. Debility of the lungs leads to giddiness and perspiration in the early hours of the morning, and a feeling like seasickness. The earth of the spleen is overcome by the wood of the liver and causes loss of appetite, lassitude of spirit, and soreness in the limbs."[96]

We know that Qin Shi is suffering from retribution for sexual transgression with her father-in-law, yet her symptoms, with the exception of uterine bleeding, are exactly the same as those of the longing maiden Daiyu.[97] Further, Skybright, a maid who is said to look and act just like Daiyu, is said to have died specifically from *nü'er lao*—girl's (virgin's) consumption.[98] In other words, the thing that separates Daiyu's and Skybright's illness from Xifeng's and Qin Shi's is sexual experience, and their illnesses manifest differently only in which emotions are being repressed and where the blood comes out.

Of all those amorous souls waiting in the Land of Illusion at the beginning of *Story of the Stone* to be reincarnated in the realm of red dust, these young women waste away. Their consumptive illnesses, like those of earlier heroines, have both karmic and retributory aspects, even if they seem less susceptible to invasion by ghosts, demons, or worms than those of their literary predecessors. The story makes clear that licentiousness and passionate thoughts are punished as one transgression: "The fact of the matter is that all these noble ladies to whom you refer hail from the Skies of Passion and the Seas of Retribution [*qingtian niehai*]. Since olden times their sex has been under a natural obligation to remain pure, pure from licentiousness [*yin*], pure even from the infection [*zhanran*] of passion [*qing*]."[99] The narrative makes it clear that Daiyu's illness (like Qin Shi's) is improper. Grandmother Jia says of her diagnosis, "If her illness is of a respectable nature, I do not mind how much we have to spend to get her better. But if she is suffering from some form of lovesickness [*xinbing*], no amount of medicine will cure it, and she can expect no further sympathy from me either."[100] The meaning of consumption as constructed by the traditional case casts doubt on Daiyu's character in the eyes of Grandmother Jia. Consumption in *Story of the Stone* is a disease of women with an overabundance of repressed passion and longing, the symptoms of which cause Daiyu to be all the more desirable.[101] Thus, while she has no power and is not sexually active, she is a threat to the family name and family line because of her sexuality, which is apparent in the manifestations of her illness. Daiyu's case reflects the same paradox as in contemporary medical casebooks, namely that women are susceptible to consumption because it is affiliated with sex through its association with blood, which recalls menstrual blood, birth, and contamination, even if the patient is a virgin. Moreover, the condition heightens beauty and desirability (Daiyu is happy with her consumptive flush, which she says is "brighter than the peach-flower's hue").[102] We see essentially two forms of depletion disorders in the women in *Story of the Stone*, and in many medical cases: the kind that is affiliated with anger, resentment, and (sexual) transgression and that seems like the female counterpart of male sexual exhaustion and venereal disease; and the chaste, longing, repressed passion and erotic dreams (with or without demons) paralleling male seminal emission.[103]

An example of how *Story of the Stone* whitewashes sex with sentiment extends even to the protagonist Jia Baoyu. His "lust of the mind" (*yiyin*) seems to have been borrowed from the Yellow Emperor's *Basic Questions of the Inner Canon*, in which it is clearly a disease of excess, of overflow:

When pondering [*sixiang*] is without limits
When one does not get what one had longed for
When [lewd] sentiments [alternatively, excessive desire, *yiyin*] flow
  unrestrained to the outside and
When one enters the [women's] chambers excessively,
[then] the basic sinew slackens.
This develops into sinew limpness.
It also causes white overflow.[104]

In emphasizing licentiousness of the mind, rather than the flesh, the
text is further feminizing Baoyu, contrasting his condition (and seminal emission after his dream in chapter 5) with the more common
male malady of sexual excess. With the increased focus on internal
causes of disease, emotions become pathological and transgressive,
as Grandmother Jia says of Lin Daiyu's illness caused by longing.[105]
Anxieties of women having sex evolve into anxieties of women thinking about sex. Yet these cause the same illnesses, and those illnesses—
taxation vacuity, demonic infection, dreams of sex with ghosts and
spirits, coughing blood, and losing blood—are all tied up with retribution for sex.

Many doctors believed that unmarried women and widows were
prone to suffering from a "congestion [*yu*] of pensiveness." Although
a medieval medical work had already defined "demonic fetuses" as
an exclusively female disorder mostly attributed to unmarried women
and "pensive women" (*sifu*), it was not until the Ming period that
physicians widely discussed pensiveness as one of the seven emotions in relation to women's melancholy and consumption.[106] Meanwhile, it was also said that widows' and nuns' sexual dreams may
result in their specific ailments of "concretions and conglomerations"
(*zhengjia*) or "demonic fetuses."[107] Zhang Jiebin (ca. 1563–1640)
stated that unmated women, including nuns and unmarried women,
often fall into "unrestrained fantasy due to yearning for love" or
"unfulfilled wishes owing to distant love." Their hearts are shaken
by the "fire of desire" (*yuhuo*), which in turn weakens their "true
yin" and hence induces irreparable damage.[108] Consequently, some
diagnostic works dating from the Qing dynasty emphasize that a physician should treat widows and nuns with care because their symptoms are often different from those of normal women owing to their
"mostly suppressed and stagnated emotions" (*qing duo yuzhi*).[109] This
viewpoint remained influential in Qing China; typified by explaining
the menstrual blockage of unmarried women, widows, nuns, and jealous concubines in terms of their "malady due to suppressed feelings"

(*yu yi cheng bing*).[110] According to the Tang dynasty poet Li Shang-yin (813?–858), "Extreme passions truly weaken fate" (*duoqing zhen boming*), and, according to the poet and sing-song girl Yang Lai'er (fl. 874–888), "Extreme passions are the cause of many illnesses" (*duo-qing duobing*).[111] But these sentiments now reflected contemporary medical literature as well.

In the late Ming, diseases of excess, particularly sexual excess, bifurcated along gender lines. This is not surprising, given the flourishing of women's medicine and focus on reproduction. Excess led to gruesome deaths of blood flow out of the sexual organ. In the Ming, depletion caused women to become less attractive. In the case of Li Ping'er, she loses color in her face, her flesh becomes emaciated, and her radiant good looks fade.[112] There is a graphic depiction of her symptoms: her blood leakage, and inability to get off of the kang to use the restroom, and the attendant's need to change the absorbent pad she was laying on two or three times a day. There was a foul odor, and the narrator says that that she had grown so emaciated that she "did not bear looking at." Virgins who suffer from *laozhai* become more beautiful, their youth enhanced, as in the case of Lin Daiyu. Their beauty becomes etherealized rather than degraded. Even when affecting virgin beauties, consumption retained a whiff of sex.[113] It is a disease of the "meager fated" (*boming*), but "meager fated" was a code word for the most desirable young women.

In both fiction and medicine Chinese men more than women suffer from sexual overindulgence; women suffer inordinately from sexual repression and manifest bodily depletion.[114] Men actively contract *yangmei* in the brothels; women passively fall prey to seductive fox spirits or erotic fantasies in their dreams. Men have too much sex; women possess excessive desire and repressed passion. Depleted males, like Jia Rui, often appear as pale, weak, and fragile as female ghosts and sickly women—the two literary tropes of hyperfemininity.[115] Thus, in his *Medical Case Histories of Stone Mountain* (Shis-han yi'an, 1531), Wang Ji's preference for restoratives may have been implicitly as much about restoring the masculinity of his male patients as they were explicitly about treating their depleted bodily resources.[116] This implicit intention would bolster the argument that Zhu Zhenheng's earlier doctrines of "yang surplus and yin deficiency" aligned the medical body with neo-Confucian metaphysics and a new construction of literati masculinity.[117] Wang Ji also recommends self-cultivation only to his male patients, as an antidote to their

overindulgence in sex, alcohol, and diet.[118] Women are neither susceptible to such excesses nor capable of moral self-cultivation.[119] This rec-
ommendation echoes the apologies for fiction in novel prefaces, which
suggest that the (male) reader can use fiction to cure his ills, even by
observing the plights and diseases of unfortunate female characters.

Understanding certain illness as metaphor in the premodern period
is a difficult prospect because maladies such as depletion disorders
were so overdetermined in the medical literature. Cases such as *Plum
in the Golden Vase* and *Story of the Stone* thwart such an investigation because they not only incorporate sophisticated understandings
of elite medical texts and the medicine of systematic correspondences
but also integrate kinds of vernacular medicine practiced by itinerant
physicians, monks, *yinyang* masters, and midwives. While one character or even the narrator might make clear to the reader their belief
that one or another diagnosis is correct, the novel taken as a whole
tends to embrace almost every aspect and signification of the illnesses
they portray. These novels are certainly by and for "literati" and, as
many scholars have demonstrated, contain a complex structure and
fantastic degree of engagement with all manner of other texts, but
that does not necessarily mean that the "low" medicine represented
in these novels—the *zhuyou ke* demonology, flying corpses, and consumption worms—was an object of derision.[120] Rather, modern readers often underestimate the degree to which demons, ghosts, and
chong were real etiological factors. Vernacular knowledge held that
retributory illnesses really were the result of a past life's deeds imping-
ing on the events of the present, or, for that matter, the logic of the
universe that meets out poetic justice, often in the form of illness.

In the gendering of depletion disorders, men had depleted semen
and women had depleted blood, but when those women with depleted
blood were unmarried young women, their depletion was not depletion due to blood loss but marked by it. Venereal disease in premodern Chinese medical and entertainment literature, though more
complicated than simple person-to-person transmission, was still a
fairly straightforward instance of retribution at work on the body.
Medicine construed women as more complex bodies, more difficult
texts to read, and requiring a more sophisticated kind of reader. But
consumption was a disease that resisted being read, in the sense that
it required multiple readers: elite physicians to read pulses, doctors to
read emotions, fortune tellers to read the future, and exorcists to read
disturbances in the unseen world. Consumption was often read as a

disease of *qing*. As such, its etiologies changed as definitions of *qing* changed. In this sense it was extremely contagious, spreading though and across all kinds of texts.

Of course *chuan* can also mean "to transmit" in the nonmedical sense. Many medical texts contain this word in their titles, and some of the terms for "rumor" include it, too, as in "transmitted to each other" (*xiangchuan*) and "to transmit and speak" (*chuanyan*). For instance, when news of Pan Jinlian's lasciviousness spread among the monks in *Plum in the Golden Vase*, "one told the other [*yige chuan yige*] until none did not know."[121] Female emotion and thought were contagious, all of these beautiful, sickly characters making so many female readers sickly.[122] Fear and fascination of women having sex, or being consumed by longing and repressed desire, also spread from text to text, until none did not know.

CHAPTER 6

Contagious Texts

Inherited Maladies and the Invention
of Tuberculosis

The *jiaoshu* [top-ranking courtesan] Lin Daiyu hails from Songjiang.
When I met her years ago in Tianjin, her bright eyes and skill in the art
of love had already established her as a top courtesan of incomparable
fame. Shortly afterwards she established herself in Shanghai, and her fame
soared to new heights. During the past ten years, everyone who happened
to come to Shanghai from high-ranking official to noble lord, from poet to
scholar, considered her the number one. While well-versed in the literary
arts, and skilled in poetry composition and singing, this *jiaoshu* is particularly skilled in social intercourse and knows the art of pleasing. Those
critics who sneer at her, reproach and slander her, do so not on the basis of
having observed her behavior but on the basis of rumors. In truth, nothing in her behavior needs to be concealed. But [the harm is done by] those
who discuss [her case] without being able to make the distinction between
black and white [truth and falsehood]. As a result they have eclipsed her
virtue instead of making it known. This is what I find so lamentable.[1]

This letter to Li Boyuan, the political novelist and publisher of the
early twentieth-century newspaper *Entertainment*, printed on the
front page, protested Lin Daiyu's low ranking in the annual flower
election—the rankings of Shanghai's best courtesans hosted by the
newspaper. There was, in the last decades of the nineteenth century
and first decades of the twentieth, a succession of famous courtesans
in Shanghai who took the moniker Lin Daiyu.[2] Many sequels to *Story
of the Stone* were written in this period, and many of them sought to
recast or reincarnate Lin Daiyu as a strong primary wife.[3] The original figure of Daiyu upset social order by her status as consumptive
orphan and her affiliated actions of dying for passion and challenging the Confucian status quo. If sequels often sought to eliminate or

mollify traumatic antinomies caused by making *Story of the Stone*'s Daiyu more domestic and responsible, these depictions of the courtesan Daiyu did the opposite.[4]

These courtesan Daiyus were path-breaking figures, public women who elevated their own status by claiming for themselves the roles of professional public entertainer, fashion icon, and arbiter of taste.[5] Lin Daiyu in particular was widely written about in newspapers, guidebooks, and travel essays.[6] Daiyu the courtesan also paradoxically features in numerous fictional works of the period, among them Zhang Chunfan's 1910 novel *Nine-tailed Turtle* (Jiuwei gui). The courtesan Daiyu was Daiyu liberated. She was beautiful and pitiable, like the original Daiyu, but now even more widely admired and desired.

Unlike the original Daiyu, who suffered from consumption, the courtesan Lin Daiyu had syphilis. The trend that Lin Daiyu started in Shanghai of applying dark makeup around the eyes and penciling in eyebrows with charcoal (her trademark) was likely in part an effort to cover up scars left by syphilis and eyebrows that had fallen out.[7] Tabloids presented conflicting images of Lin Daiyu, particularly as she aged. They described her as "lonely" and living in "miserable conditions" even as they enumerated her many jewels.[8] If in the nineteenth century "every languishing young lady imagined herself a Daiyu," in the modern era, it was no less the case for fashionable, modern young women to imagine and admire the courtesan Daiyu.[9] Daiyu's (evolving) character type was itself a tainted inheritance for women. While the courtesan Daiyu was only the most recent image in a long lineage of Daiyu models for women, and thus was always in part a figure of nostalgia, she was often represented in novels and media that were in many ways globalized. Courtesan novels were serialized in Western-style periodicals and newspapers, they moved about the foreign concessions of Shanghai, and they adopted and incorporated Western fashions and technologies into their texts. The courtesan Daiyu was a new threat to a new social order, with her body, with her attitude, and her popularity: "Every stinking man who talked of the courtesan quarters was saying Lin Daiyu, Lin Daiyu."[10] In the early decades of the twentieth century the figure of Daiyu was modern and nostalgic, familiar and dangerous. If the iconic image of the Shanghai courtesan gave way to the disease-carrying, publicly visible, disorderly, and victimized "pheasant" prostitutes who walked the streets of 1940s Shanghai, the courtesan Daiyu still had years to exert her influence on the conception and formulation of the modern woman as circulating publicly, cut off from but a threat to family, embodying independence, sexually alive, and living with illness.[11]

TRANSMITTING PAST KNOWLEDGE IN THE PRESENT

Vernacular texts such as newspapers and fiction continued to transmit fusty medical knowledge well after medical officials had repudiated it in the early decades of the twentieth century.[12] Records of people passing the illness (*guolai*), for instance—the practice by which one cures oneself of a disease by having sex with a stranger and infecting them with it—persisted in China until at least 1937. The problem with stories about passing or selling sickness, according to the prominent twentieth-century writer Zhou Zuoren (1885–1967), is that they not only disseminate false medical knowledge; they make for bad literature. Zhou questioned whether the falsity of information carried in a story could be divorced from its (poor) quality as fiction. According to him, though these stories might come from the weighty brushes of the ancients or appeal to the general taste, "they have no basis in fact" and "in the interest of truth they should be rectified."[13] But more so, "even judged as anecdotal literature [*suibi wenxue*], there is nothing to recommend them."[14] Fiction and stories, at least in the modern period, had some responsibility to tell the truth either through a kind of realism that challenges false but very real practices, or by simply disseminating true, scientific information. But why did these stories about "selling the sickness" persist? Zhou argued that it has to do with a fundamental salaciousness (*xiangyan*) and eccentricity (*liqi*) in the Chinese psyche.[15] He wrote that the Chinese have historically gotten overwrought about sex, that so many of their stories' descriptions "begin with wasp waists and end with tiny feet." But the Chinese, wrote Zhou, are also eccentrics at heart, by which he meant that they are interested, as are all humans, in tales of outlandish things. But, he claimed, the Chinese have a particular ability to discard whatever truth might be found in tales of romance or the marvelous—they "eat scabs without regard to the flow of blood" (*shijia buxi liuxue*).[16] That is, they have an unhealthy penchant for fiction without regard for its use or function. They took the fiction for reality and were not able to benefit from fiction because they were not interested in becoming talented readers.

Perhaps readers had become accustomed to gleaning much of their scientific knowledge from novels. Zhou blames readers of modern fiction for having an overdeveloped willingness to suspend disbelief, but Li Yu and others had been accusing their readers of doing the same thing for centuries.[17] Zhou's critical discourse of literature's failure to be modern by transmitting new information and challenging received wisdom would have been familiar to seventeenth-century century readers of fiction criticism. The problem for Zhou was not just in literature's failure to clearly represent scientific knowledge but also in readers' inability to read for it. Readers of modern fiction were looking for entertainment, and were not themselves scientific; rather, they were desultory, wanton, and careless.

The present was being infected by stories from the past. Premodern medical knowledge of all kinds was latent in modern Chinese fiction. Granted, premodern medical knowledge of all kinds continued to be practiced by many kinds of doctors well into the Republican period, if the manuscripts contained in the Berlin collection are a fair sample. Yet many works of vernacular literature or film that strove to be modern or that were appreciated because they were modern, foreign, or "scientific" were infected by what came before.

Certain diseases are often believed to be conditions of modern times. The fact that some diseases appear to be modern derives in part from the emergence of the biomedical concept of contagion. The germ theory of disease began to take shape in the 1880s,[18] and quite a few Chinese fictional works from the last decades of the nineteenth century and the first decades of the twentieth address contagion as an emblem of modernity—a diagnosis that conditions subjectivity and an agent that defines borders and spheres of interaction. Contagion undermines old conceptions of illness and contributes new biomedical perspectives. It changes the way we think about all sorts of daily practices and interactions, including coughing, shaking hands, and the use of toilets, because blood, feces, sputum, and breath come to be perceived as potential vectors of disease transmission. Practices that might spread a particular illness become associated with all illnesses. Infectious disease passes among people who come into contact with one another or are part of the same group, and contagion defines social groups by those same pathways of transmission. These pathways link people not only in space but also in time. As revolutionary, modern, and Western a notion as contagion was in China, its effects on medicine and literature had close ties to the past.

Illness in modern Chinese fiction from the fin de siècle period through the Second World War, like depictions of illness in premodern fiction, is typically more about having an illness than about contracting one. The concept of contagion did not appear to be revolutionary to many modern authors; instead, it functioned merely as a useful way of pointing out just how ignorant, tragic, or uncivilized many of their fictional subjects were. Literary works typically focused more on processes of contamination than on contagion. Some of Chinese fiction's most famous modern characters are marked by their illnesses—in fact, they are often marked *as* modern by their illnesses. The representations of these characters' illnesses are indebted to traditional fiction, and the ultimate cause of their illnesses is often a tragic inheritance from their ancestors. Chinese fictional depictions of tuberculosis from the late nineteenth and early twentieth centuries in particular reflect an overlapping set of understandings of contagion (*chuanran*), including not only the modern, biomedical understanding of the concept, but also a set of more traditional understandings as developed within Chinese medicine, fiction, and religion. Modern sickness is described in terms of traditional medicine, and tradition itself is identified as that which makes moderns sick. For characters in modern Chinese literature, traditional Chinese culture is the contagion, and the traditional family is the vector.

TUBERCULOSIS, CONTAGION, AND TRANSLATION

Tuberculosis (TB, *feijie he*) was *the* paradigmatically modern illness in fictional and medical literature in the fin de siècle period, yet TB is described in modern Chinese literature as moving between people according to all three traditional notions of *chuanran*: pouring (*zhu*) or dyeing (*ran*), sex, and contact with the sick. If external causes of depletion disorders had been internalized in the late Ming, subjugated to emotions as *the* cause of consumption, they returned in the modern period attached to metaphors of the "new" tuberculosis. In traditional literature that discussed disease, there are many illnesses that share symptoms and treatments with *laozhai* consumption. Most of them evoke infection by ghosts, demons, or ancestors: exhausted sacrifice (*laoji*), corpse infection (*shizhu*), worm infection (*chongzhu*), ghost infection (*guizhu*), "innocence" (*wugu*), and so on. The infectiousness of premodern diseases that share symptom sets with what modern medicine calls tuberculosis was described as early as the Jin dynasty by Ge Hong. He called these diseases corpse infection (*shizhu*) and pointed out that the disease could be passed from a dead person to other members of the family and could cause the extermination of the entire line."[19] In his fourth-century book *Master Who Embraces Simplicity* (Baopuzi), he describes corpse demons as having the form of worms.[20] Although the disease had demonic origin, its treatment was pharmaceutical rather than ritual. According to Ge Hong, ghost or demon infestation is the same as corpse infestation, the last in a group of five types of affliction caused by different sorts of pathogens known as "corpses" (*shi*). Corpse infestation brings along a host of accompanying demons and ghosts to cause harm. The disease undergoes a prodigious number of transformations, and comprises thirty-six or even ninety-nine varieties in all.[21] These beliefs were alive and well in the first decades of twentieth-century China. To give an example from the Berlin medical manuscripts, one healer records, "27th day: the patient has met the unsettled spirit roaming in the west who has sent out the demon responsible for consumption disease [*laobing gui*], named Du Shifu. . . . The demon sits behind the door in the house. Revealing this will be very auspicious. There is no need to pay [the demons] money to send them away."[22]

Traditional notions of contagion did not completely disappear with the dissemination of germ theory, even in the truth-telling fiction of the most informed moderns. One reason for this may be the shared symptom sets of traditional depletion disorders and the seemingly modern, Western, consumptive illnesses. The coincidence of these maladies encouraged mutually reinforcing portrayals of them. In the early years of the twentieth century, the translation of romantic writers, while not at all systematic, was voracious and pervasive. These writers often portrayed tuberculosis as a particularly "modern" disease—not in its etiology but in its effects. In 1899, Lin Shu (1852–1924) translated Alexandre Dumas fils's *La Dame aux Camelias* into classical Chinese.[23] The original story describes the most beautiful, popular, and charming courtesan in Paris, Marguerite Gautier, and her love affair with an aristocrat, Armand Duval. Armand comes to love Marguerite because of her pure and seemingly virginal yearning for true love. Armand's father intervenes to salvage his family's reputation. Marguerite nobly and tragically leaves Armand and, pining for him, dies of consumption. Despite being rendered into classical language, Lin Shu's *Chahua nü* (Lady of the camellias) became incredibly popular with modern readers.[24] Many believe its attractiveness to have been a result of its very modernity, its newness, and its foreignness: "The amazing popularity of [*La Dame aux Camelias*] in China also reflects the romantic sensibilities of a whole generation gradually liberating itself from traditional values and inhibitions."[25] But these new, foreign works also reflected deeply held native beliefs.

Associations with Western consumption, "thought to produce spells of euphoria, increased appetite, and exacerbated sexual desire," were taken up by the new generation of Chinese writers.[26] As Zhang Gongrang (1904–1981), himself a former consumptive, put it, "consumptives have especially strong sexual requirements."[27] Those Chinese heroines who suffered from consumptive depletion disorders in the Ming were tied to sexual activity, but in the Qing these patients suffered from passionate longing rather than passionate activity. In the modern period, Western metaphors and biomedical notions complicated the representation of these illnesses even further. One example of this is the overlap of metaphors across diseases. For instance, in European fiction and essays, syphilis and consumption often compelled their victims to feverish creativity and great writing activity.[28] Zhang asserts that "consumptives seem to be especially intelligent, and especially sensitive. . . . From ancient times, great writers and poets, like Dante, Goethe, Gorky, Lu Xun, and even our own Lin Daiyu, have all had lung disease."[29] Ironically, the fusing of modern Chinese associations of tuberculosis with imported associations with syphilis portrays the Republican-era consumptive as suffering from a complex very much like those we find in novels and medical literature of the late Ming, such as *Plum in the Golden Vase*'s Li Ping'er. Capacity for emotion, evidenced by feverish writing, typifies modern metaphors of tuberculosis in May Fourth literature, as does the conflation of sexual experience with chastity, fiction with reality, and the past with modernity.

In the Chinese translation of *La Dame aux Camelias* the interplay between the virgin and the courtesan, which is essential in the Western text, disappears, and the emphasis is placed instead on the protagonist's purity and moral superiority.[30] With the introduction of terms such as "propriety" (*li*) and "chastity" (*zhen*) into the Chinese text, Marguerite becomes familiar. More generally, the process of translation "is literally the process by which a Chinese reader recasts the foreign as familial."[31] But with Marguerite—especially in light of her becoming less sexualized, more chaste, more virtuous, and thus more like the archetypal suffering beauties of the Chinese tradition—it is also the familiar that is presented as foreign. In the case of *Chahua nü*, this is accomplished in part by the loose translation but also by the romantic quality of the original text.

Lin Shu's Marguerite is beautiful and full of desire and passion but is not able to express her passion fully. Although Marguerite and Armand's many sexual encounters are often shortened, removed, or rewritten in the Chinese version, her consumption is conditioned by her desire and her inability to express it. Toward the end, in letters to Armand, she writes that she "coughs blood all the time."[32] Lin Shu's Chinese translation reads, "The doctor has forbidden me to write. Sitting thus and thinking only makes my fever worse."[33] TB, in other words, is not only a disease of romantics but also of intellectuals. Moreover, it recalls not just the excessive emotion of depletion disorders but the stagnation, consumption, and dreams that result from pensiveness and literary activity.

Marguerite closely resembles Lin Daiyu in other ways as well: in the fact that her illness heightens her unlucky (or *boming*, "meager-fated") condition, in her beauty, and in the tragedy of her death.[34] The tubercular body is concealed in favor of the tubercular metaphor; we witness the coughing of blood, the willowy waist, the flushed cheeks, and the feverish forehead, but the paroxysms and the strained face of the illness and of sexual intercourse are absent from the Chinese version. Daiyu similarly suffers from a disease of (unexpressed) passion that literally consumes her—with her inner heat manifesting itself though the expectoration of blood.

La Dame aux Camelias employs concepts of contagion rhetorically and metaphorically. First, Marguerite and Armand are surrounded by a culture and society that they frequently describe using metaphors of disease. Armand describes himself as a parasite of love, and characterizes vices as diseases: "when I was cured of Marguerite, I would be cured of gambling."[35] He also describes love in terms of disease, "the habit of seeing me—or rather the need to see me—which Marguerite had contracted."[36] Marguerite describes a luxurious apartment, "the whole place furnished in a manner that would take a hypochondriac's mind off his ailments."[37] Disease is coupled with decadence, as asceticism is coupled with the cure. Second, contagion is applied to elements that are not medical pathogens. When Marguerite is out with her other lovers, Armand feels ill, and when he retaliates out of jealousy, Marguerite's illness worsens. Thus, they alternately infect each other, with Marguerite's death resulting in Armand's illness. This culture of sickness and the ability to infect each other with real or imagined disease highlights the individual's subjectivity among and in contradistinction to healthy bodies.[38]

The Chinese version of the novel lacks or twists most of this sort of discourse. There is much discussion of Marguerite's illness, but very few "parasites," little "infection," and no "contagion." There is one instance in which Armand mentions how he is "infected by love" (*zhanlian*), and another in which Marguerite specifies that she is not, but for the most part, it is Marguerite who is sick, not the world she inhabits and by which she is infected.[39] There is no *chuanran* in *Chahua nü*, but there are a few instances of *zhan*. Meaning "to infect, stain or moisten," *zhan* recalls the traditional link between moist environments, miasmas, and infection. Similarly the links between consumption, desire, and reading and writing are preserved in—or at least reintroduced into—the Chinese version, with Marguerite being forced by her doctor to stop writing letters, and with her tears moistening (*zhan*) the page.[40] Marguerite says that her consumption is both the cause and the result of her obsession with letters. In general, the world of *Chahua nü* is less infectious than that of *La Dame aux Camelias*, and the Marguerite of *Chahua* is ill more due to her inner life—her thinking, her writing, and her feeling—than is her French counterpart, who is sick because "her past ["life of dissipation, balls, and even orgies"] appeared to her to be one of the major causes of her illness."[41] Like the protagonist of the original novel, the Chinese Marguerite is subject to a heightened sensitivity, and her illness "continued to stir in her those feverish desires which are almost invariably a result of consumptive disorders."[42] Marguerite's consumption in *Chahua* becomes more about desire and less about sex, more about her personality and less about her circulation in a sickly world. Her attachment to letters points to this circulation and to a removal from it. Her illness, like her writing, hints at a previous life of love and intimacy, which has now been replaced by passionate longing.

So how did the Chinese Marguerite get consumption? She does not contract it through sex or sin, as in the French version, but rather she manifests it as a latent symptom of her congenital predisposition to desire. In Lin Shu's translation, Marguerite writes, "Today I am very sick. I may die of my illness. I am terribly weak and have had the illness for a long time. I know I cannot endure—like my mother who also died because of consumption. She bequeathed to me the origin of this illness. It is the family legacy that was left to me."[43] The mode of transmission reveals the degree to which the illness is intertwined with her personality. Marguerite's consumption appears to be congenital, and either is part of her personality or conditions it. Armand even says of her condition, "It is not illness, it is Marguerite."[44]

The aspects of contagion that transform premodern consumption into modern tuberculosis, namely germs or bacilli, did not get translated in Lin Shu's version of La Dame aux Camelias. Instead, traditional medical beliefs and traditional medical metaphors are used to translate modern or foreign medical discourses. But there were many modern and Western metaphorical aspects to Marguerite's consumption that did get translated. The most important of these is that Marguerite was of a lower economic class than many fictional consumptives of her day in China. Tuberculosis was, after all, called a "rich-man's disease" (fugui bing).[45] Although it was now a disease also available to the lower classes, consumption continued to be associated with refinement and sensitivity. It made the lower class more attractive, and brought the conditions of boredom and decadence, with which it was associated, to less affluent romantics and intellectuals.

Daiyu has always been sick; Marguerite has always been sick. Both are passionate, careless about the adverse effects they know their actions will have on their health. The difference is retribution (bao). Daiyu suffers from karma. She has a debt of tears from a previous lifetime which she must pay through a consumptive death, the tears giving way to the heat, dryness, and blood of exhausted longing. Marguerite (at least in the Chinese translation) suffers from hereditary.[46] She has inherited her illness from her family, from her remembered past. She, too, is a passionate and frail beauty, predisposed to illness, but she acts on her passion. It is her feverish circulation among people that activates her latent illness—but that is what makes her consumption modern. Either way, Marguerite and Daiyu both inherit their consumption, and other modern characters seem to get it from them.

THE CASE OF QIU LIYU

That tuberculosis was conflated with venereal disease in the early modern period makes sense given its metaphorical implications of class, circulation, and passion. This conflation is further interesting because of the early associations of depletion disorder with sex, passion, and longing. One modern example of this comes from the opera The Predestined Affinity of Sickness and Jade (Bing yu yuan chuanqi), first published in 1907 and performed frequently in the twentieth century.[47] It is the story Chen Qi, from Anhui, who is traveling in Guangdong looking for a relative. He loses his money and accepts a proposal from a matchmaker to marry into a wealthy local family. The Qiu family has plans to take him in so that their daughter, Liyu, can pass her congenital *mafeng* on to him and cure herself. Chen is delighted when he sees that Qiu Liyu is exceptionally beautiful. She falls in love with him and vows not to pass the illness to him. They hatch a plan, tell everyone that they have consummated the marriage, and Chen escapes back to Anhui. Meanwhile Liyu develops the illness and is expelled by her family. She begs her way to Anhui, finds Chen, and is warmly accepted by his family, who are grateful that she saved their son's life. She is aware that she has become a burden to them, though, and decides to commit suicide by drinking wine from a vat into which a poisonous snake has fallen. Unexpectedly, her disease is cured. The happy couple then returns to Guangdong and cures many *mafeng* patients with their viper wine.[48]

There are many traditional themes deployed to accentuate the tragic features of the custom of passing the illness. Qiu's beauty and virtue, her tragic fate of being born with a fatal disease, her selfish family, the serendipitous cure of viper wine, the miraculous effect of selfless suicide, and so on were all topoi common in traditional fiction and drama.[49] This terrible, traditional practice of *guolai* is combated by the virtue of Qiu Liyu. While the author points to the dangers of backwardness, he also systematically uses modern medical terms, such as translations of the Western terms "hygiene" (*weisheng*) and "microorganisms" (*mei jun wei shengwu*).[50] But it is not modern medicine that cures Liyu; it is her virtue as a sexually contagious virgin, the abandonment of her family's tradition of spreading disease, and her disciplined self-control that cures her.

Liyu is a modern enough woman to be able to cure not just her disease but the family and traditions that originated and sustained it. Chen falls in love with Liyu's natural, unbound feet. Although she is from the south, she is not uncivilized; she is a liberated, modern woman. Chen says to himself, "If she is not a Guanyin of the southern seas, she must be a woman literatus of Western Europe." Chen asks if the virtuous but sexually contagious Qiu Liyu is "another Camellia of France."[51] She is wise, almost foreign, but also familiar. She is a liberated woman with traditional virtues. She has a sexually transmitted disease but the virtues of a consumptive virgin.

It is difficult to believe that the title of the play *The Predestined Affinity of Sickness and Jade* is not referencing the title by which *Story of the Stone* was known in Shanghai from its first edition published by Tongwen Shuju in 1884 through the early decades of the twentieth century: *The Predestined Affinity of Gold and Jade* (Jin yu yuan).[52] The formulation is a strange one, though, since in *Predestined Affinity of Gold and Jade* the "jade" refers to the hero, Jia Baoyu, and the "gold" to the Confucian heroine, Xue Baochai. In *The Predestined Affinity of Sickness and Jade*, the hero and heroine have been replaced by the heroine ("jade" now referring to Qiu Liyu) and the illness (*bing*). This is the affinity of the heroine and her illness. In recalling *Story of the Stone* and Marguerite (and the woman European literatus), the author and audience must have had some sort of Lin Daiyu in mind, but a more active one, and a more Confucian one. For all of its modern medical rhetoric, the effective medicine in this story is not modern but traditional and sympathetic, with like curing like. The modern, female protagonist of the story is a chimera of old and new. She evokes Daiyu, but as soon as she is cured she returns to the backward south to cure those who engage in traditional practices.

THE CASE OF MISS SOPHIE

"Miss Sophie's Diary" (Shafei nüshi de riji), Ding Ling's (1904–1986) popular 1928 story, presents another consumptive heroine, this one intended to be distinctly modern. This story uses a robust medical discourse to describe love, in the style of the Western *La Dame aux Camelias*, and presents the heroine as a truly liberated woman. In fact, while Sophie's disease confines her in some ways (for instance, it prevents her from having a job), it also liberates her in others (it encourages reckless behavior). Sophie falls in love with a beautiful but soulless man from Singapore, the first man she has fallen for since her previous homoerotic relationship. She lives alone in Beijing, away from her parents, in a series of dreary, plain rooms. She breaks from traditional social norms, but as a result often feels lonely, isolated, insecure and melancholy, miserable and degraded.

Sophie presents a typical example of the modern tubercular. There seem to be two basic ways of talking about TB in modern Chinese fiction. On the one hand is the lover—the passionate, sensitive iconoclast who suffers consumption as an extension of lovesickness, repression, or exhaustion. On the other is the alienated modern citizen—whose experience of tuberculosis is through melancholy, weakness, and masochism. Sophie is both of these. Tuberculosis (*laobing*), was an old illness, and giving it modern meaning could not entirely erase the old associations. Sophie describes herself and her world as thoroughly modern—she masturbates regularly, and speaks of infection and nervous headaches. In her first diary entry, she describes reading advertisements in the newspaper about lawsuits over divisions of family property, ads for 606, venereal tonics, cosmetics, announcements of the latest shows at the Kaiming Theater, and the Zhengguang Movie Theater listings. That 606 (Salvarsan), a treatment for syphilis, should be so casually named reveals that venereal disease and its tonics were as much a part of modern life as cosmetics, movies, and the fragmentation of the family. At the same time, however, modern subjects such as Sophie and Qiu Liyu conflate high and low class, lovesickness and venereal disease. Sophie has a disease of refinement but portrays her consumption as a venereal disease—something that happens to people who circulate in society without regard to health or decorum. Sophie remains tied to the past. She talks about her fear of ghosts going back to when her uncle read her stories from *Strange Stories from Liaozhai* (Liaozhai zhiyi, 1766) and how even exposure to scientific textbooks in school did not assuage her still real fear of ghosts. She also discusses her friend Yunjie, who used to sing arias from *The Peony Pavilion* before she died from loving "that ashen-faced man." Sophie's lovesickness recalls Yunjie's, a traditional malady of young, unmarried women.

"Miss Sophie's Diary" also uses modern medical vocabulary. Although Sophie often refers to her condition obliquely as "my illness," she also uses the modern medical term imported from Japan, *fei jiehe* (which was based on the term "nodule" or "tubercle" *jiehe*), and twice uses the generic term *feibing* (literally, "lung disease"), which was the term for TB preferred by Chinese authors in the modern era. At one point she remarks, "I've never figured out what it is in me that they love: Do they love my arrogance? Do they love my temper? Do they love my tuberculosis?"[53]

Despite the modern terminology for her disease, Sophie brings Lin Daiyu to mind. Like Daiyu, Sophie also claims that her diary, rather than being a record of her life, is "the sum of all my tears."[54] The refrain that runs through the story—"I've always wanted a man who would really understand me"—might as well have come from Daiyu's lips.[55] Daiyu cannot escape the house, or her self-pity. Sophie at least escapes her house. Also like Daiyu, Sophie's consumption is bound up with her unexpressed passion. Marguerite may have developed consumption from her engagement with other bodies, but it causes her to fall in love with Armand and to withdraw from the world—entering it only through the circulation of letters. Sophie engages with other bodies *after* she contracts TB. What should be debilitating for her inspires a careless life. Sophie is careless and wanton, but she is still a Daiyu, perhaps more like her courtesan iteration at times than the girlish original character of *Story of the Stone*, but much like both.[56] The modern figure is sick and careless, but, like Daiyu, we do not know if her sickness is exacerbated by carelessness (as when Daiyu becomes determined to die by ruining her health) or if it was contracted through carelessness. What we do know is that the modern subject who is sick and careless draws heavily and directly on age-old concepts found in fiction and medical literature.[57]

Like Marguerite, Sophie is frequently bored, and her awareness of that state underscores her modern condition: "There remained little else to do except to sit and sulk all by myself, by the heater. The trouble was, even sulking became routine."[58] Sophie is decadent, and though she lives in cheap apartments, she constantly engages in reflective self-pity. In her self-awareness and in her financial condition Sophie is a modern subject. It is because she expresses her desire explicitly that she is modern. In the first lines of the story, Sophie refers to "boiling her milk" for the third time—a reference to masturbation. Satisfying herself in this regard ties her to the passionate, longing, consumptive beauties who preceded her, but doing something about it shows that she is a semiliberated, modern woman: "In order to save myself from the temptation of sensuality and the disintegration it brings, I'm going to Xia's place tomorrow morning."[59] Sophie's course of treatment, however, is primarily traditional: she takes the bitter medicine prescribed to her, though it does no good, and she receives from her doctor the same advice given to Marguerite—to "eat and sleep a lot, and not to read or think."[60] She sees a Western doctor, but he only indicates that her situation is hopeless.

The paradox of debilitation and inspiration that comes with consumption makes it the perfect condition to describe the quasiliberated woman in 1920s and 1930s China, who was only partially freed from the traditional and institutionalized modes of womanly behavior.[61] Sophie has an ambivalent attitude toward sex. She is critical of friends who "suppress the expression of their love," suggesting that she herself would not be so restrained, but she also worries that her own actions are not those of a "respectable woman."[62] She defiantly proclaims her passionate desires, yet does not feel free to indulge them. Her sexual desires and her tuberculosis function analogously and in tandem—both are powerfully destructive forces, deeply subversive of physical and mental well-being, and both may result in either annihilation or liberation.[63] Sophie and Marguerite use their illness as an excuse when attempting to dismiss a man who has come to call. In this way, the culture of illness found in Dumas is apparent in Ding Ling, as a way of giving young women power, control, and agency.

Perhaps most interestingly, we never learn how Sophie contracted TB. She speaks as though it has been with her a long time, perhaps since birth, and it appears to be manifested through her repressed passion, her anger, and her melancholia. She is, in other words, a modern woman with an old disease. At the same time, however, her illness helps make her that which can *chuanran*—that which can circulate and stain. She can be the infectious element that is passed between people, infecting them: "Jianru got sick because of me. I think that's great. I'd never refuse the lovely news that somebody had gotten sick on account of me."[64]

Tuberculosis in the modern era tends to be depicted as an affliction one *has*, not a disease one *gets*. But perhaps as a way of highlighting that it is only certain types of people and characters (creative types and lovers) who suffer it, having TB in Chinese fiction generally suggests the manner in which it was contracted. Like the terms *chuan* (transmit), *ran* (dye), and *zhan* (stain), consumptive disorders like *lao* were often categorized in medical texts as "pouring [*zhu*] illnesses."[65] In the Sui and Tang periods, some *zhu* disorders were called *guizhu* ("ghost pouring" or "demon influx"), or *shizhu* ("corpse pouring out"), and these were classed as disorders of the lungs *lao* or *laozhai*. In turn, many modern scholars often translate them as, or affiliate them with, tuberculosis. *Zhu* disorders are caused by pollution, incited by death or demons. Some contend that a person could be contaminated by proximity to death or demons; others give the patient more agency and responsibility for *zhu* illness that inevitably resulted from disturbing the world of demonic forces.[66] Sophie's fear of ghosts, her ambivalent stance toward the past, her (actual or perceived) sexual and moral transgressions, and her inauspicious, careless existence suggest that her consumption is not only reflective of her personality but punishment for it.

Even with its modern name, tuberculosis still has many traditional associations in "Miss Sophie's Diary." Sophie does not seem
to have so much contracted tuberculosis so much as it has always
been part of her, like her temper or her arrogance; the story emphasizes not how she got tuberculosis but rather how she exacerbates it
through repressed or unexpressed passion. Sophie is the kind of person who *has* TB and who wears the disease like an ornament. This
mode of "transmission"—the predisposition to tuberculosis—seems
innate, or inherited: "Perhaps I was born a hardhearted woman, and
for this I fully deserve my share of sorrow and distress."[67] Although
tuberculosis has often been portrayed as a disease of lovers who perhaps contract it through intimate contact, it is just as often depicted
as the result of a passionate mind struggling to liberate itself from
traditional cultural and social structures. The modern representation of tuberculosis in China has as much to do with national concerns and patriotic striving as with amorous dispositions. Sophie
represents the culmination of decades of metaphorical discourse
that has associated the modern with sexuality, passion, and the city.
She is also an example of a new kind of tubercular, who explicitly
works against traditional social expectations. And yet, she is also
an archetypical consumptive. She is a virtual orphan, and her individuality, solitude, and repressed passion—which all contribute to
her illness—are a result of her having been being separated from
her family. This is the common image of the tubercular patient in
modern Chinese fiction—one who leaves her parents but who has
figuratively inherited the disease from them. The multiple origins
of Sophie's lung disease are seemingly reflected in the varied newspaper items she reads in her first diary entry: disputes over family
inheritance, romantic films, and tonics for venereal disease.

Sophie is archetypal in that she is a culmination of the aspects of
the tubercular patient in premodern Chinese literature, particularly
vis-à-vis her status as a woman. But many of her traits find expression in other fictional TB patients. A brief survey of these patients
includes Wang Wenxuan in Ba Jin's *Cold Nights* (Hanye, 1947) and
Ba Jin's other tubercular characters in *Ward Four* (Disi bingshi,
1946) and *Family* (Jia, 1933), marked by melancholy and alienation;
Lu Xun's Little Shuan in "Medicine" (Yao, 1919), the victim of a
backward nation; Lu Ling's Chunzu from *The Rich Man's Children*
(Caizhu de ernümen, 1948), repeatedly betrayed by patriotic causes;
Qin Shou'ou's Qiu Haitang in *Begonia* (Qiu Haitang, 1941), betrayed

by patriotic causes as well; Su Qing's character in her *Ten Years of Marriage* (Jiehun shinian, 1944), who, like Sophie, experiences tuberculosis as a side effect of freedom from an arranged marriage and traditional life; a young woman who is the arranged wife rejected for a modern woman in Feng Shulan's "A Virtuous Woman" (Zhenfu, 1926); the narrator in Yu Dafu's "Shining Paper Money" (Zhibi de tiaoyue, 1930), who has an ambivalent attitude toward his rural family and their traditional values; and Yu's ailing and nostalgic writer in *Blue Smoke* (Qingyan, 1923) "both western Imperialism and the failings of an atrophied and feeble Chinese society, hobbled in tradition and lethargy."[68] Tuberculosis in Chinese literature has always been a symptom of a deeper malaise, usually functioning as a metaphor for a continually thwarted sensitive mind, a benighted populace, or an enfeebled nation.[69]

Sophie, in some ways, is a lens through which to understand tuberculosis in cultural elites. Many authors of fiction, such as Lu Xun, Zhang Tianyi, Jiang Guangci, Xiao Hong, and Yu Dafu, were suffering from tuberculosis in the 1920s and 30s. These writers fit popular conceptions of literati (*wenren*) as being both refined and shameless. Successful authors of the 1920s, in the (sarcastic) words of Zhang Kebiao, had to "like modern, fashionable clothes, have gourmet tastes, indispensable habits of drinking and smoking, peripatetic residences, gamble and patronize brothels, have debts, an illness (especially tuberculosis or syphilis), and the ability to chat and meditate."[70] Readers felt authors' lives were romantic, and that *wenren* should recount their amorous liaisons, but these tubercular authors were generally not just romantic about romance (with the notable exception of Lin Shu)—they were romantic about modernity, and struggling against tradition. Nor did these authors contract tuberculosis in the old way. Many premodern and early modern cases of TB, both in fiction and in medical literature, suggest that it is pining—passion without action—that results in illness. This is the kind of consumption (*xulao*, "depletion exhaustion" or "depletion wasting") that burns from the inside and consumes the patient as a fire consumes fuel. Premodern consumption is a wasting disease, in which the sufferer does not waste himself, does not throw himself away, but is consumed.[71] Modern authors' tuberculosis, by contrast, signified the sort of refinement that used to be respected but by this time was seen as increasingly decadent and backward.[72]

TRANSMITTED CORPSES

Rarely are we told explicitly in modern literature how characters or authors contracted tuberculosis.[73] Mostly we are shown how they live and die with it, and what the symptoms signify. Sophie and the Marguerites have it congenitally, inherited from their parents either as a predisposition to passion or as a tainted inheritance. They suffer from the kind of TB that recalls depletion taxation (*xulao*), a burning caused by longing and confinement, suppressed and unexpressed passion—a form of the illness that evokes important and old literary uses while pretending to be imported from the West.

But modern fiction also invokes another aspect of TB as a contagious condition—namely that of "corpse-transmitted consumption" (*chuanshi lao*). Corpse-transmitted wasting is an ancient belief that dead things can emit "worms" (*chong*) that can infect the nearby living and make them sick.[74] If elite medicine increasingly represented the etiology of depletion disorders as essentially internal issues of emotion and thought, vernacular medical tradition and religious texts consistently represented them as having distinct exogenous origins.[75] Manuscripts discovered at the Mawangdui archaeological site make clear that elite medicine before the second century BCE held that bugs and demons played a decisive role in the generation of disease.[76] The medicine of systematic correspondences, codified in the *Yellow Emperor's Inner Classic* and the basis of the vast majority of medical texts for the next two millennia, simply ignored bugs and worms as pathological agents, and it was not until the late nineteenth and early twentieth centuries that tiny living things also termed "bugs" (*chong*) were once again acknowledged as disease agents, this time under the auspices of germ theory. But vernacular medicine, and the literature of pharmacology and recipe books, consistently transmitted concepts of bug pathology. Writings on exorcism (*jiezhu wen*) related to talismans and texts placed in tombs ward off evil discuss pouring (*zhu*) disorders within the framework of the "world of demonic forces" (*sha*) of religious Daoism and the Yinyang masters.[77] One of these texts, the "Middle Book of the Most High Three Corpses" (Sanshi zhongjing, late Tang) states,

> In the abdomen of every person dwell three corpse demons and nine worms which can cause great harm. They ascend to heaven on the *gengshen* day to make a report to the Celestial Thearch [Tiandi]. They record and report their host's culpability in detail, cutting short his "life-register" [*shengji*], reducing his allotment of prosperity, and causing his untimely death [accordingly]. After the host dies, the *hun* soul ascends to heaven, and the *po* soul descends to the earth, while

(a)   (b)

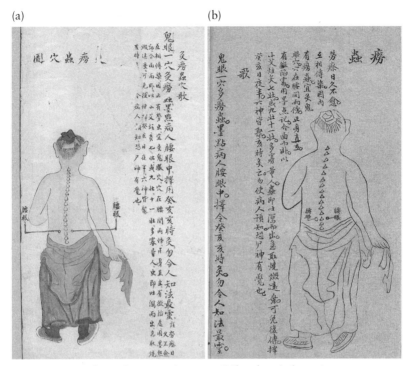

Figures 6.1a, 6.1b. "Consumption worm" (*laochong*) charts in two acumoxa manuscripts: (a) "The lumbar eyes (*yaoyan*) point, also known as ghost eyes (*guiyan*), is located on either side of the lumbar midline, in the two depressions that can be seen in the small of the back when the patient is standing upright. Moxibustion with small moxa cones at the lumbar eyes point can be used to treat lingering consumptive diseases (*laozhai*)"; from *Record of Sovereign Teachings* (Chuanwu lingji lu). (b) A description of treatment of consumptive worm disease (*laochongbing*) or lung worm disease (*feichongbing*), noting that such illnesses belong to the dual category of lung disease / tuberculosis (*feibing*) and worm disease (*chongbing*); *Master Zou's Acupuncture and Moxibustion* (Zou shi zhenjiu). Wellcome Library, London.

the Three Corpse Demons wander around and are known as ghosts [*gui*]. These ghosts expect sacrifices during the four seasons and eight festivals. If the sacrifices are not rich enough, they will cause disasters, produce various illnesses, and damage human lives.[78]

These corpse demons and corpse worms are agents of retribution. Even if they, like other bugs, disappeared from the discourse of elite medicine, the depletion diseases discussed in vernacular medical texts, fiction, and encyclopedias recalled them.[79]

The retribution implied by depletion disorders caused by bugs or worms also evoked death pollution. Chao Yuanfang (fl. 605–16) describes four of these related conditions in his *Treatise on the Origins and Symptoms of Diseases* (Zhubing yuanhou lun, 1378),

> When a person's age-fate [*nianming*] is weak and he attends a funeral, his mind suddenly experiences fear of the inauspicious [*wei'e*]. The corpse worms [*shichong*] in his body, who by their nature dislike the inauspicious, are subjected to a malign influence and provoke a chronic illness. . . . Whenever he enters a place of mourning, the disorder always breaks out. Consequently, it is called mourning corpse [*sangshi*]. . . . When a person comes into contact with or approaches a corpse, the corpse qi enters his abdomen; together with the corpse worms within his body, it causes a disorder. . . . Consequently, it is called corpse qi [*shiqi*]. . . . Whenever a person dies of a *zhu* disorder [*bingzhu*], whoever comes to his house contracts the disorder [*ranbing*] and may himself pass away. That person may then pass along [the illness] to others. This is therefore called death pouring [*sizhu*]. . . . When a person approaches a corpse, if his body is depleted [*xu*] he will receive the corpse's qi. It will dwell in his connecting vessels and bowels. . . . Therefore the disorder is called mourning infection [*sangzhu*].[80]

Although Dr. Ren's diagnosis of Li Ping'er in chapter 54 of *Plum in the Golden Vase* repeatedly makes it explicit that her disease is *not* of exogenous origin, once she dies, she is extremely contagious, dangerous, and polluting. Ximen Qing is told by the Daoist Master Pan to stay out of the sickroom while Ping'er is dying, lest he bring catastrophe upon himself, and another of his wives says to him, "Have you no compunction about crying that way face to face with a corpse? You run the risk of being contaminated by the evil qi from her mouth."[81] It is also due to the contaminating power of corpses that Lady Wang orders to have Skybright's body taken immediately to the cremation site in *Story of the Stone*. She says, "The girl died of consumption [*nüzi lao si*], you mustn't keep the body in the house, whatever you do."[82] Skybright was the young, beautiful maid that novel commentators believed to be a "shadow" of Lin Daiyu, both of whom are labeled by the novel as "meager-fated" (*boming*). Despite the fact that those invariably beautiful, unmarried young women are meager-fated because of karmic retribution for some past sin, they are paradoxically figures of sympathy, since there is nothing they can do in this life to escape their plight. The *Arcane Essential Prescriptions from the Imperial Library* (Waitai miyao, 752) of Wang Dao shows

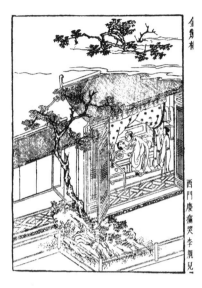

Figure 6.2. Ximen Qing weeps face to face with Li Ping'er's corpse in the novel *Plum in the Golden Vase*. From Xiaoxiaosheng, *Jinping mei cihua*.

that *chuanshi* was the same as "bone steaming," and also known as "innocence" (*wugu*).[83] Hong Mai called the disease "generational disease corpse transmission" (*shibing chuanshi*), making it clear that consumption was a generational disease, inherited from the family.[84]

Beginning in the final years of the Later Han, the concept of inherited culpability (*chengfu*) starts to show up in religious Daoist writings, such as *The Scripture on Great Peace* (Taiping jing, Late Han dynasty).[85] This notion suggests that disorders that pour (*zhu*) are essentially the result of the wrongdoings of ancestors transformed into a force that brings misfortune upon the descendants. *The Scripture on Great Peace* maintains that when ancestors are not able to exculpate or redeem themselves within their lifetime, their descendants will repay all debts.[86] In this sense *chengfu* is a sharing of fate, a transmission of burdens. Certain "crimes may have been committed by only a few persons in earlier times, but the consequences involve later generations of the offender's families and neighborhoods."[87] Vengeful demons, corpse worms, and corpse qi threaten the family of the deceased, and also those who live in the same area.[88] As a result, with regard to *zhu* disorders, the concept of *chengfu* illuminates the premodern Chinese conception of *chuanran*, which is often closer to the terms "to transfer" or "to transmit" than "to contract" or "to infect." A well-known passage from the Daoist canon *Master*

Red-Pine's Almanac of Petitions (Chisongzi zhangli) from the Six
Dynasties period states that when "a certain deceased has done misdeeds, causing uninterrupted disorders, there is no end to death; and
there is no end to transmission of disease [*ranbing*] until the entire
family is subdued by terror. . . . The living belong to Heaven, the dead
the underworld; life and death follow different roads. Do not disturb
anybody!"[89] The sin of the deceased is hereditary. This culpability
cannot be abolished; it can only be redirected: "Other inauspicious
calamities are diverted and implanted into the passersby."[90] Thus,
from meager fate, from relation to wrongdoers, or simply by living
next to them or having bad luck, *zhu* is able to find a way in.

The etiological narrative of corpse-transmitted consumption
involved worms or bugs moving out of a corpse and into a new, living body. As the result of presumed serial infections by these worms,
several members of one family often suffered and eventually died
from the same wasting disease.[91] The *Great Mirror of the Medical
Lineage*, in recording a prescription for transmitted corpse, records,
"If the patient has *laozhai* for many days, it can give rise to evil
worms (*e'chong*), which, once the body dies, are transmitted [*chuanran*] by chance to those nearby, even to the point where it wipes out
an entire family [*miemen*], and it is called 'transmitted corpse consumption' [*chuanshi lao*]."[92] Gong Tingxian writes, "When there are
worms within the internal organs eating into the heart and lungs,
it is called consumption [*zhai*]. In this case it is 'transmitted corpse
bone-infesting consumption' [*chuanshi zhugu lao*]. Working their
way from top to bottom, [the worms] pass from the bones to the
flesh, and there are even some that destroy whole households."[93] A
robust understanding of consumption, like the examples presented
in premodern novels, uses symptoms to describe personality (depletion from overexertion, burning from an inner passion) and also
etiologies to hint at karmic burdens and outcomes (inherited culpability, bugs, worms, and demons).

These wasting worms behaved differently from modern germs.
Only after the patient died were the worms thought to move out of
the corpse, hence "transmitted corpse" or perhaps "corpse-transmitted" consumption. These worms did not attack people simply
because of proximity or touch (unlike many demons or ghosts). They
attacked family members specifically, and the basis of the worms'
transmission was the idea of shared guilt or collective responsibility for the entire lineage. Since the act of transmission by worms

took place only after the original host had passed away, this process resembles the inheritance of property, or debt, from deceased family members. In other words, people were aware of the communicability of consumption among family members, but they attributed this phenomenon to lineage membership. This was not transmission by contact; it was a hereditary stain, a literal "pouring out" (*ran*) of immoral disease from the dead parent into the living child. It was a depraved inheritance.

During the antituberculosis movement of the 1930s, some medical authorities used the term "corpse transmission" (*chuanshi*), though modern doctors generally tried to avoid using traditional medical terms for fear of confusing patients.[94] Apparently the medical authorities felt that because traditional habits were responsible for the great incidence of tuberculosis, traditional terminology had to be used to combat those habits. For Ge Chenghui, a graduate of Yale medical school, the combination of family habits such as sharing meals, sharing the bed, and, in particular, sleeping with the windows closed due to a traditional fear of wind as a cause of illness provided the tuberculosis bacillus with a perfect opportunity to spread within the self-contained space of the extended family, closed off to the outside world. Thus Ge wrote in 1935, "If one member of the family is infected, soon enough half the family succumbs. Hence the name 'corpse-transmitted consumption' was given to tuberculosis in the past.[95] Ge was likely trying to employ traditional medical terminology to enhance the possibility of acceptance of the notion that the family—a group of people living in close proximity, sharing indoor space, food, and air—was the source of contagion. Yet in employing the traditional notion of corpse transmission, Ge invites the conflation of modern notions of contagion with traditional conceptions of disease transmitted though heredity and a shared guilt, and thus shared punishment for the transgressions of the entire lineage.[96]

This concern with heredity transmission—of the pouring of disease out of the past and into the present—raised concerns about race and eugenics, which was expanded upon in discussions of venereal disease and plague in literature. The May Fourth movement and subsequent developments killed traditional Chinese culture, but its corpse continued to transmit disease and infect those who were guilty of sustaining its links to the modern world, and of sharing this tainted heredity. For many tubercular authors and characters, the lesson of their illness was that the past is dead, but not inert.

TREATING TUBERCULOSIS

Tuberculosis is, of course, a very real disease, and from the 1920s to the 1940s was the leading cause of death in China.[97] In the 1920s, more than 850,000 people died of TB each year, most of them between the ages of twenty and thirty-five.[98] In the 1930s, 1.2 million people died of TB in China every year. The degree of incidence among the Chinese was thought to be significantly higher than among Westerners (though the data is not reliable). Many Chinese and Western doctors believed that ethnic Chinese at home and abroad were contracting and dying from TB at epidemic rates, and tuberculosis quickly came to be viewed as a particularly Chinese problem.[99] An early Republican manuscript titled "Taxation Disease, Consumption" (Laobing laozhai) includes thirty-six recipes, most of which are for treating *laozhai* and lung disorders; another late Qing manuscript devoted to *laozhai* includes twenty-three recipes for consumption and includes a poem on "blood loss consumption" (*shixue lao*).[100] In 1929, a health manual written in simple Chinese noted in its section on tuberculosis that "people say that nine out of ten people have consumption [*lao*]; truly, too many Chinese are dying of tuberculosis! [*fei laobing*]."[101]

A few medical studies found TB rates to be higher among wealthy patients than the poor, higher among hospital patients in private rooms than those in wards, and much higher among professionals than among laborers.[102] It was suggested that this was because these wealthier patients spent too much time indoors, or because they had enough money to live out traditional ideals such as the large, multigenerational family, or because their morbid sensibility or delicate constitution that made them more susceptible to tuberculosis.[103] However, studies that found incidence of tuberculosis to be particularly frequent among the wealthy and refined relied on statistics that were gathered in hospitals, and neglected the many who did not seek treatment, or who were not admitted.[104] The repurposing of the traditional category of literati in the modern period as being both elite and subversive, even debauched and outcast at times, seemed to be reflected in data showing the decadent rich suffering more from tuberculosis than the uneducated masses, and at other times, provided (culturally) powerful but (financially) poor authors of fiction the impetus to find or create a new illness by which to identify themselves.

Many health experts involved with the antituberculosis campaigns in China entertained the idea that crucial differences existed between tuberculosis in China and in the West.[105] The China Medical Commission of the Rockefeller Foundation reported in 1914, "The most destructive and wide-spread diseases of China at present are tuberculosis, hookworm and syphilis."[106] Unlike the typical Western tubercular patient, who was seen as either a target of romantic agony or a poor victim of the ills of industrial society, for instance, the typical Chinese was often someone still capable of enjoying a traditional lifestyle, and who embodied Chinese aesthetics.[107] The foregrounding of rich patients and their lifestyles had the effect of rejecting social class as the major characteristic of Chinese tuberculosis patients.[108] There were cultural moments in the early modern period that seem to indicate acceptance of Western metaphors, for instance, in *The Bureaucrats* (Guanchang xianxing ji, published serially in 1901–6), compared to the Western soldiers, the Chinese soldiers are all slovenly, poorly outfitted, have bad posture, and are suffering from tuberculosis or opium addiction. "Those with TB didn't care at all about contagion, spitting wherever they pleased, and the opium addicts all wiped tears from their eyes."[109] But we might understand this not to be agreement that tuberculosis occurs more commonly in the poor but rather that it occurs more commonly in the Chinese, particularly as identified by the unhygienic act of spitting.[110]

The foregrounding of rich patients and their literati-inflected lifestyles suggests a rejection of the European concept of tuberculosis as a social problem of modern industrialization and emphasizes tuberculosis in China as a problem of family and culture.[111] In early twentieth-century China, meanwhile, tuberculosis afflicted not only city dwellers but also people living in the countryside. The most popular way of explaining how tuberculosis had spread to the countryside was to blame local practices, particularly the daily habits and rituals of traditional family life. Foreign doctors believed Chinese families were unusually intimate and typically blamed the traditional ideal of several generations living under one roof for the spread of the disease.[112]

Even when tuberculosis was presented in Chinese literature as a paradigmatic modern, Western disease, it was still tied to China's past. It was commonly depicted as a hereditary disease, one of lineage transmission—a congenital disease brought on not by karma but by the sins of the parents and of their parents. Although this particular depiction of TB in literature waned in the 1920s and 1930s, a strikingly similar representation began to be disseminated by medical authorities and the antituberculosis movement, suggesting that the most important way to combat the disease was at the level of the family, instead of with public measures.[113] That the family—the most fundamental unit of traditional culture—was to blame made tuberculosis a marker of tradition and not a marker of modernity, as it was in Europe. As a metaphor, therefore, tuberculosis in China symbolized not the pathological cost of modernity but rather the weight of traditional habits and family structures, which prevented China from entering the modern, individualistic world.

Modern science supported the metaphors that grew up around tuberculosis. A traditional fear of wind supported the family vector theory of contagion.[114] Vitiated air marks the modern, Western tuberculosis patient, suffering in small, dark spaces that stink. In the West, there was a modern desire to open the windows, to have better air, to bring the outdoors in. Sophie has this desire too; she talks about her cramped, dingy living conditions, and as her diary progresses from winter (December 24) to spring (March 28), she increasingly looks forward to the weather warming up so that she might go to the western hills, or south. Seeking better air but at the same time being afraid of its power as a vector of contagion serves as a model for cultural reformers' challenges in bringing bacteriology to China.

The concept of the modern tubercular as someone suffering from traditional culture seems to oppose the representation of the disease by May fourth writers as one of iconoclastic modernity. It calls into question the fact of May Fourth writers' own tuberculosis and undermines their project and the significance of their sacrifices. Under the microscope of Western medicine, the bodies of writers such as Lu Xun are infected with hereditary diseases that eat or burns them from within while political conflict and the wages of modernity directly inscribe their bodies with pain. Modern authors in China are betrayed by modern learning; they are diagnosed as sick by the very scientific thinking they thought would cure China. They secretly know that they are guilty of causing their own infection because of a passionate attachment to old metaphors, or because of a shared responsibility for what they have inherited. Lu Xun describes the backwardness and corruption of traditional medicine and medical practitioners in what essentially amounts to an inherited malady model of modern Chinese medical historiography.[115] Tuberculosis as a family disease, contracted through heredity, shared guilt in a lineage, or traditional

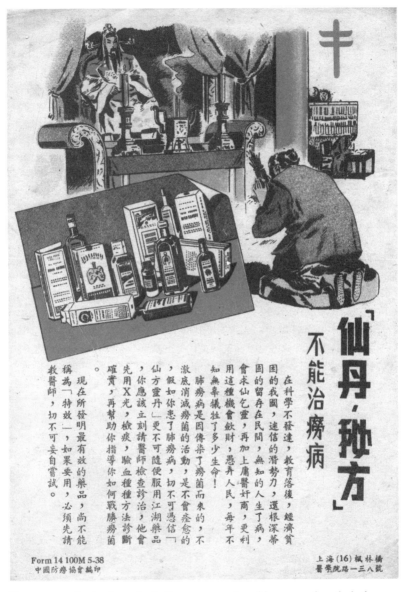

Figure 6.3   Anti-tuberculosis flyer, 1940s. An old woman kneels before an altar and prays for health, with a poster inset that advertises traditional nostrums and quack remedies, while at the same time referring to TB as *lao-bing*. National Anti-Tuberculosis Association of China, Shanghai. Collection of the National Library of Medicine, National Institute of Health, Bethesda, MD.

cultural practice, suggests that the project of Western medicine in China is not only futile but also irrelevant.

Institutional medicine and cultural reformers both identified Chinese tradition as the source of tuberculosis and acknowledged its contagiousness and its multiple modes of infecting, pouring into, and staining Chinese moderns. These various sources of medical knowledge, alike in their attitude toward tubercular contagion, contributed to a sense that the condition of modern Chinese subjectivity was a pathological one, but also a shared one. Chinese moderns viewed themselves as white cloth, *predisposed* to dyeing, and ultimately bearing a pathological stain. They had inherited constitutional susceptibility to disease that made them vulnerable and exposed to this infectious pouring from the environment, from the family and from the past.

Zhou Zuoren blames fiction for the continued belief in premodern medical notions despite the flourishing of new medical literature based on Western science, such as the *Dictionary of Chinese Pharmacology*, newly published in 1937. He writes, "The reason why present-day Chinese pharmacologists disavow germ theory and put their trust in a novelist who lived more than a century ago is none other than that they are captivated by the marvelous nature of his explanations."[116] Zhou goes on to lament the continued influence of premodern thought: "Over the generality [of writings] which delight in the bizarre and tell of retribution I can only sigh. I sense they are of no small consequence, but have no antidote to prescribe."[117] As modern consumptives inherited their diseases from the past, from Chinese tradition itself, such traditional medical notions were being kept alive in the scientific age by readers' attachment to premodern fiction.

ai er bu shang le er bu yin 哀而
  不傷樂而不淫
aiye 艾葉
an 暗
aza zheng 醃臢症

Badou Dahuang 巴豆大黃
Bai Shiying 白石英
baibiandou 白扁豆
baibing zhuzhi yao 百病主治藥
baicao shuang 百草霜
baidingxiang 白丁香
baihuashe 白花蛇
bangzi qiang 梆子腔
bao 報
baojuan 寶卷
baomen 飽悶
Baopu zi 抱樸子
baoying 報應
baoying chuang 報應瘡
Beijing chuanlai 北京傳來
bencao 本草
Bencao beiyao 本草備要
Bencao bieshuo 本草別說
Bencao chunqiu 本草春秋
Bencao gangmu shiyi 本草綱目
  拾遺
Bencao ji 本草記

Bencao jiyao 本草妓要
bian 便
Bian du 便毒
Bian du deng zheng 便毒等証
bianwen 變文
bianyi 辨疑
bie 鱉
biji 筆記
bingzhu 病注
bixie 辟邪
bixie meiwu e 辟邪魅忤惡
boming 薄命
busicao 不死草
buyang 補養

cai 財
caibu zhi zhan 採補之戰
Caizhu de ernümen 財主的兒女
  們
cansha 蠶沙
Caomu chunqiu lingyi zhudiao
  草木春秋 鈴醫諸調
Caomu zhuan 草木傳
caowu 草烏
caoze yi 草澤醫
chang sixiang 長思想
changchuan chuanlai 娼船傳來
Changsheng dian 長生殿

Chao Yuanfang 巢元方
chen 臣
Chen Cheng 陳承
Chen Qi 陳綺
Chen Qirong 陳起榮
Chen Tong 陳同
Cheng An 誠庵
chengfu 承負
chijiao daxian yubiao zhongzi
    wanfang 赤腳大仙魚鏢種子
    丸方
chinüzi 癡女子
chiren shuomeng 癡人說夢
Chishui xuanzhu 赤水玄珠
Chisongzi zhangli 赤松子章曆
chixiaodou 赤小豆
chong 蟲
Chongxiu zhiyao 崇修指要
chongyao 蟲咬
chongzhu 蟲疰
chouchang 丑唱
choufeng chumai 仇風出賣
Chu Renhuo 褚人獲
chu xiesui 除邪祟
chuan 傳
chuanhoupu 川厚樸
chuanqi yeshi 傳奇野史
chuanran 傳染
chuanran buyi 傳染不已
chuanshi 傳屍
chuanshi lao 傳屍癆
chuanshizhu 傳屍疰
chuanshi zhugu lao 傳屍注骨癆
Chuanya 串雅
chuanyan 傳言
chufa 初發
chunqian bing 春前病
Chunxiao mixi tu 春宵秘戲圖
chunyao 春藥
chunyi yao 春意藥

Ci Gu 慈姑
cihu 刺虎

Da Ji 大戟
da laoer wan 打老兒丸
dafeng xuanchuang 大風癬瘡
dafengzi 大風子
Dai Baoyuan 戴葆元
daixia 帶下
daiyi 待醫
damafeng 大麻風
danbai 旦白
danfang 單方
danggui 當歸
Dangkou zhi 蕩寇志
daotiejin 倒貼金
Daquan tongshu 大全通書
diaobai 吊白
diaojiaosha 吊腳痧
diding 地丁
dingchuang 疔瘡
dingxiang 丁香
Disi bingshi 第四病室
donger buxie 動而不瀉
doubaicao 鬥百草
doucao 鬥草
douchi 豆豉
Doupeng xian hua 豆棚閒話
douzhen 痘疹
Du Ji 杜稷
Du Shifu 杜世福
duanyu wan 斷欲丸
duoqing duobing 多情多病
duoqing zhen boming 多情真薄
    命

e zhi yu cheng chuang 惡指欲成
    瘡
e'chong 惡蟲
e'chuang 惡瘡

e'jiao 阿膠
e'qi 惡氣
Erke paian jingqi 二刻拍案驚奇

fabing 法病
faming 發明
Fan Bie zaofan 番鱉造反
Fan Biezi 番鱉子
fanglao tuxue 房勞吐血
fangshi 方士
fangshu 方書
fangzhongshu 房中術
fanmen 煩悶
fanzei 反賊
feijie he 肺結核
Feilong zhuan 飛龍傳
feishi 飛屍
feng 風
fenglai 風癩
fengren 風人
fengyue 風月
Fengyue baojian 風月寶鑑
fenzhongchong 糞中蟲
fu 賦
fufang 附方
fugui bing 富貴病
fuqian 膚淺
Furen daquan liangfang 婦人大
    全良方

Gan Cao 甘草
Gan Cao heguo 甘草和國
Gan Sui 甘遂
ganchuang 疳瘡
Ganfu touqin 甘府投親
ganhuo 肝火
ganran 感染
ganzheng 疳症
gewu 格物
Gong Juzhong 龔居中

Gong Xin 龔信
gong'an 公案
gongli 攻利
gu 蠱
Gua Zhi'er 掛枝兒
Guaizheng qifang 怪症奇方
Guangdong chuang 廣東瘡
Guangnan 廣南
guantong qimai 貫通氣脈
Guanyin jiuku fang 觀音救苦方
Guanyin liu 觀音柳
Guanyin puji fang 觀音普濟方
gui 鬼
guiji 鬼疾 / 鬼擊
guijiao 鬼交
guijing 鬼精
guimei 鬼魅
guiqi 鬼氣
guisui 鬼祟
guitai 鬼胎
guizhu 鬼注 / 鬼疰
gujing 古鏡
gumo wan 古墨丸
guobao 果報
guofeng 過瘋
guolai 過癩
guolao 國老
guzheng 骨蒸
guzheng zhi ji 骨蒸之疾
guzhenglao 骨蒸勞

Hai Zao 海藻
haijinsha 海金沙
hailin de 害淋的
haipiaoxiao 海螵蛸
haishi 海石
hao wanming 好丸名
heiqi 黑氣
heishen wan 黑神丸
heishu 黑書

heixianmao 黑仙茅
Heshouwu zhuan 何首烏傳
honglian 紅蓮
Honglou huanmeng 紅樓幻夢
Honglou meng tu yong 紅樓夢
    圖詠
Hongniang 紅娘
Hongniang mai yao 紅娘賣藥
hongniangzi 紅娘子
Hou Shuihu 後水滸
houpu 厚樸
hu 胡
hu feng 護封
huaji 滑稽
huaming liulü 花明柳綠
huang 黃
Huang Dan 黃丹
Huang Lian 黃連
Huang Qi 黃芪
Huang Qin 黃芩
huangbai 黃柏
huangbing 黃病
Huanhun ji 還魂記
huaxie bu jin 滑泄不禁
huimin yaoju 惠民藥局
Huizhou 徽州
Hujiao 胡椒
hun 魂
hundun 混沌
hundun bian wei wenming 混沌
    變為文明
hushen 護身
huxiang chuanran 互相傳染
huyou 護幼
huzhang 虎杖

jian 賤
Jiang Shiquan 蔣士銓
jianghu yi 江湖醫
jiao 角

jiaohun 叫魂
jiaoqi 腳氣
jiaoshu 校書
jiase shanghan 夾色傷寒
jiaxun 家訓
jie 竭
jie fanxiaoyu 解煩消鬱
Jie Shuihu zhuan 結水滸傳
Jiehun shinian 結婚十年
jiexuan 疥癬
jiezhu wen 解注文
jifabei 及發背
Jigong zhuan 濟公傳
jijie 集解
Jin Lingzi 金鈴子
Jin Shengtan 金聖歎
Jin Shihu 金石斛
Jin Yingzi 金櫻子
Jin Yinhua 金銀花
Jin yu yuan 金玉緣
jinbuhuan 金不換
Jinchai yihuo 金釵遺禍
jing 精
jing er chu 精而出
Jingbao 京報
Jinghong ji 驚鴻記
jingqi manxie 精氣滿泄
jingxu 精虛
Jingyan fang 經驗方
jingyan liangfang 經驗良方
jingzhong hanre tong 莖中寒熱
    痛
jinqiang budao 金槍不倒
jinshen 謹身
jinyao 禁藥
Jisheng bacui fang 濟生拔粹方
jiuling 酒令
jizhuakui 雞爪葵
Ju Hua 菊花
Jue Mingzi 決明子

juhong 橘紅

jun 君

kesou laozheng 咳嗽勞症

kewu 客忤

keyi shuixing keyi yubing 可以睡
　醒可以愈病

kongqing 空青

kouchuang 口瘡

kufan 枯礬

kuicai 葵菜

kuxiao shuo 苦孝說

laimai **來**脈

lanji wan 爛積丸

Lantai guifan 蘭台軌範

lao 勞 (depletion)

lao 癆 (depletion disorder)

lao sunxue zhi bing 勞損削之病

laobing 勞病

laobing gui 癆病鬼

laochong 癆蟲

laoji 勞祭

laoqie zhi zheng 勞怯之症

laozhai 勞瘵 / 癆瘵

laozhai huanzhe zhi huishengshu
　癆瘵患者之回生術

laozheng 勞瘵

leishu 類書

li 俚

Li Guochang 李國昌

Li Lou 李樓

Li Ruding 李如鼎

Li Shangyin 李商隱

Li Ting 李廷

Li Zhuowu 李卓吾

lian 楝

liancai 憐才

Liang Qichao **梁**啟超

liangtoujian 兩頭尖

lianrui 蓮蕊

liao yuanji 療冤疾

Liaodu geng 療妒羹

liaozhu 療疰

liji 痢疾

Liming 黎明

Lin Daiyu 林黛玉

Linchuan meng 臨川夢

Lingxian pingkou 靈仙平寇

lingyi 鈴醫

Lingyuan fangquan 靈苑方泉

Linlan xiang 林蘭香

Linzheng zhinan yi'an 臨證指南
　醫案

lipu 曆譜

liqi 離奇

liqu 俚曲

lishu 曆書

liu 留 (leaves behind)

liu 溜 (dribbling)

Liu Chun 劉純

Liu Jinu 劉寄奴

Liu Yu 劉裕

liuyu qiqing 六慾七情

liyang chuanran 癘瘍傳染

longgu 龍骨

Lu Dahuang 路大荒

Lu ji 鹿記

Luo Guanzhong 羅貫中

Luohan song 羅漢松

Lüye xianzong 綠野仙蹤

Luzhen 魯珍

mafeng 麻風

Mai Mendong 麥門冬

maibing 賣病

maijue 脈訣

mailuo 脈絡

mailuo guantong 脈絡貫通

majing 馬經

Mao Xihe 毛西訶
Mao'er Xi 貓兒戲
Meichuang milu 黴瘡秘錄
meng jienei 夢接內
meng yu guijiao 夢與鬼交
mi jue bu ke qing chuan yu ren
 秘訣不可輕傳於人
Miaoyu 妙玉
Mituo seng 密(彌)陀僧
miemen 滅門
mifang 秘方
mimenghua 密蒙花
ming 明
Mingyi lun 明醫論
Minjia zachao 民家雜鈔
minjian yanfang qiu xianglin 民
 間驗方救鄉鄰
mituoseng 密陀僧
mo 墨
Mu Tong 木通
muse er wang 慕色而亡

Nan Shi 南史
Nanshan jing 南山經
naosha 硇砂
neiyi 內醫
nian huanong liulin 拈花弄柳淋
niangao qisheng jiuwu seyu 年高
 氣盛久無色欲
nianming 年命
niekong cao 躡空草
niniao qulai 溺尿去來
niuma 牛馬
nü'er lao 女兒癆
nüeji 瘧疾
Nüxian waishi 女仙外史

Pan Jinlian 潘金蓮
Pang Chunmei 龐春梅
pengsha 硼砂

pi 癖 (hobby/habit/mania)
pi 癖 (hardness/stone)
Pinhua baojian 品花寶鑑
Pinghe 平和
pipa 枇杷
Pipa ji 琵琶記
po 魄
Puji fang 普濟方

Qi Dezhi 齊德之
Qian bencao 錢本草
qiangyin yi jingsui 強陰益精髓
qianjin dan 千金丹
qianli fumai 千里伏脈
qiemai 切脈
qili san 七厘散
Qilu deng 歧路燈
Qin Shi 秦氏
qing 情
qing duo yuzhi 情多鬱滯
qingchi 情癡
qingfen 輕粉
qinghao 青蒿
qingji zhiyang 情寄之瘍
qingtian niehai 情天孽海
Qingwen 晴雯
qingzhi 情志
qinpu 芹圃
Qinpu xiansheng 芹圃先生
Qinpu Xiansheng de yide 芹圃先
 生的医德
qishang 七傷
qisiren bu changming 氣死人不
 償命
Qiu Changchun 丘长春
Qiu Haitang 秋海棠
Qiu Liyu 邱麗玉
qiukui 秋葵
qiuyi zhibing 求醫治病
qiwei 氣味

qixu 氣虛
qizheng qizhifa 奇症奇治法
quanying 全嬰
qubing 祛病

ran 染
ranbing 染病
rancheng 染成
ranyi 染易
rechuang 熱瘡
relao 熱勞
ren 仁
rendong 忍冬
rengui 人傀
renma pingan san 人馬平安散
renshen 人參
Renzhai zhi zhi 仁齋直指
renzhang 人瘴
renzhongbai 人中白
renzhonghuang 人中黃
rishu 日書
riyong leishu 日用類書
ruxiang 乳香
ruyi 儒醫
Ruyijun zhuan 如意君傳

Sang ji sheng zhuan 桑寄生傳
sangshi 喪屍
sangzhu 喪注
sanhuangsan 三黃散
sanqi 三七
sanshi bao 三世報
Sanshi zhongjing 三屍中經
se yaofang huanle 色藥方歡樂
sebing 色病
selao zhi si 色癆之死
seyu liangfang 色欲良方
sha 煞
Shan Bao 單豹
shanbao 善報

Shangbao 商報
shanghan 傷寒
Shen Fan 沈璠
Shenbao 申報
shenfang 神方
shengji 生籍
shengjin dan 勝金丹
shenmiao zhi fang 神妙之方
Shennong bencao jing 神農本草
　經
shi 士
shiba fan 十八反
Shibao 時報
shibing chuanshi 世病傳屍
shibo 世薄
shichong 屍蟲
shichuan 食傳
Shidao Gu 石道姑
Shi'er lou 十二樓
Shihu xiangyao 石斛降妖
shijia buxi liuxue 嗜痂不惜流血
shijing 失精
shijiu wei 十九畏
shijunzi 使君子
shiming 釋名
shinü 石女 (stone maiden)
shinü 實女 (solid maiden)
shiqi 屍氣
shiquan dabutang 十全大補湯
shiru 師儒
Shiwu bencao 食物本草
shixue lao 失血癆
shiyi 市醫 (city doctor)
shiyi 世醫 (generational doctor)
shizhu 屍疰 (注)
shouhun 收魂
Shu bencao 書本草
shufu 書符
Shuihu zhuan 水滸傳
shuiqin 水芹

Shuowen jiezi 說文解字
Shuoyue quanzhuan 說嶽全傳
si nanzi bu de 思男子不得
si seyu busui 思色欲不遂
sida jingang 四大金剛
sifu 思婦
Siku quanshu 四庫全書
sini tang 四逆湯
sixiang 思想
Siyan maijue 四言脈訣
songyan dan 松煙丹
suibi wenxue 隨筆文學
Suitang yanyi 隋唐演義
Sun Derun 孫德潤
Sun Yikui 孫一奎
suosha 縮砂

taichan 胎產
Taichan xinshu 胎產新書
Taiping jing 太平經
taiyi 太醫
Tan Ze 談則
tanghuo shaodang 湯火燒蕩
tian bao chuang 天報瘡
tian pao chuang 天皰瘡
Tian Xianzi 天仙子
Tiandi 天帝
tianluo 天羅
tiansigua 天絲瓜
tianwang buxin dan 天王補心丹
Tianzhu Huang 天竺黃
Tiesha Shen Luzhen xiansheng
    yi'an 鐵沙沈魯珍先生醫案
tieshan san 鐵扇散
tonglü 銅綠
tongqing 銅青
tongshen jinjie 通身筋節
tongsheng 通勝
tongshu 通書
tongyou 桐油

tongzibian 童子便
Tu Long 屠隆
tufuling 土茯苓
Tuoseng xi gu 陀僧戲姑

Waike Jingyi 外科精義
Waike xinfa yaojue 外科心法要
    訣
waishi 外史
Waitai miyao 外臺秘要
waiyi 外夷
Wang Ang 汪昂
Wang Boliang 王伯良
Wang Kentang 王肯堂
Wang Linheng 王臨亨
Wang Mengying 王孟英
Wang Ren'an 汪訒庵
Wang Shizhen 王世貞
Wang Tao 王燾
wang wei ru 枉為儒
Wang Weilu 汪為露
Wang Xiangxu 汪象旭
Wang Xifeng 王熙鳳
Wang Yongjian 王永健
wangyuesha 望月砂
Wanhua lou 萬花樓
Wanli 萬曆
wanshengjiao 萬聲嬌
Wanshou tang 萬壽堂
Wanshou xianshu 萬壽仙書
Wei Lingxian 威靈仙
wei'e 畏惡
weisheng 衛生
Weixian chuanlai 濰縣傳來
weizhan 帷站
wenbu 溫補
Woxian Caotang 臥閑草堂
wu 巫
Wu Bian 無邊
Wu Wushan 吳吳山

wuchuan 屋傳
Wudang quan 武當拳
wugu 無辜
wuhuang san 五黃散
wujia bao 無價寶
wujia baozhen wan 無價保真丸
wujia wan 無價丸
wujin san 烏金散
wujin wan 烏金丸
wujin zhi 烏金紙
wulao qishang 五勞七傷
wulingzhi 五靈脂
wushaoshe 烏梢蛇
wuxing 五行
wuyang wan 烏羊丸
wuzang xu 五臟虛

xiagan 下疳
xiaji yile yi tanjing 下己遺了一
　灘精
xiangchuan 相傳
xiangran 相染
xiangru'er 香薷兒
xiangyan 香艷
xianren zi tuoyi 仙人自脫衣
xiao chou po men 消愁破悶
Xiao Guanlan 蕭觀瀾
Xiaoqing 小青
xiaoshuo 小說
Xiaoyou 孝友
Xiaren 俠人
Xibao 錫報
xiebai 薤白
xie'e qi 邪惡氣
xieqi 邪氣
xieqi jiaogan 邪氣交感
xiesi wangdong zhi zheng 邪思妄
　動之症
xiesui 邪祟
Xihu Diaoshi 西湖釣史

Ximen Qing 西門慶
Ximen Qing tanyu de bing 西門
　慶貪慾得病
Xin Xiaoshuo 新小說
xinbing 心病
xinfu xieqi 心腹邪氣
xingming shi 星名詩
xinguang tipang 心廣體胖
xinqi xu er sheng huo 心氣虛而
　生火
Xinxinzi 欣欣子
xinxue haojin 心血耗盡
Xiong Damu 熊大木
Xiong Zongli 熊宗立
xionghuang 雄黃
xiuzhi 修制
xixin 細辛
xu 虛
Xu Chunfu 徐春甫
xu er duomeng 虛而多夢
Xu Mingyi lei'an 續名醫類案
Xu Shifan 徐士範
Xu Zeng 許增
Xuanze tongshu guang yuxia ji
　選擇通書廣玉匣記
Xue Lizhai 薛立齋
xueji 血疾
xueji dafa 血疾大發
xuemai jingluo 血脈經絡
xuexu 血虛
xuhan 虛寒
xulao 虛勞
xulao fare 虛勞發熱
xulao jingjie 虛勞精竭
xulao mengxie 虛勞夢泄
xure 虛熱
xushi 虛實
xusun 虛損

yagan 牙疳

Yan Shifan 嚴世蕃
Yan Song 嚴嵩
yanfang mifang 驗方秘方
Yang Lai'er 楊萊兒
Yang Xiuwan 楊琇頑
Yangchong yaoyin 樣蟲藥引
yangmei 楊梅
yangmei chaung 楊梅瘡
yangmei du chuang 楊梅毒瘡
yangmei feng 楊梅風
yangmei gan xie 楊梅疳瀉
yangmei jiedu 楊梅結毒
yangmei lixiao xiang 楊梅立消香
yanguo 驗過
yangsheng 養生
yanyu 讞語
Yao wang 藥王
yao yinzi 藥引子
Yaochaji 藥茶記
Yaohui tukao 藥會圖考
Yaohuitu 藥會圖
Yaohuituqupu 藥會圖曲譜
yaoming shi 藥名詩
Yaoshe chuxian 妖蛇出現
Yaowu suoyin caomu chunqiu 藥
物索隱草木春秋
yaoxing bangziqiang 藥性梆子腔
yaoxing ge 藥性歌
yaoxing xi 藥性戲
yaoying 搖影
Ye Tianshi 葉天士
yemingsha 夜明砂
yeqin 野芹
yeshi 野史
yezhang 業障
yi 醫, 毉
yi nai renshu 醫乃仁術
Yi Zhizi 益智子
yi'an 醫案
Yibuquanlu 醫部全錄

yichuan 衣傳
yige chuan yige 一個傳一個
yijing lao 遺精癆
yijing lun 遺精論
yijing mengxie 遺精夢泄
yilin 醫林
yin 淫 (sexual desire)
yin 銀 (silver)
yincang yaoming 隱藏藥名
Yinglie zhuan 英烈傳
yingongshu 陰功書
yinguo 因果
yingyan liangfang 應驗良方
yinhan 陰寒
yinqi 陰器
yinsang 淫喪
yinshui siyuan 飲水思源
yinxie zhi ren 淫邪之人
yinxu 陰虛
yinyang 陰癢
yinyang shui 陰陽水
yinyang yi 陰陽易
yinyi 淫醫
yiseng suochuan 異僧所傳
Yisheng tang 義盛堂
Yishu zachao 醫書雜抄
Yixue juyu 醫學舉隅
yiwei jishi zhi dao 以為濟世之道
yixue 醫學
yiyin 意淫
yizhi 益智
yong yi 庸醫
yongju 癰疽
Yongxi yaofu 雍熙藥府
yongxin guodu 用心過度
you shi wei zheng 有詩為證
youchou silü 憂愁思慮
Youxi bao 遊戲報
youxiao 有效
youyu 憂鬱

yu 欲
Yu Bo 虞博
Yu Chu xinzhi 虞初新志
Yu niang 俞娘
yu nanzi er bu ke de 欲男子而不
可得
yu taiguo 欲太過
Yu Wanchun 俞萬春
yu yi cheng bing 鬱抑成病
Yu Zhizi 預知子
Yuan Hongdao 袁宏道
Yuan Hua 芫花
yuanji 冤疾
yuanjia 冤家
yuannie 冤孽
yuannie zhi zheng 冤孽之症
yuanqi 元氣
yuanye 冤業
yuanye zhi zheng 冤業之症
yuanzhi 遠志
yuhuo 慾火
Yuji weiyi 玉機微義
yujiang 玉漿
yujie 鬱結
yujie buzu zhi bing 鬱結不足之
病
yujie yu zhong er busui 鬱結於中
而不遂
yukou 魚口
yunu 鬱怒
yuyi 禦醫
yuzheng 郁症

zao 燥
zao hundun er po tianhuang 鑿
混沌而破天荒
zaokai hundun 鑿開混沌
zaomen 燥悶
zhai 瘵
zhan 沾

zhang 瘴
Zhang Chao 張潮
Zhang Lu 張潞
Zhang shi 蟑史
Zhang Shushen 張書紳
Zhang Xinzhi 張新之
Zhang Zhupo 張竹坡
zhangbu 帳簿
zhangchuang 杖瘡
zhangqi 瘴氣
Zhangui zhuan 斬鬼傳
zhanran 沾染
Zhao Boyun 趙柏雲
Zhao Xuemin 趙學敏
zhaohun 招魂
Zheng En 鄭恩
zheng ren 正人
zhenbian 針砭
Zhengdao 證道
zhenguai 鎮怪
zhengjia 癥瘕
zhengwu 正誤
zhengyin haobo 徵引浩博
Zhengzhi zhunsheng 證治準繩
zhi humei fang 治狐媚方
zhi huofu 知禍福
zhi yebing fang 治噎病方
zhibing douxiao 治病都效
zhiguai 志怪
zhimu 知母
zhishang tanbing 紙上談兵
zhizhu 蜘蛛
Zhizi 栀子
Zhizi douzui 栀子鬥嘴
zhong'e 中惡
Zhongguo yaoxue dacidian 中國
藥學大詞典
Zhou Yi 周義
Zhou Zhigan 周之幹
zhongzi 種子

zhongzi fangfa 種子方法
zhu 疰 or 注
Zhu Xi 朱熹
zhuangyang dan 壯陽丹
Zhubing yuanhou lun 諸病源候
論
zhulan gen 珠蘭根
Zhulin Yeshi 株林野史
zhuqi 助趣
zhusha 朱砂
zhuti 豬蹄
zhuyi 諸夷

zhuzhi 主治
zi 子
Zi Shiying 紫石英
zidi 子弟
zisuye 紫蘇葉
Zongjilu 總記錄
zou moru huo 走魔入火
zoufang yi 走方醫
Zu Taizhi zhiguai 祖台之志怪
Zuixing shi 醉醒石
zuoshi 佐便

NOTES

INTRODUCTION

1. Lu Yitian (*jinshi* 1836), *Lenglu yihua*, 286. Wang Qiongling (*Qingdai de sida caixue xiaoshuo*, 421) cites the same story, "Prescriptions for Injuries from Scalds and Burns."

2. Lu Yitian's *Medical Discourses from Cold Hut* is still in print today.

3. For the relation between the late-Ming novel *Plum in the Golden Vase* and the daily-use encyclopedia, see Shang Wei, "Making of the Everyday World."

4. At least, the same prescription appears there. See chapter 3, this volume.

5. See, e.g., Wang Qiongling, *Qingdai de sida caixue xiaoshuo*, 365ff.

6. For more on the early modernity of this period, see Struve, *Qing Formation in World-Historical Time*; and Hay, *Sensuous Surfaces*, 13–14.

7. Widmer, "Huanduzhai," 77ff.

8. When discussing dramatic works, this study focuses on texts rather than performance history.

9. Flueckiger, *In Amma's Healing Room*, 2–4.

10. Barnes and Hinrichs, *Chinese Medicine and Healing*, 1.

11. Unschuld and Zheng, *Chinese Traditional Healing*, 73.

12. See Xu Zeng, quoted in Unschuld and Zheng, *Chinese Traditional Healing* (which catalogues the manuscripts in the Berlin collection and gives a description of each), 78. See also Zhao Xuemin, "Fanli" (Statement of general principles), in *Chuanya quanshu*, 7. Some of the Berlin manuscripts show that itinerant healers could display a great deal of familiarity with medical theory (Unschuld and Zheng, *Chinese Traditional Healing*, 88).

13. The 1593 text is *juan* 4 of Wang Wenmo's *Scattered Gold Recipes to Help Mankind* (Jishi suijin fang), titled "Extraordinary recipes of all sorts based on secretly transmitted skills of immortals" (Michuan shenxian qiaoshu gese qifang).

14. Zhao Xuemin, "Fanli," in *Chuanya quanshu*, 7.

15. See Unschuld and Zheng, *Chinese Traditional Healing*, 77–106.

16. "Book on Selling Plasters" (Mai gaoyao shu), SBB Slg. Unschuld 8011. I refer to the Berlin manuscripts by title (if there is one) and shelf number, since most do not have an identifiable author, compiler, or copyist.

17. See Sima Qian's biography of Bian Que. Sima Qian, *Shiji*, 2793 (Mair, *Hawai'i Reader*, 177).

18. See chapter 1, this volume; and Leung, "Yuan and Ming Periods," 129–60. The Qing did have an imperial academy of medicine, but it trained doctors who would be employed in the palace.

19. Chao, "Ideal Physician." Hymes, "Not Quite Gentlemen?," 51ff.

20. On the emergence of *ruyi* between the Song and Yuan periods, and on their distinctive styles of praxis, see Hymes, "Not Quite Gentlemen?"; Scheid, *Currents of Tradition*; Chen Yuanpeng, "Liang Song de 'shang yi shiren'"; Leung, "Medical Learning"; Furth, "Producing Medical Knowledge" and "Physician as Philosopher"; and Chu Pingyi, "Song, Ming zhi ji de yishi yu ruyi."

21. See Hinrichs, "Pragmatism."

22. Hymes's term; see his "Not Quite Gentlemen?."

23. Wu Qian et al., *Yizong jinjian*, preface, 16. I follow Yi-Li Wu, *Reproducing Women*, 41.

24. Wu Yi-Li, *Reproducing Women*, 55. Many scholars have argued convincingly that medicine was becoming increasingly professionalized in the Ming and Qing. In these periods, it was not sociolegal institutions but expert practice and cultural norms that defined professional identity. See Unschuld, *Medical Ethics*; Chao, "Ideal Physician"; Furth, "Producing Medical Knowledge"; and Hsiung, "Facts in the Tale."

25. *Flowers in the Mirror* was known to contain "simple prescriptions" (*danfang*) for easy dissemination, and Lu Yitian refers to the okra salve as such. Even though women were excluded from the elite medical training that relied on transmission from master to disciple, they sometimes received training as doctors within clans or lineages so that they could care for young or female family members. Some were even summoned to the palace to treat female members of the imperial household. By the late Ming, highly educated women doctors from elite families began authoring medical writings in the learned tradition (Cass, *Dangerous Women*, 52–57; Furth, *Flourishing Yin*, 285–98; Leung, *Leprosy*, 126–27).

26. Elite status was also claimed by doctors who situated themselves within a lineage of medical practitioners.

27. For a detailed discussion of these schools, see Hanson, *Speaking of Epidemics*; and Scheid, *Currents of Tradition*.

28. Many "vernacular" medical texts (and fictional ones, too) were composed in a simple classical Chinese that would have been equally as accessible to the marginally literate as a complicated vernacular.

29. Unschuld, *History of Ideas*, 7, 50; Strickmann, *Chinese Magical Medicine*, 1–58.

30. In some cases, "figurative logic" might be a better descriptor of the nature of a correspondence but is subsumed by the more general category "literary logic."

31. These hand-copied medical manuscripts, in a collection at in the Berlin State Library (Staatsbibliothek zu Berlin), have been catalogued by Paul Unschuld and Zheng Jinsheng in *Chinese Traditional Healing*. Their book

summarizes the contents of each manuscript. The manuscripts themselves have not been published, although at the time of this writing most of the manuscripts in the collection have been made available on the library's website at http://digital.staatsbibliothek-berlin.de/ (accessed May 27, 2015).

1. BEGINNING TO READ

1. Furth, *Flourishing Yin*, 23.

2. E.g., ibid.

3. The line between elite and vernacular medicine was not always clear or even static. These are only the causes listed by *Systematic Materia Medica*, 3.51, 51.25 (in citations of this text, the first number refers to the *juan*, and the second to the entry within that *juan*).

4. Unschuld and Tessenow, *Huang Di nei jing su wen*, 180–83.

5. Unschuld and Zheng, *Chinese Traditional Healing*, 10.

6. E.g., the *Systematic Materia Medica* cites poetry over 300 times.

7. E.g., the *Systematic Materia Medica* entry on *danggui*, 14.01.

8. E.g., *zhanghui xiaoshuo* was used for traditional novels, to indicate their particular chapter structure, and *changpian xiaoshuo* for the modern novel, to indicate its comparative length.

9. Some of this poetry is "mimetic" (composed, written, recited, or read by characters in the narrative, as opposed to being quoted by the narrator). Also, some of the poetry is doggerel.

10. "Poetry" here also includes parallel prose, the set-piece descriptions of which were often attacked by commentators.

11. See Plaks, *Four Masterworks*, chapter 6.

12. There are many kinds of Chinese novel, including what Wilt Idema calls "chapbooks," which, based on their simple language (often simple classical Chinese), were likely for the moderately literate. Their literary value (and how clearly to draw a distinction between chapbook and novel) is a matter of scholarly debate, but their popularity, as judged by sheer number published, is not.

13. An example of the "anonymous author" issue is the veritable slew of novels attributed to Luo Guanzhong (ca. 1330–ca. 1400), the putative author of *The Three Kingdoms* (Sanguo zhi yanyi, 1522). This attribution problem speaks to the demand for authors on the part of readers. Commentary editions went out of their way to present authorial figures for their novels, such as Jin Shengtan attributing *Outlaws of the Marsh* (aka *The Water Margin* [Shuihu zhuan]) to Shi Nai'an and the Wang Xiangxu commentary edition attributing *Journey to the West* (Xiyou ji) to Qiu Changchun. Some commentators created a nameless figure for the author, as did Zhang Zhupo for *Plum in the Golden Vase* (aka *The Golden Lotus* [Jinping mei]). Of the six "great novels," however, none was published under a pseudonym. The closest is *Plum in the Golden Vase*, whose Xinxinzi ("Master of Delights") preface claimed the author was "the Scoffing Scholar."

14. Meir Shahar argues that vernacular novels became a major vehicle through which knowledge of the Daoist and Buddhist pantheons and local

cults were propagated. See Shahar, "Vernacular Fiction," 184–211. Precious scrolls (baojuan), long narrative texts of Buddhist content divided into chapters and written in prose and ci verse, were another vehicle for such transmission, since many were written precisely to propagate a particular sect.

15. The entire idea of defining "literati" to describe the shi involves a circular rhetoric. The term "literati" was originally used by Robert Burton in his Anatomy of Melancholy (1620), as borrowed from Matteo Ricci's Latin term to describe the shi in China, a group for which there was no close equivalent (such as gentry) in Europe. Nonetheless, Hucker defines shi as "a broad generic reference to the group dominant in government which also was the paramount group in society; originally a warrior caste, it was gradually transformed into a non-hereditary, ill-defined class of bureaucrats among whom litterateurs were most highly esteemed" (Dictionary of Official Titles, 421). Fang Yizhi (1611–1671), for instance, defined the shi "as a group that lie between the various officials and the ordinary people" (Fushan wenji qianbian, 3.8a). Fang thought that the majority of customs and values of the ordinary people came to them from the literati. He also felt that literati practices were both crucial and in decline, and wrote that there were increasingly many who regarded the acquisition of literary skills as a "means of tricking the world and achieving success" (3.8b).

16. Zhang Xinzhi makes these later kinds of comments as well in his commentary on The Story of the Stone (e.g., chapter 51). See Feng Qiyong, Bajia pingpi.

17. See Zeitlin, "Literary Fashioning of Medical Authority."

18. After the fall of the Ming, sequels (xushu) became common, and they clearly served the purpose of commentary in correcting or emphasizing certain aspects, subjects, narrative schema, or "errors" of the original work. See Huang, Snakes' Legs. Medical texts too, produced sequels to augment, explain, or correct previous editions.

19. The "fiction" category here includes dramatic works. See Chia, Printing for Profit, chapter 5; Brokaw, Commerce in Culture, 514–23; and Hegel, Reading Illustrated Fiction, 148–50.

20. Chia, Printing for Profit, 186.

21. Brokaw, Commerce in Culture, Appendix G. See also Hegel, Reading Illustrated Fiction, 143–44, 149.

22. Widmer, "Huanduzhai," 81–100; Unschuld, History of Pharmaceutics, 170.

23. Widmer, "Huanduzhai," 80; Chia, Printing for Profit, 230–34.

24. See, e.g., the biographies of Doctor Xiong Zongli (1409–1482) and of his great-grandson Xiong Damu (active mid-sixteenth century) in Chia, Printing for Profit, 226.

25. For a detailed study of the Jianyang printing business, see Chia, Printing for Profit.

26. For instance, characters in The Story of the Stone use almanacs on 1.15, 42.562, 48.642, 62.851, 77.1080, 86.1213, 97.1336, 99.1359, 100.1375, 102.1397, 114.1528, 116.1550, and 120.1600.

27. Smith, Chinese Almanacs, 28.

28. Ibid., 22–23.

29. BSS Slg. Unschuld 8649 "Records in a Jade Casket" (Yuxia ji). Alternately, it is possible that this title means that the information in the manuscript came from the almanac *Records from a Jade Casket* (Yuxia ji).

30. Such as BSS Slg. Unschuld 8157, 8467, 8670, and 48011.

31. E.g., BSS Slg. Unschuld 8480 "Casual Notes on Medicine and Pharmaceutics" (Yiyao biji) and 8823 "Miscellaneous Records of Good Recipes" (Liangfang zalu).

32. Unschuld and Zheng, *Chinese Traditional Healing*, 787. One manuscript from the 1930s (BSS Slg. Unschuld 8145 "A Complete Book with Guidelines Published in Chinese News Media" [Zhongguo xinwen zhidao quanshu]) is composed almost exclusively of prescriptions and medical information copied from newspapers and their advertisements. Many of these prescriptions, like the one for cholera, were influenced by Western medicine.

33. BSS Slg. Unschuld 8145 (Zhongguo xinwen zhidao quanshu) is particularly concerned with the dangers of sexual intercourse and contains a hybrid of Chinese traditional theories and Western physiological knowledge in a section titled "A Way toward Longevity by Curbing Desires" (Jieyu changshou fa). Unschuld and Zheng, *Chinese Traditional Healing*, 1090.

34. BSS Slg. Unschuld 8033 ("A Collection of Wondrously Effective Remedies" [Souji shenxiaofang]), dating from 1932–45, includes a clipping from a newspaper discussing the treatment of cholera pasted next to a prescription for cholera in the manuscript. Unschuld and Zheng, *Chinese Traditional Healing*, 48.

35. The category of printed dramas was also increasingly popular in this period, and can under traditional rubrics be included with novels under the umbrella term *xiaoshuo*. For a number of reasons, these contained a narrower range of intertexts than did full-length chapter novels.

36. Shang Wei, "Making of the Everyday World," 63–92.

37. Hanan, "Sources," 60ff.

38. Shang Wei, "Making of the Everyday World," 63–92.

39. Just as often, intentional changes were made when passages were copied into novels.

40. For instances of both, see chapter 3, this volume.

41. See Wang, Cheng-hua, "Art in Daily Life," 6–10; Oki Yasushi, "Bunka no kenkyu," 103–7; Shen Jin, "Tushu zhi liutong yu jiage," 101–18; Yu Yaohua, *Zhongguo jiageshi*, 766–830; Brokaw, *Commerce in Culture*, 550; Chia, *Printing for Profit*, 252.

42. "This Dr. Yang was a well-known quack who was a steady customer for four-ingredient soup, which he gave for toothache, and three-yellows powder, which he gave for stomach problems. His behavior was not very exemplary, and his character even worse. He was a pushy man who insinuated himself into people's homes and then carried tales about other men's wives all over town, so most people kept a distance from him, but Chao Yuan felt an affinity for him and always called him when a doctor was needed." Xizhousheng, *Xingshi yinyuan zhuan*, 2.9a–b.

43. Xizhousheng, *Xingshi yinyuan zhuan*, 2.11a. *Seeking No Help* was a generic term for these encyclopedias, in addition to the individual titles they might have had.

44. It very well may have been that the simple classical language found in some encyclopedias was easier for the marginally literate to read than the dense vernacular of novels.

45. Bréard, "Knowledge and Practice," 305–29.

46. Chen Yuanpeng, "Liang Song 'shang yi shiren' yu ruyi,'" chapter 4; Hymes, "Not Quite Gentlemen?," 16–20.

47. Unschuld and Zheng, *Chinese Traditional Healing*, 18.

48. Ibid., 4. For the *Yizong jinjian*, see Wu Qian et al.

49. This section is indebted to a number of observations made by Idema in "Diseases and Doctors, Drugs and Cures."

50. Ibid., 39.

51. An epidemic is featured at the beginning of *Outlaws of the Marsh* (Shuihu zhuan), but little direct description is involved, and the problem is not handled "medically."

52. As when Wei Jing helps Qin Qiong in *The Romance of the Sui and Tang Dynasties* (Suitang yanyi, 1695).

53. E.g., Qin Hui in *The Life of Yue Fei* (Shuoyue quanzhuan, 1684).

54. E.g., *Marriage Destinies to Awaken the World*; *The Unofficial History of a Female Immortal* (Nüxian waishi, 1711); *Humble Words of an Old Rustic*; *The Illustrious Heroes* (Yinglie zhuan, 1643); *and Fairy Traces in a Mundane World* (Lüye xianzong, 1771?).

55. *Qing*, sentiment, has been discussed in great detail by Huang (*Desire*), Yu (*Rereading the Stone*), Li (*Enchantment and Disenchantment*), and others.

56. Zheng En, in *Tale of the Flying Dragon* (Feilong zhuan), for instance, is warned not to overindulge in sexual intercourse even after he is married.

57. The most famous example is Ximen Qing in *Plum in the Golden Vase*, who dies from ceaseless ejaculation. There are many other examples, such as *The Lord of Perfect Satisfaction* and *Coarse Stories from Zhulin* (Zhulin yeshi, mid-seventeenth century?); *The Carnal Prayer-mat* (Rou putuan, 1657); *The Unofficial History of a Female Immortal*; *Three Women Named Lin, Lan, and Xiang* (Linlan xiang, mid-eighteenth century?); *Humble Words of an Old Rustic*; and *The Precious Mirror for Ranking Flowers* (Pinhua baojian, 1849).

58. E.g., *The Sobering Stone* (Zuixing shi, ca. 1650) and *Idle Talk under the Bean Arbor* (Doupeng xian hua, late 1660s).

59. See Zeitlin, *Historian*, 61–97.

60. Sivin describes the medical practice in "Emotional Counter-Therapy." Fiction abounds with characters that die from excessive anger or laughter, and novels such as *Story of the Stone* and *Humble Words of an Old Rustic* feature characters that treat those dangerous conditions by provoking corresponding emotions.

61. The two most famous doctors in *Romance of the Three Kingdoms* (Sanguo yanyi), Hua Tuo and Yu Ji, treat poisoned wounds almost exclusively.

It is curious that the type of doctor they represent is not treated explicitly, as is another famous historical doctor, Cheng Ying of *Orphan of Zhao* (his status as "doctor" changes in different versions of the story).

62. The novels *Marriage Destinies, Humble Words of an Old Rustic,* and *Three Women Named Lin, Lan,* and *Xiang* describe this practice.

63. Li, *Bencao gangmu,* 26.06.

64. Ibid., 35.23.

65. On the "reintegration" of apotropaic medicine into the more elite practice based on systematic correspondences, see Unschuld, *History of Ideas,* 189–228; and Unschuld and Zheng, *Chinese Traditional Healing,* "Introductory Essay."

66. Sutton, "Shamanism," 222–23.

67. Unschuld, *History of Pharmaceutics,* 25.

68. "There is a beast here whose form resembles a wildcat with a mane. It is called the *Lei* and is both male and female. Eating it will cure jealousy." See Yuan Ke, *Nanshan jing* chapter, entry 6.

69. Unschuld, *History of Ideas,* 194–212; Peterson, *Cambridge History of China,* 9:444.

70. Unschuld, *History of Ideas,* 216.

71. See Nappi, *Monkey and the Inkpot,* 81; Murray and Cahill, "Recent Advances," 1–8.

72. Li, *Bencao gangmu,* 8.16.

73. Cao Xueqin, *Honglou meng,* 120.

74. *Story of the Stone* 3.56.87.

75. *Story of the Stone* 4.98.372. There were both refined and coarse versions of each kind of soul. In Ding Yaokang's *Sequel to the Plum in the Golden Vase* (Xu Jinping mei, 1660), for instance, two different spiritual souls of the same dead person get into a fight.

76. In 1768, when *Story of the Stone* was being written, there was a pandemic of soul stealing. See Kuhn, *Soulstealers,* 1–29.

77. Though it is also true that a person who merely fainted was often said to have "died" (*si*).

78. "Calling the soul" refers both to a sorcerer calling a soul away from the body, and calling a soul back to the body, as a devoted parent might do when a child's soul has been frightened away.

79. There are different versions of the Qin Zhong story, with more or less emphasis on demons. A "Red Inkstone" (Zhiyan zhai) comment claims that the inclusion of demons that are coming to take him to King Yama of the underworld are not to be taken at face value (as, he implies, they might be in ordinary or popular fiction).

80. "An Easy View on Medical Formulas" (Yifang bianlan), SBB Slg. Unschuld 8453. Quoted in Unschuld and Zheng, *Chinese Traditional Healing,* 1815.

81. Wang Ji's *Stone Mountain Medical Case Records* (Shishan yian), Jiang Guan's *Cases from Famous Doctors, Arranged by Category* (Mingyi lei'an), and the case histories of Zhou Zhigan and Sun Yikui were all published in the sixteenth century. See also Grant, *Chinese Physician,* 53.

82. The case histories of many renowned physicians reappear in the Berlin manuscripts. Ye Tianshi's *Compass Guide for Clinical Situations: Medical Case Histories* (Linzheng zhinan yi'an) seems to have been particularly popular.

83. Zeitlin, "Literary Fashioning of Medical Authority," 169ff.

84. Xu Dachun, *Huixi Yian*, 19a–b. The case is the followed by an addendum, presumably by Xu Dachun, of the prescription for regrowing the penis in fifty days.

85. Li, *Bencao gangmu*, 14.21.

86. The practice of medicine was generally unregulated by the state, with the exception of notes in the (at least Ming and Qing) legal codes providing for the prosecution of intentional or unintentional malpractice leading to death. Unofficial regulation and market competition is discussed in chapter 3, this volume.

87. *Chloranthus spicatus* (Thub.).

88. Unschuld and Zheng, 1817.

89. BSS Slg. Unschuld 8071, "Complete Book on Drugs" (Quan yaoshu); Unschuld and Zheng, *Chinese Traditional Healing*, 905.

90. Most manuscripts with tonic formulas originated in larger cities. In rural regions, people who wrote medical manuscripts for their own practice tended not to record tonics, since they were called upon exclusively to treat existing ailments.

91. Unschuld and Zheng, *Chinese Traditional Healing*, 1818.

92. Zhao Xuemin is most famous for his *Addendum to Systematic Materia Medica* (Bencao gangmu shiyi), in which he added 716 new items that Li Shizhen had not included. *Strings of Refined [Therapies]* (Chuanya) was a long list of empirical methods and prescriptions from a personal friend, Zhao Boyun, who was an itinerant physician. Published in 1759, it created a tremendous stir among the ranks of regular scholar-physicians and revealed the parallel world of secretly transmitted medical knowledge. Portions of its text are frequently copied into the Berlin medical manuscripts.

93. Unschuld and Zheng, *Chinese Traditional Healing*, 1818.

94. "Excerpts Copied from Various Medical Books" (Yixue zachao), SBB Slg. Unschuld 8484.

95. In some of the tales of the strange, it seems likely that what appears fantastic to us (e.g., the habits of ghosts) was presented as practical information.

96. Unschuld and Zheng, *Chinese Traditional Healing*, 1817–18.

97. Li, *Bencao gangmu*, 40.10.

98. Ibid., 50.6. My translations follows, with slight variations, Nappi, *Monkey and Inkpot*, 116.

99. Ibid., 52.37.

2. READING MEDICALLY

1. The title is a reference to the Han-dynasty historian Sima Qian and his willingness to believe fantastic stories.

2. Yue Jun, "Chi nüzi," in Yisu, 347.

3. In his preface to *Fodder for the Ears*, Yue Jun writes that he has simply recorded what he has heard during his wanderings, "wild words not worth attending to. I do not believe in them at all; others do." Like the eleventh-century poet Su Shi (from whom he borrows the terms "listening wildly" and "talking wildly"), Yue Jun seems to be more interested in their appeal than their veracity. Ibid., 1.

4. Jiang Shiquan's (1725–1785) play *Dreams of Linchuan* (Linchuan meng, 1774?) tells the story of a woman so taken with *The Peony Pavilion* that she becomes lovesick for its author, Tang Xianzu, and dies.

5. Yue Jun, *Fodder for the Ears*, 347.

6. Zeitlin, "Shared Dreams," 129. Xiaoqing's biographers and the "Xiao-qing lore" they created (Dorothy Ko's term, *Teachers of the Inner Chambers*), generally framed Xiaoqing as a devotee of *Peony Pavilion*, who styled herself after the heroine Du Liniang, who dies of lovesickness. Xiaoqing also appears in about seventeen late-Ming and Qing dynasty plays. Pan Guang-dan both took exception to and perpetuated the Xiaoqing myth well into the modern period. See Lee, *Romantic Generation*, 190–99. For Xiaoqing and reading, see Berg, *Women and the Literary World*, 129–68.

7. On Miss Yu of Loujiang see Xu Fuming, *Mudan ting yanjiu ziliao kaoshi*. Miss Yu also is a featured character in Jiang Shiquan's *Dreams of Linchuan*, a play about Tang Xianzu, his readers, and literary history. On the parallel to Shen Yixiu's daughter, Ye Xiaowan, see Ko, *Teachers*, 196–97. See also Idema and Grant, *Red Brush*, 497–542. Lisa See wrote a novel based on the "three wives" titled *Peony in Love* (New York: Random House, 2007).

8. Wang Yongjian, quoted in Zeitlin, "Shared Dreams," 128.

9. Zeitlin, "Shared Dreams," 128.

10. Usually only the most famous scenes were performed. There are no clear records of a complete performance before 1999 at Lincoln Center. See Swatek, *Peony Pavilion Onstage*, 1–29.

11. But one actress is said to have died in the midst of acting a scene from the play. Lam, "Matriarch's Private Ear," 382.

12. Tang in his preface mentions three "sources" for his play (at the same time that he does not mention the proximate source, which was preserved in miscellanies in both *huaben* and *chuanqi* form). In the play itself, he mobilizes the emperor to vouch for Liniang's story when Du Bao resists. See Lu, *Persons, Roles, and Minds*, 97–144.

13. Some, of course, insisted that the "three wives" commentary was written by Wu Wushan. Zeitlin, "Shared Dreams," 175–79.

14. Zeitlin, "Shared Dreams," 130.

15. Zeitlin, "Shared Dreams," 130. Widmer writes that early stories of Xiaoqing (e.g., the Zhi Ruzheng text that was in existence by 1626) state that her reading of *Peony Pavilion* was a factor in her early death, although the exact way in which it harmed her is unclear ("Xiaoqing," 115).

16. Men died from reading fiction too, but those deaths are usually described as being caused not by excessive emotion, but by overindulg-ing—the literary equivalent of a medical issue common to men who frequented brothels.

17. Many prefaces to collections of women's poetry speak of the dangers faced by a woman who was both beautiful and talented. See, e.g., Wang Qi, *Chidu xinyu chubian*, 2.

18. Zeitlin, "Shared Dreams," 143. Widmer writes, "Judging from contemporary comments on historical female readers, once a woman was no longer young and charming, the dangers from reading seem to disappear" ("Xiaoqing," 127–28).

19. Furth, "Blood, Body, Gender," 48.

20. Accounts in fiction of death from strong emotions were not new in the Qing; examples include death from anger in chapter 4 of *The Sobering Stone* (Zuixing shi); in *A Tower for the Summer Heat* (Shi'er lou) a young wife dies of lovesickness during the absence of her husband (*juan* 9); in *Silent Operas* (Wusheng xi), a father dies of rage over his son's bad behavior (*juan* 8); in chapter 2 of *Tower of Myriad Flowers* (Wanhua lou), Di Qing's grandmother dies after she is told her daughter has committed suicide, and in chapter 61 Chen Pin laughs himself to death when his archrival is executed.

21. Sivin, "Emotional Counter-Therapy," 19; Chen Hsiu-fen, "Between Passion and Repression," 63–65; Unschuld, *History of Ideas*, 215–23; Scheid, *Currents of Tradition*, 164.

22. Grant, *Chinese Physician*, 137.

23. Gong Xin quoted in Hsiu-fen Chen, "Between Passion and Repression," 55.

24. Kuriyama, "Epidemics, Weather, and Contagion," 4.

25. On the "cult of qing," see Ko, *Teachers*, 68–112; and Santangelo, *Sentimental Education*, 186–206.

26. Joy, anger, grief, pondering/thinking/brooding/obsessing, sorrow, fear, fright. These are sometimes confused with the seven emotions often discussed in Confucian texts: joy, anger, sorrow, fear, love, hate, and desire.

27. Xu, *Huixi yi'an*, 90. Trans. in Unschuld, *Forgotten Traditions*, 12. The six excesses refer to the following environmental factors that turn harmful if they enter the human organism in excessive, or unbalanced, amounts: wind, cold, heat, dampness, dryness, and fire.

28. For a history of this notion, see Kuhn, *Soulstealers*, 96–118.

29. In one *Systematic Materia Medica* formulation, "Excessive grief diminishes the Vital Energy ... Overexertion consumes the Vital Energy ... Excessive anxiety makes the Vital Energy stagnate ... Excessive Heat causes the Vital Energy to leak." Physical factors can also cause emotions; *Bencao gangmu*, 14.09 records the excessive anger of a woman due to adverse ascending of malignant blood stasis. Eating hot food may cause pent-up excessive anger, as in *Bencao gangmu*, 26.01.

30. Grant, *Chinese Physician*, 3–19.

31. Quoted in Hanson, "Depleted Men," 298. These perceived differences between men and women in medical literature were seen as differences of kind (women's bodies are more complicated, susceptible to different maladies) and also degree (women are more prone to excessive emotions and less able to prevent them from resulting in illness).

32. Ko, *Teachers*, 99–103.

33. I use the term "consumption" to translate a variety of depletion disorders that generally have the same symptom sets of premodern, European consumption: frailty, weakness, weight loss, sleeplessness, expectoration of blood, feverishness, flushed cheeks, etc. Since it is often the result of excessive emotion or passion that consumes bodily resources, the translated term captures some of the illness mechanism. The emotion "sorrow" was linked to the pulmonary system as early as the first century BC.

34. Hawkes, *Story of the Stone*, 16. Dore Levy and Chi-hung Yim have both written in detail about Daiyu's illness, Levy from a metaphorical perspective, and Yim from the standpoint of medical theory and foreshadowing. See also Schonebaum, "Medicine in *The Story of the Stone*," 172–79.

35. In chapter 42, the traditional, dutiful Xue Baochai lectures Daiyu about the ethical dangers of reading fiction and drama.

36. Lin Daiyu did not die from reading fiction, but it contributed to and symbolized her overemotionality. She shows that she is a sophisticated reader of many kinds of literature, but fiction and drama raise her expectations with regard to her future and her marriage above what is likely, and provide a kind of code that she shares with Baoyu, leading to episodes of intimacy and painful misunderstanding.

37. Tang Xianzu, "Ku Loujiang nüzi," 654–56; Zeitlin, "Shared Dreams," 129.

38. A prime example of such a complaint is Zhang Xuecheng's comment on *Romance of the Three Kingdoms* being dangerous because it mixed history and fiction. Another way this problem was spoken of was using the phrase "speaking of dreams to the foolish" (*chiren shuomeng*), since they take dream for truth.

39. A clear reflection of the effect of the novel was that brigands adopted the nicknames of figures from *Outlaws of the Marsh*. This novel was banned at the end of the Ming precisely because of this.

40. Quoted in Brokaw, *Ledgers*, 164.

41. This is one of the main complaints in Liang Qichao's famous 1902 essay "On the Relationship between Fiction and the Government of the People" (Lun xiaoshuo yu qunzhi zhi guanxi).

42. Written by Wu Bing (?–ca. 1647), this play is about the orphan Xiaoqing, who at sixteen becomes the concubine of a much older man. The man's wife is jealous. Xiaoqing is abused by the wife, who locks her in the inner courtyard, where she is completely alone. She reads *Peony Pavilion* in solitude every night, becomes sick, and dies. She then returns to life. The scene from this play that has remained in the performance repertoire is the one in which she enacts reading *Peony Pavilion* and comments on the play.

43. Chen Yong, "Chusanxuan congtan," 349–50.

44. Quoted in Rolston, *Traditional Chinese Fiction*, 170.

45. Ibid.

46. *The Story of the Stone* is quite a long novel, almost 2,500 pages in English translation. Thus, reading it seven times in a month would require a significant effort.

47. Jia Rui misunderstanding of how to properly use the mirror (mentioned in chapter 1, this volume).

48. *Story of the Stone*, 1.12.251.

49. Those in the mirror are referred to simply as "people," but I use "demon" to be consistent with the many ghosts and demons in *Story of the Stone* who are drawn to, or metonymic of, excessive passion, such as those who try to drag Baoyu into the Ford of Error in his dream in chapter 5.

50. Keith McMahon summarizes traditional literary thought (more precisely the "pornoerotic tradition") on male/female differences with regard to sex by saying that the male was exhaustible and the female inexhaustible, a belief Chinese medical thought did not promote (*Misers, Shrews, and Polygamists*, 195). The binary in both medical traditions that finds men overspending bodily resources and women internalizing emotion was likely (in part, at least) a reflection of the circulation of men outside of the house, with the women cloistered within it.

51. *Honglou meng*, 7.

52. To some, both *Plum in the Golden Vase* and *Story of the Stone* use a seductive surface to draw readers in so that they can be delivered a message, but for other readers (such as Jia Rui) this does not work (they never wake up).

53. Baochai makes this point explicitly in chapter 42 of *Story of the Stone* when she reprimands Dai-yu for reading fiction:

Even boys, if they gain no understanding from their reading, would do better not to read at all; and if that is true of boys, it certainly holds good for girls like you and me. . . . A boy's proper business is to read books in order to gain an understanding of things, so that when he grows up he can play his part in governing the country. . . . Not that one hears of that happening much nowadays. Nowadays their reading seems to make them even worse than they were to start with. And unfortunately it isn't merely a case of their being led astray by what they read. The books, too, are spoiled, by the false interpretations they put upon them. They would do better to leave books alone and take up business or agriculture. At least they wouldn't do so much damage.

Zhang Zhupo makes similar remarks in his "How to Read *Jinping mei*" (*dufa*) essay.

54. In some editions it is the mirror itself that speaks the reproof.

55. Grandmother Jia, in *Story of the Stone*, seems to think too much reading, regardless of content, is bad for someone such as Baoyu.

56. This recipe occurs in a number of the Berlin medical manuscripts, but it is clearly copied from a printed text. One records the source as the "Subtle Discourse on the Preservation of Life" (Yuan [Yi] sheng weilun), written by the Ming author Li Shicai. See Unschuld and Zheng, *Chinese Traditional Healing*, 1401, 2191.

57. Thanks to Volker Shied for this reference.

58. *Complete Works of Ding Yaokang* 2:2.

59. Ibid.

60. Hu Hsiao-chen, "In the Name of Correctness," 78.

61. The postulation that Wang Shizhen was the author grew out of a suggestion by Shen Defu (1578–1642) in his *Random Gatherings from the Wanli*

Era (Wanli ye huo bian, 1606), 222. This notion is also mentioned in the prefatory Xie Yi essay in *Plum in the Golden Vase*, as it is in many chapter-ending comments. This is the same Wang Shizhen who wrote a preface to *Systematic Materia Medica*, recommending it to the emperor.

62. For instance, the legend was well known to Lu Xun, who taught it (as legend) in his lectures at Beijing University and records it in the 1934 printed edition of his lectures. Lu Xun, *Zhongguo xiaoshuo shilue*, 221–22.

63. Zhou Zuoren writes in 1937, "It is popularly believed that illness can be cured by magic. People write 'evil wind for sale' [*choufeng chumai*] on a piece of paper, wrap it round a coin, and leave it by the roadside. . . . I have personally met with such things" ("Tan guolai," 94). Other accounts of this practice record that "selling sickness money" would be collected from each member of a family on New Year's Eve and thrown out of the front gate, which then remained locked until dawn on New Year. Whoever picked up the scattered money would get the illness that had been destined for the family (Esherick, *Ancestral Leaves*, 134).

64. Some accounts refer to the essence of this worm as the *gu*.

65. For more on *gu* poison and its prominent role in medical and demonological literature, see Unschuld, *History of Ideas*, 46–50.

66. Li Shizhen discusses *gu* poisoning at length in *Systematic Materia Medica*, and medical manuscripts offer remedies for it as late as late Qing and early Republican era. BSS Slg. 8799 ("Text on Nourishing Life" [Yangsheng shu]) and BSS Slg. 8217 ("Extraordinary recipes for convenient use" [Jianbian qifang]), respectively.

67. Both Ming and Qing legal codes explicitly recorded punishments for those who engaged in *gu* poisoning.

68. The majority of the characters in the first twenty (of one hundred) chapters of *Plum in the Golden Vase* come from the *Outlaws of the Marsh* (Shuihu zhuan), as does most of the overall plot, but *Plum in the Golden Vase* is nonetheless an original work by a single author.

69. *Analects*, 3.20. *Jinping mei cihua*, preface (*xu*) 1a–2b. *Plum in the Golden Vase*, 3.

70. Zhu Xi, preface to *Zhongyong* in *Sishu Jizhu*, 4a.4. The *Unofficial History of the Scholars* chapter comments employ the same or similar language as Zhang Zhupo's commentary: "From the prologue in the first chapter one can see how the arteries and veins of the entire book are finely interconnected" (chap. 1, n. 1); "The writing really has tendons and sinews that articulate its entire body" (repeated twice; chapter 6, note 7, and chapter 47, note 4). "Chapter Comments" in Rolston, *How to Read*, 252–90.

71. A similar phrase relating the threads of the plot to the circulatory system was used by Li Kaixian (1501–1568) to describe *Outlaws of the Marsh*. See *Plum in the Golden Vase*, 1:456n5.

72. Following Zhang, the Woxian Caotang commentator on *The Unofficial History of the Scholars* (Rulin waishi) employs the terms "channels and veins" (*mailuo*) and "tendons and sinews that articulate the entire body" (*tongshen jinjie*). The Zhang Xinzhi (fl. 1828–1850) commentary on *The*

Story of the Stone (1881) similarly employs the term "channels and arteries" (*laimai*) in describing the reader's role as "distinguishing clearly the important channels and arteries" in order to "obtain results." Discussion of "channels" (*mai*) also appears in geomancy, and this usage, literally "hundreds of miles of concealed channels," might refer to geomancy (the body of the earth) rather than to the human body.

73. "Zhupo Dufa," section 52, in *Zhang Zhupo piping diyi qishu*, 20b. Roy, *Plum in the Golden Vase*, 232. Likely unbeknownst to Zhang, he was commenting on the Chongzhen (Xiuxiang) edition of *Jinping mei*, whose first chapter differs radically from that of the *Jinping mei cihua* edition.

74. Part of the motivation to make the reader concentrate on rhetoric (*wen*) over actual content (*shi*) in Zhang Zhupo (and in Jin Shengtan before him) has to do with the perceived problematic nature of the content of the novel(s).

75. Most likely, Zhu Xi, along with other leading thinkers of the twelfth century, believed this circulatory system to consist of twelve vessels that transported blood, qi, and possibly other substances from the chest and head to the extremities and organs, and vice versa. By the time the notion of circulation was applied to fiction, both the popular form of literature and the medical terms used to describe it were more complex. See Unschuld, *History of Ideas*, 189–228.

76. Wu Jingzi, 13.1b. The early seventeenth-century short story collection *A Needle for Embroidering Mandarin Ducks* (Yuanyang zhen) employs similar language (*Story of the Stone*, 108–11).

77. Manuals on such arts as chess and garden landscaping also contributed technical vocabulary and illuminating anecdotes to criticism of Chinese fiction. See Rolston, *How to Read*, 14.

78. Zhang Yanhua, *Transforming Emotions*, 63. This story does not seem to appear in historical accounts. In Zhou's biography in the *History of the Three Kingdoms* (Sanguo zhi, comp 285–97), for instance, it just says that he died of illness.

79. Wu Jingzi, *Unofficial History of the Scholars*, chapter 3. Overjoy is treated with fright when his fearsome butcher father-in-law slaps Fan Jin in the face and he regains his senses.

80. Sivin discusses this text in "Emotional Counter-Therapy," 5–6. Earlier texts remark on "curing emotions with emotions." *The Scholar Serving His Kin* (Rumin shiqin, compiled 1217–21) contains some such cases, and its compiler, the physician Zhang Congzheng (1156–1228), was well known to employ this healing method. See Zhang Yanhua, *Transforming Emotions*, 72–74.

81. From Sivin, "Emotional Counter-Therapy," 2.6.

82. See Zhu Zhenheng, *Danxi xinfa*, 5:483. This medical case is also recorded in Wu Kun, *Yifang kao*, 202–3. See Chen Hsiu-fen, "Between Passion and Repression," 56. The famous former Han physician Chunyu Yi also records treating a woman suffering from "wanting a man yet not being able to get one" (*yu nanzi er bu ke de*). Sima Qian, *Shiji*, 105:2808–9.

83. Wu Kun records a case of a young man suffering from similar derangement and idiocy as a result of sorrow and resentment. See Sivin, "Emotional Counter-Therapy," 10–11.

84. Yuan Hongdao, "Wenchao," 14. I follow Naifei Ding, *Obscene Things*, 84.

85. *Jinping mei cihua* 1b.3. I follow David Roy, with minor changes, *Plum in the Golden Vase* 3.

86. Quoted in *Plum in the Golden Vase*, 430.

87. Ibid., 364–65.

88. Hawkes, *Story of the Stone*, chapter 23.

89. Li Yu also writes in *Casual Expressions* that that which one's nature (*benxing*) loves obsessively is an antidote to illness because "where there is obsession, there is life itself" (*Li Yu quanji*, 2.348).

90. Cao, *Honglou meng*, 2005, 6; *Story of the Stone*, 50

91. I follow Shuen-Fu Lin in Rolston, *How to Read*, 286.

92. Li, *Bencao gangmu*, 3.51, 3.52.

93. Ibid., 18.01, 31.02.

94. E.g., Li, *Bencao gangmu*, 31.02; 33.13.

95. For the history of these terms, see Wile, *Art of the Bedchamber*, 19–23.

96. Wu, Yi-li, "The Bamboo Grove Monastery," 60.

97. A short list of entertainment literature concerned with excessive sex would include *The Startled Swan* (Jinghong ji, 1590 preface) the main late Ming southern drama to treat the story of Yang Guifei and a major influence on *Palace of Lasting Life* (Changsheng dian, completed 1688). *The Startled Swan* features An Lushan procuring aphrodisiacs for Tang Ming Huang (scenes 11 and 12). The novel *Marriage Destinies to Awaken the World* depicts Zhenge having a miscarriage because of the aphrodisiacs Chao Yuan brought (chapter 4). In *Humble Words of an Old Rustic*, Su E takes aphrodisiacs by mistake and falls ill (chapter 17). *A Precious Mirror for Ranking Flowers* also features a scene describing aphrodisiacs and their dire consequences (chapter 58), to say nothing of *Plum in the Golden Vase*, *The Carnal Prayer-mat*, *Coarse Stories from Zhulin*, and so on.

98. Medical texts copied for use in urban areas often featured patent medications with fixed formulas printed in *fangshu* or available at large pharmacies. Unschuld and Zheng, *Chinese Traditional Healing*, 2447.

99. That aphrodisiacs and tonifying medicines were similar if not the same medicines is evident as late as the 1843 *The Illusion of the Story of the Stone* (Honglou huanmeng), which rewrites Jia Baoyu as a sexually and romantically successful lover who has six wives. A friend of his from the south gives him an aphrodisiac to keep him from "harming himself" (Huayue chiren, *Honglou huanmeng*, 19.288–9).

100. SBB Slg. Unschuld 8167, under the heading "pills the led to the beating of an old man," *da laoer wan*; 1141–42), and SBB Slg. Unschuld 8429, in which the same prescription appears under the heading "priceless pills to safeguard the true [essence]" (*wujia baozhen wan*). Unschuld and Zheng, *Chinese Traditional Healing*, 1753–54.

101. Unschuld and Zheng, *Chinese Traditional Healing*, 1534.

102. The foreign monk who gives Ximen the aphrodisiac proclaims its tonifying affects:

If used for long, your appetite will be insatiable;
It will stir your testicles and stiffen your organ.
In a hundred days your hair will regain its color;
In a thousand days your stamina will be augmented.
It will strengthen your teeth and brighten your eyes;
And its dangers:
If you are not able to believe these claims,
Mix it in with rice and feed it to your cat.
For three days it will indulge itself without restraint;
On the fourth day it will be too overheated to stand it.
A white cat will be transformed into a black one,
Its excretory functions will stop and it will die. (*Plum in the Golden Vase*, 3.200)

103. The monk has a purple head, sunken eyes, wears a flesh-colored gown, has a trickle of jade-white mucus dribbling from his nose, and so on. Commentary points out the similarity to a penis: "Now, what does he look like?" (*Zhang Zhupo piping diyi qishu*, 49.12a).

104. Xiao Jing refers to Juzhong as such. (*Xuan Qi jiuzheng lun*, juan 6).

105. Unschuld and Zheng, *Chinese Traditional Healing*, 2373.

106. The "Biblio Materia Medica" seems to belong to a parodic genre, along with the likes of *Materia Medica: Prostitutes of Essentials* (Bencao jiyao, 1754), a Japanese book imitating Wang Ang's *Materia Medica: Provision of Essentials* (Bencao beiyao, 1694) and expounding the nature, use, and effects of prostitutes in Edo-era Japan; and the "Money Materia Medica" (Qian bencao, mid-Qing), a piece written in the style of a pharmaceutical monograph elaborating on the effects of the "drug" money.

107. Zhang Chao, "Shu bencao," *juan* 12, 40a–41b.

108. Ibid., 41a–b

109. Zhang Chao, in spite of his own warnings, published a collection of short literary language fiction (*chuanqi*): *New Tales of Yu Chu* (Yu Chu xinzhi, eighteenth century).

110. Fei Cidu (Fei Mi, 1623–1699) was a member of a counter-neo-Confucianism movement and was a strong advocate of practical knowledge.

111. Three of the people mentioned are military leaders, two good, one bad. The good ones are likened to the proper use of novels as medicine. Growing up, Han Xin and Yue Fei were both poor, fatherless, and self-taught. Zhao Kuo, on the other hand, was the son of a general, widely read in military strategy, but without military experience. Wang Anshi (1021–1086) saw in the *Rites of Zhou* (Zhou li) an all-encompassing system for realizing the common good, though he was criticized by many Southern Song commentators for this belief.

112. Ibid., 41b.

113. Ding, *Obscene Things*, 108.

3. VERNACULAR CURIOSITIES

1. Zhang Jun, *Qingdai xiaoshuo shi*, 131. Columbia University, Harvard University, and the National Library of China have editions that they date to this period on the basis of its Kangxi-era (1661–1722) publisher, Zuile Tang. Sun Dianqi also records that it is a work of the Kangxi period, as does Wang Qingyuan. Zhao Chunhui claims the author was Wang Jia (zi, Jieren; 1610–1684) ("zuozhe chutan," 83).

2. Tian Zhiwen, *Caomu chunqiu yanyi*, 25; Ōtsuka, *Zōho chūgoku tsūzoku shōsetsu*, 155–56.

3. Zhu Yixuan, *Zhongguo gudai xiaoshuo*, 621; this volume is recorded in *Zhongguo tongsu xiaoshuo zongmu tiyao*, 570.

4. Wang Qingyuan et al., *Xiaoshuo shufang lu*, 87. See also Ōtsuka Hidetaka, *Zōho chūgoku tsūzoku shōsetsu*, 155–56.

5. There are two editions that Wang Qingyuan is unable to date, one that employed woodblock printing, and one that was printed lithographically, a technology introduced into China in the late nineteenth century. The latter may also date to this late Qing era, when popular fiction from the Ming and Qing was published en masse in Shanghai. See Pan Jianguo, "Metal Typography," 562–70.

6. Among the medical texts that predate the *Caomu chunqiu yanyi* and have similar titles are Ji Han's *Observations of Herbs and Woods in the South* (Ji Han nanfang caomuzhuang), Taiqing's *Herbal Prescriptions* (Taiqing caomu fang), Lu Ji's *Book of Herbs* (Caomu shu), and Ye Ziqi's *Herbs* (Caomu zi).

7. *Caomu chunqiu yanyi*, "zixu," 1a–b.

8. Ibid., 1a.

9. Bartholomew, "One Hundred Children," 71.

10. *Story of the Stone*, chapter 62, 211.

11. See Shang Wei, "*Jinping mei*," 194.

12. West and Idema, *Orphan of Zhao*, 219–20.

13. Li, *Bencao gangmu*, 14.01. Li Shizhen also quotes Chen Cheng (fl. 1086–1094), *Materia Medica with Additional Comments* (Bencao bieshuo) as saying, "When both blood and vital energy are displaced, *danggui* can lead them back and bring peace to the overall condition. So the name *danggui*, 'should come back,' can be explained as blood and vital energy 'should go back to their original places.'"

14. Li, *Bencao gangmu*, 12.10. Although *Story of the Western Wing* predates *Systematic Materia Medica*, I use it for the sake of consistency and because it quotes many texts prior to the Yuan, when the play was written.

15. Li, *Bencao gangmu*, 40.4.

16. Ibid., 12.03.

17. I follow the translation of West and Idema, *Story of the Western Wing*, 220, with minor changes.

18. Wang Shifu, *Jiping jiaozhu xixiang ji*, 137.

19. Ibid., 137.

20. According to *Story of the Western Wing* commentators, many *sanqu* "conceal the names of medicines" (*yincang yaoming*), and all with didactic intent. Ibid., 138.

21. At first glance, the *Story of Mr. Sangji* by the Ming author Xiao Guan-lan (early sixteenth century?) appears to be a person's biography. However, almost every phrase employs the name of a drug. The first few sentences read, "Mr. Sangji [tree fungus], a man of Changshan [*Radix dichroae febrifugae*], was kind and straightforward [*houpu; magnolia officinalis*] toward others. When young, he had far-reaching ambition [*yuanzhi*; milkwort], he attended school and read several hundred books [*baibu; stemona*], as he got older, he became extraordinarily intelligent [*yizhi; Alpinia oxyphylla*, a type of ginger]."

22. *Li Zhuowu pingben Xiyou ji*, 28.4b.

23. *Plum in the Golden Vase*, chapters 33 and 61 (2:269–70 and 4.38–39).

24. Chen Jingji sings one such poem in *Plum in the Golden Vase*, 2.271.

25. Tian Zhiwen, *Caomu chunqiu yanyi*, 25.

26. The Berlin Medical Manuscript collection has a copy, in the back of which is written information about real estate in the area, including how much land was occupied by a school, and how much it paid in fees for jour-nals and newspapers in 1931 and 1932. Unschuld and Zheng, *Chinese Tra-ditional Healing*, 912–20. The China Academy for Traditional Chinese Medicine has a copy of the drama *Illustration of Numerous Pharmaceutical Drugs* (Yaohui tu), dated 1935.

27. Rhythmic-block melodies (*bangzi qiang*) was a form of local opera found in Shangxi, Henan, Hebei, Shandong, and so on. I generally use the words "drama," "play," and "opera" interchangeably because I focus on con-tent, audience, and the written text without regard for literary merit or generic distinctions.

28. Seven of the 881 medical manuscripts in the Berlin collection copy these plays, though some are missing one or two scenes.

29. Unschuld and Zheng (*Chinese Traditional Healing*, 175) call them this.

30. Ibid., 921.

31. Disseminating medical information was a widely recognized form of philanthropy that allowed one to demonstrate personal virtue and concern for humanity. See Wu, *Reproducing Women*, 75–81.

32. Shang zhijun et al., *Lidai zhongyao*, 470, 504.

33. Unschuld and Zheng, *Chinese Traditional Healing*, 1312.

34. The earliest edition of a medical play that I have been able to find is a Yaohui tu edition dated 1840, unless it is for some reason spurious. Lu Dahuang included a version of *Caomu zhuan* in his edition of *Pu Songling's Works* (Pu Songling ji, 1962), though no copy exists from that period. See Jia Zhizhong, "Questioning the authorship of *Caomu zhuan*," 26–27.

35. Unschuld and Zheng, *Chinese Traditional Healing*, 2647.

36. The *Yixue juyu*, "Medical learning, Comprehension by analogy," has a different plot but the characters and the style is similar to those of the *Caomu chunqiu*. The *Yaoxing xi*, has essentially the same plot but recasts some of the characters (Gancao falls ill after his encounter with four robbers, etc.).

37. The surname Jin is likely from a vernacular name for the plant identi-fied by Li Shizhen, *jinchai shihu* ("Shihu in the shape of a hairpin"). Li, *Ben-cao gangmu*, 20.01.

38. By which I mean a body of a politic nature as well as a politic of a bodily nature.

39. Unschuld and Zheng, *Chinese Traditional Healing*, 177.

40. The name Guolao for Gancao was first recorded in the *Additional Records of Famous Physicians* (Mingyi bielu), according to *Systematic Materia Medica*. Li Shizhen quotes Tao Hongjing, "Gancao is a principal drug among all the drugs. . . . It is also called Guolao or 'the imperial instructor.' Gancao is similar to the imperial instructor, who is not the monarch, but the monarch follows his instructions. Hence the name Guolao." Li, *Bencao gangmu*, 12.01.

41. The *shiba fan* also circulated in poetic form to aid memory, such as "the 18 [substances whose effects are known to] oppose each other, in rhyme" (*shiba fan ge*), recorded in the medical manuscripts.

42. Li Liangsong, *Zhongguo chuantong wenhua*, 330–31.

43. In Chinese medicine, all drugs are toxic to a certain extent, and originally toxicity was a measure of efficacy or power (Cullen and Lo, *Medieval Chinese Medicine*, 327. "Toxic" refers to undesirable or unpleasant side-effects, or simply to the powerful effects of the drug.

44. The distinction between 密陀僧 and 彌陀僧 is lost in some manuscripts, and in the novel version of *Caomu chunqiu*, suggesting that later editors and copyists were less concerned with linguistic play than were the author(s).

45. Unschuld and Zheng, *Chinese Traditional Healing*, 177–78.

46. *Caomu chunqiu*, act 1. Unschuld and Zheng, *Chinese Traditional Healing*, 178.

47. Unschuld and Zheng, *Chinese Traditional Healing*, 179.

48. Ibid.

49. Quoted in Leung, "Medical Instruction," 145.

50. The "white in man" refers to the white sediment in human urine, good for treating (in various versions of the play) mouth sores. *Systematic Materia Medica* also records that it is a cure for consumptive corpse transmission (*chuanshilao*). Li, *Bencao gangmu*, 52.11. Different versions of the play recommend somewhat different drugs, but all of them are in keeping with the form of the particular aria (in this case some form of excrement).

51. Unschuld and Zheng, *Chinese Traditional Healing*, 182 (with small modifications).

52. One play has "stomach" instead of "heart," which must have been a change made by a copyist with a knowledge of medicine.

53. Unschuld and Zheng, *Chinese Traditional Healing*, 181 (with small changes).

54. Ibid., 182. Dragon bones were usually fossilized animal bones, perhaps from elephants (mammoth), rhinoceros, hipparion (ancient three-toed horses), gazelles, or cows.

55. Jia and Yang argue that the language of the plays was so simple and clear that they must have been meant for performance. If not, they were clearly meant to be read by the broadest possible readership. *Qingdai yaoxing ju*, 458, 492.

56. *Caomu chunqiu*, act 10.

57. Unschuld and Zheng, *Chinese Traditional Healing*, 181.

58. Unschuld, *History of Pharmaceutics*, 230–32. The "Story of Flowery Knotweed" (Heshouwu zhuan) of the Tang dynasty is a political allegory composed around a person bearing the name of a an innocuous plant that has risen to become a much-cherished pharmaceutical substance in Chinese traditional medicine; readers in later times failed to see the original purpose of the author, Li Ao, when he selected a plant without pharmaceutical effects to convey his political message.

59. Wudang, a small mountain range in the northwestern part of Hubei Province, is known historically for its many Daoist monasteries. Wudang is also known as the home of a number of Chinese martial arts (*Wudang quan*). In the modern period, Chinese martial arts have generally been categorized as belonging to Shaolin or Wudang.

60. Presumably the author chose Hujiao (pepper) as the name for the foreign country because *hujiao* was produced in countries to the west of China. *Hu* also is a general marker for things foreign. Li Shizhen says *hujiao* is produced in countries in the Nanfan area, as well as southern Yunnan, and he quotes Tang Shenwei as saying that it comes from Mojiatuo (Madhyadesha; northern India) to the west.

61. Li, *Bencao gangmu*, 28.10.

62. In the *Systematic Materia Medica*, Jin Yinhua is found as an alternate name for *rendong*, and Jin Lingzi is known as *lian*.

63. Li, *Bencao gangmu*, 8.14.

64. Described in chapter 14.

65. Somewhat paradoxically, it also evokes the doctor Sun Simiao, who according to legend rode a tiger.

66. Li Gao quoted in Li, *Bencao gangmu*, 17.01.

67. Wang Kentang, *Zhengzhi zhunsheng* (Guidelines for treating illness) 29b–30b. Wang quotes the doctor Liu Zonghou (Liu Chun) in retelling this story. The citation comes from his *Subtle Meanings of the Precious Machine* (Yuji weiyi), 50 *juan*, completed in 1396. For Liu's original quotation, see Liu Chun, *Yuji weiyi* (Siku Quanshu edition), *juan* 43:3b–4b. Wang argues that these drugs are appropriate only for stagnations of blood, not for loss of blood or qi. Thanks to Yi-Li Wu for providing this reference.

68. By "popular," I mean that they are employed hundreds of times in prescriptions listed in *Systematic Materia Medica*; "infrequently" means that they occur fewer than twenty-five times. In Li, *Bencao gangmu*, Shihu is known as Jinchai.

69. Wu Cheng'en, *Xiyou ji* (Renmin Wenxue edition), 831.

70. Monkey is not necessarily a quack, but he does represent an antiestablishment attitude toward medicine (consistent with his carnivalesque character). He says of the medical officials that they are all idiots (Wu, *Xiyou ji*, Renmin Wenxue edition, 831).

71. *Xiyou zhengdao shu*, 69.7b.

72. Zhang Shushen, *Xinshuo xiyouji* commentary, 69.8a.

73. *Wujin san* is a prescription for prenatal and postnatal illness mentioned by Li Shizhen from the "*generally helpful prescriptions (puji fang)* that refers to soot as "hundred grass frost." It also calls for the urine of a boy.

74. Urine from a white horse (*baimani*) is recorded in Li, *Bencao gangmu*, as being good for treating a number of diseases, including abdominal hard masses (caused by overeating), as well as those in the breast.

75. *Li Zhuowu pingben Xiyou ji*, 14a–b. The prefatory material in this commentary edition stresses the large number of "joking" comments in it, but this particular statement seems accusatory, if also funny.

76. Wu, *Journey to the West*, 276.

77. Li, *Bencao gangmu*, 5.15. Sourceless water was particularly good for treating hot diarrhea. Sourceless water is one of forty-three different kinds of water discussed in the *Systematic Materia Medica*. The medical official says that sourceless water is taken from a well, which is also what Li Shizhen says, but Monkey contradicts him, saying that sourceless water is rainwater that has never touched the ground, perhaps parodying the adage "When you drink water, think of the source." *Bencao gangmu*, under "sourceless water," also mentions that the *Strategies of the Warring States* (Zhanguo ce) records that Doctor Changsang Jun fed his student Bian Que "water from the upper pond" (*shangchishui*), and after that Bian Que could see clearly the Five Viscera (Liver, Heart, Spleen, Lungs, and Kidneys) and the Six Bowels (Gall Bladder, Stomach, Large Intestine, Small Intestine, Urinary Bladder, and Sanjiao [Triple Burner]) of his patients. Monkey also recalls another diagnostic master, Sun Simiao, the "medicine king," who used the technique of "dangling the thread" to read the pulses of the king while sitting in another room.

78. Unschuld and Zheng, *Chinese Traditional Healing*, 1497.

79. Ibid., 930.

80. Ibid., 950.

81. Ibid., 930. *Mo*, or *wujin*, good for stopping treating bloody feces, urine, coughing blood, nose bleeds, seminal emission, *kewu* ("visitor's hostility) and *zhong'e* ("struck by the malign"), postpartum blood loss, and melancholy. Black ink *mo* was made using soot from burning pine, which perhaps explains the alternate name "pine smoke" for "black gold."

82. Goldschmidt, *Evolution of Chinese Medicine*, 173–98.

83. Li Yu, *Wusheng xi*, 93–106.

84. Ibid., 333. This is effectively the opposite of the treatment for the "stone virgin"; see chapter 4 of this volume.

85. Jue Mingzi is also compared to Chen Ping (and Zhuge Liang) in *Caomu chunqiu yanyi*.

86. It seems that the commentators on *Xiyou ji* were not among the group of readers who were familiar with medicine. They repeatedly mention that the author "must have read *Nanjing* and *Maijue* every day in order to know how to take the pulses so well" and that "this medicine reflects a thorough knowledge of *bencao* literature."

87. I am not alone in my belief that *Caomu chunqiu yanyi* is far inferior to the *caomu* plays in terms of the depth of pharmaceutical content. Zhijun, Qianlian, and Jinsheng, *Lidai zhongyao wenxian jinghua*, 504. It may be that the novel was written first, with the plays developing what they found in the novel into more entertaining and sophisticated literature, and therefore a

more useful medical information delivery system. It may also have been that the proliferation of the plays in the late Qing caused a revival of interest in the novel.

88. Li, *Bencao gangmu*, 15.21.

89. Ibid., 35.47.

90. Ibid., 17.01.

91. Some might say that Li Shizhen was actually classifying the important natural world, since he includes a discussion of some objects, such as crickets, which were not used as medicines but were, Li explains, relevant, since people kept them for fighting or singing. Nappi, *Monkey and Inkpot*, 53.

92. Metailie, "*Bencao gangmu* of Li Shizhen," 223–24.

93. Liu Dabai, *Du He Dian*, 211–18. Originally published in the newspaper the *Dawn* (Liming).

94. Idema and Haft, *Guide to Chinese Literature*, 228.

95. Mentioned by Lu Xun in volume 12 of collected works, *Lu Xun quanji*, 12.229. Mao Dun called it a symbolic novel in the style of *Flowers in the Mirror*.

96. The only medicines that are used to treat ailing characters are fantastical, such as "Immortal grass" (*busicao*), which cures all ailments, but even this seems to have had no special significance. *Busicao* revives the Han soldiers from all sorts of illnesses, but is also an alternate name for Mai Mendong, a drug cast in this novel as one of the evil, invading generals—another example of the chaos this novel brings on itself.

97. One reader began underlining all of the characters' names in red ink but gave up before finishing the first chapter. Jiang Hong, *Caomu chunqiu yanyi* edition in the Columbia University Library.

98. One obvious reason is that because there was money to be made reprinting all kinds of texts (as a result of lithography and new mass market), many previously obscure texts got reprinted.

99. Du Ji, *Caomu chunqiu yanyi*, 1.

100. "Seeking out the hidden" appears in commentaries from quite early on and became particularly prominent in the late Qing and early Republic in allegorical or roman à clef commentaries of novels. Rolston, *Traditional Chinese Fiction*, 78.

101. Cf. chapter 2, this volume, for traditional novels that also claimed to alleviate melancholy and engender enlightenment.

102. Ding Yaokang, *Xu Jinping mei*, "Fanli," 8.

103. Xizhou sheng, *Xingshi yinyuan zhuan*, "Fanli," 7, 8.

104. See Yang Yu-Chun, "Re-orienting *Jinping mei*," 205–12.

105. And it is still available today.

106. Many modern editions excise them and put in their place the phrase "two first-rate and wonderful aphrodisiacs," as in the 1981 Renmin Wenxue edition. *Xingshi yinyuan zhuan*, 881.

107. Reprinted in chapter 36 of *Flower Shadows behind the Screen* (Gelian huaying). Soon after *Sequel to Plum in the Golden Vase* was banned in 1665, a revised version of it was published, titled *Flower Shadows behind the Screen* (Gelian huaying, late seventeenth century), which strategically

deletes all the passages with political associations, such as those concerning the Jurchen invasion. The narrator's discussions of karmic retribution are also omitted, removing many of the concepts fundamental to Ding Yaokang's original version.

108. See, e.g., Gong Tingxian, *Wanbing huichun*, 438.

109. E.g., Xu Qilong, *Xinke quanbu*, 20:135; Xu Sanyou, *Wuche bajin*, 18:87, 109; Yu Xiangdou *bu qiu ren*, 26:503.

110. Wu Huifang indicates that all Wanli-era encyclopedias include one volume named "Fengue." However, by the Chongzhen period, only one encyclopedia includes a *"fengyue"* chapter. It then disappeared, and is not found in Qing encyclopedias ("Minjian Riyong leishu," 111).

111. Handlin-Smith, *Art of Doing Good*, chapter 4; Wu Yi-Li, "Qing Period," 161–208; Scheid, *Currents of Tradition*, chapter 2.

112. Unschuld, *Medical Ethics*, 62–114.

113. Chen Hongmou, *Xunsu yigui*, 26a.

114. BSS Slg. Unschuld 8288, "Miscellaneous Hand-copied Notes from People's Homes" (Minjia zachao), for instance, contains many long passages copied from the novel *The Romance of the Three Kingdoms* (Sanguo zhi yanyi).

115. SBB Slg. Unschuld, 8503. "A Guide to Medications for Treating the Foreign Bug" collects all references to medical and pharmaceutical knowledge in this novel *Record of Wiping Out Bandits* (Dangkou zhi), which was also known as *Supplement to the Shuihu [zhuan]* (Hou Shuihu), and also as *Conclusion of the Shuihu zhuan* (Jie Shuihu zhuan).

116. Widmer, "Modernization without Mechanization," 65–68.

117. Wang Qingyuan et al., *Xiaoshuo shufang lu*, 18–162.

118. Shahar, *Crazy Ji*, 268n1. These dates are all from Wang Qingyuan, *Xiaoshuo shufang lu*, 1–184.

119. Just as prescriptions with figurative aspects do not seem to be practical, ala Baochai's "cold fragrance pills" in *Story of the Stone*.

120. Lu Yitian, *Lenglu yihua*, 223.

121. Medical cures are discussed in Li Ruzhen, *Jinghua yuan*, 26.3b–4a, 27.1a, 27.3b–4a, 29.1b–3b, 30.1a–2a, and 95.1b–2b.

122. *Colloquies on the Novel* (Xiaoshuo Conghua), published in *New Fiction* (Xin xiaoshuo) between 1903 and 1905. Quoted in Hsia, "Scholar-Novelist," 463n26. Ying, *Wanqing wenxue congchao*, 211.

123. Li, *Bencao gangmu*, 16.10.

124. Quoted in Wang Qiongling, *Sida caizi*, 420.

125. Wrote Xiaren, who contributed a series of notes on fiction to Liang Qichao's (1873–1929) journal, *New Fiction*. Quoted in Hsia, "Scholar-Novelist," 463.

126. Li Ruzhen, *Jinghua yuan*, chapter 9.

127. Sun Jiaxun, *Jinghua yuan gongan bianyi*, 98.

128. Mid-Jiaqing period medical works *Jiji danfang* and *Heshi jisheng lun* also record this prescription, changing its name to "Ping'an san."

129. Xu Dachun, *Xu Lingtai yixue quanshu*, 401.

130. The medical manuscripts have many examples of the type "secret instructions, must not be given to others indiscriminately" (*mijue buke qing*

chuan yu ren). Some private lists of recipes have a seal printed at the end of each formula stating, "Keep secret [*hu feng*]!" The relationship of the names Li Ruzhen and Li Shizhen is unclear but could not have been lost on the author of *Flowers in the Mirror*, or on those of his readers who were interested in his medical prescriptions.

131. Chen Yiting, "Kan Li Ruzhen de yiyao yangsheng guan," 165–69. The prescription for "five yellow power" (*wuhuang san*) of chapter 91 does stem from recipe books. The Ming dynasty work *Formulas for Universal Benefit* lists it, as does *Selected Materials for the Preservation of Health* (Jisheng bacui fang, 1315). The prescription was comprised of *huangdan*, *huanglian*, *huangqin*, *dahuang*, *huangbai* (Chinese cork tree), and *ruxiang* (frankincense), for "curing wounds inflicted by a stick *zhangchuang* decreasing swelling, drawing out pus, and reducing swelling." The prescription in *Flowers in the Mirror* is the same, but with the addition of *xionghuang* (realgar), perhaps in yet another attempt by novelists to outdo their predecessors by adding more. To include this prescription with the major ingredients all containing the word "*huang*" also ties it to *caomu* literature, word games, and the literary logic employed in them to entertain and delight.

132. See Huang, "*Xiaoshuo* as 'Family Instructions,'" 67–91.

133. Li Ruzhen, *Jinghua yuan* (Renmin Wenxue edition, 27. 124–25).

134. Ibid., 126.

135. The manuscript of "On Seasonal Diseases. All [Therapy] Patterns Prepared for Use" ([Shibing lun. Beiyong zhufa], SBB Slg. Unschuld 8315) does not copy the complete prescription, though. Perhaps the copyist did not read the novel, and got the prescription from some intermediary source, or perhaps he was remarking to himself the uniqueness of the prescription by copying only the ways in which it differed from what he already knew. Unschuld and Zheng (*Chinese Traditional Healing*, 1489) date the manuscript to 1882.

136. Li Ruzhen, *Jinghua yuan*. Shu An's comment (Waseda University Library edition, 29.38a). See also Sun Jiaxun, *Jinghua yuan gongan bianyi*, 98.

137. Li Ruzhen, *Jinghua yuan*, 26.120.

138. Ibid., 55.257–58.

139. Chen Yiting, "Li Ruzhen de yiyao yangsheng guan," 165–69.

140. Zhao Xuemin, *Chuanya quanshu*, 11.

141. The case of quacks in premodern China was probably similar to that described by Roy Porter in seventeenth through nineteenth century England, where the term applied to doctors who hawked nostrums in public, i.e., "quacking in the market." Porter shows that those doctors disparaged as "quacks" in fact had the same university medical training and beliefs as their detractors, and that their medical therapies were also the same. Accusations of quackery thus cannot be taken literally as accurate assessment of what a practitioner did or was. Instead, this was a rhetorical device used by one set of practitioners to disparage another. Xu Dachun's claims similarly conveyed accusations about a self-promoter's lack of propriety, with the implication being that someone as crass as to promote himself would also not be above selling fraudulent cures. Porter, *Quacks*.

142. Unschuld, "Chinese Retributive Recipes," 328–40.

143. Unschuld and Zheng, *Chinese Traditional Healing*, 843, 1747, 1855.

144. "Cao Xueqin diagnoses illness" (Cao Xueqin kanbing). The dating of these stories is uncertain, but some are as late as the 1960s, like those in Zhang Jiading, *Tales and Legends of Cao Xueqin* (Cao Xueqin chuanshuo gushi).

145. *Systematic Materia Medica* lists *qin* as sweet, cold, and nontoxic. It is used in a variety of cures, topically for various bites and toxins, and for curing cases of pathogenic humidity and heat.

146. "Medical Virtue of Mr. Celery" (Qinpu Xiansheng de yide) in Dong Xiaoping, *Honglou meng de chuanshuo*, 56–57.

147. This likely refers to the area west of Beijing where Cao is supposed to have lived.

148. All Manchu households were placed into one of eight administrative or military divisions known as "banners."

149. "The Origins of Cao Xueqin." in Dong Xiaoping, *Honglou meng de chuanshuo*, 8.

150. When Cao Xueqin names prescriptions, there is inevitably a comment in the margins—"well-named pill" (*hao wanming*)—suggesting that the prescription's value was primarily literary and not practical. E.g., the comment on Bao-chai's "cold fragrance pill." Feng Qiyong, Qixin Chen, and Xueqin Cao *Bajia pingpi*, 159.

151. Chu Renhuo, author of the *The Romance of the Sui and Tang Dynasties* (Sui Tang yanyi, 1695), saw his own novel as a kind of moral "account book" (*zhangbu*). Chu, Renhuo, *Xiuxiang Sui Tang yanyi*, preface.

4. DISEASES OF SEX

1. *Jinping mei cihua*, 79.17b. *Plum in the Golden Vase*, 639.

2. One of the most prominent physicians of the Jin-Yuan period, Zhu Zhenheng, who is often -cited in *Plum in the Golden Vase* and other novels, wrote a preface to his "Views on Extending Medical Knowledge" (Gezhi yulun, ca. 1347) explicitly warning against the dangers of these excesses, and devoted the first two chapters to "admonitions on food and drink" and "admonitions on sexual desire."

3. For instance, the corrupt official Cai Jing's name puns on money (*cai*) and semen (*jing*); Ximen Qing leaves behind a few pieces of loose silver after an assignation with Pan Jinlian, with "leaves behind" (*liu*) punning with "dribbling" (*liu*), equating silver and semen; and there is a similar equation between excessive sexual desire (*yin*) and silver (*yin*) throughout the text, reinforcing the equation between sex and money. See Satyendra, "Metaphors of the Body"; Roy, *Plum in the Golden Vase*, vol. 1, introduction.

4. The commentator Zhang Zhupo uses the terms "retribution" (*bao* and *baoying*) to describe the author's rendering of Ximen Qing and other characters "*dufa*." See Rolston, "How to Read *Jinping mei*," 210, 214, 232, 240.

5. *Yinhan*, for instance, which can be translated as "genital coldness," is discussed in a variety of medical texts as a cause of female and male infertility.

Here, it is likely caused by yang depletion and a consequent abundance of cold. Doctors counteract *yinhan* with heating drugs (including those used as vaginal suppositories). Some of these texts refer to the malady as "*shanghan* from lasciviousness *jiase shanghan*]." As for *bian du*, there is an entire essay on *bian du* in the *Formulas for Universal Benefit* (*juan* 290) that seems to be copied from *Easy and Direct Formulas of Mr. Yang Shiying* (Renzhai zhi zhi, Song dynasty, edited in Ming, *juan* 23). The eminent Ming doctor Sun Yikui wrote an explicit comparison of *bian du* and *yangmei* (syphilis) in his *Pearls of Wisdom from the Crimson Sea* (Chishui xuanzhu, 1584, *juan* 30); and another towering Ming medical figure who explains *bian du* in detail is Wang Kentang, in his massive compendium *Guidelines for Treating Illness* (Zhengzhi zhunsheng, compiled 1597–1607, *juan* 111). *Bian du* means something along the lines of "toxic accumulation in the groin," is manifested by swelling, nodes, and sores in the region of relief. Thanks to Yi-Li Wu for these references. *Bian du* was identified by "swelling and nodes that have developed because of collections resulting from a clash of decayed essence/semen with blood." *Effective Formulas from Generations of Physicians* (Shiyi de xiaofang, 1337), quoted in Zhang Zhibin and Zhibin and Unschuld, *Dictionary*, 65.

6. For instance, Li Guijie uses the term "boils and chancres from heaven" (*tian pao chuang*), which in the Ming and Qing designated ugly sores on the skin caused by *yangmei* or *mafeng* (*Jinping mei cihua*, 74.7a, 79.18b). See Leung, *Leprosy in China*, 256n.15. Descriptions of sores accompanied by the "white turbidity" (*baizhuo*) that later became known as gonorrhea are detailed in Qi Dezhi's *Essence of Surgery* (Waike jingyi) of about 1335. Dikötter argues that while gonorrhea seems to have been known and accurately described much earlier than syphilis, "none of these infections, however, was recognized as being transmitted by sexual intercourse [until syphilis became prevalent], although Tang physicians realized that sexual promiscuity encouraged the spread of contagious disease. Called painful urination [*linzhuo*], gonorrhea was thought to be limited to penile pain during urination and viscid discharges from the urethra. According to Chinese pathology, it was a benign disease that was due to an attack of wetness-heat evil on the urinary bladder" ("Sexually Transmitted Diseases," 341; Van Gulik, *Sexual Life*, 182; Wong, "Notes on Chinese Medicine," 1918, 353).

7. Such diseases included boils and sores/ furuncle (*dingchuang*), evil sores (*echuang*), *yangmei* sores (*yangmei chaung*), leprosy (*fenglai*), scabies/ ringworm (*jiexuan*), heat sores (*rechuang*), ulcerated *yangmei* sores (*yangmei gan xie*), carbuncles (*yongju*), lumbar dorsal carbuncles (*jifabei*), leprosy with tinea and sores (*dafeng xuanchuang*), "sores all over the body which are even worse on the scrotum and both feet," and illnesses like *bian du* [*bian du deng zheng*]. Li, *Bencao gangmu*, 17.21.

8. Li, *Bencao gangmu*, e.g., 30.28.

9. Description under *dafeng zi* (Li, *Bencao gangmu*, 1.48).

10. Li, *Bencao gangmu*, 4.21.

11. *Bian du* was discussed often in the *Comprehensive Record of the Section on Medicine* (Yibu quanlu), a work of the Qing, and mentioned a few

times in the *Continuation of the Cases from Famous Doctors, Arranged by Category* (Xu Mingyi lei'an, ca. 1770), but does not seem to occur much if at all in fictional works after the Ming.

12. This story appears in *Words to Structure the World* (aka *Tales of the World's Exemplars*; Xingshi yan, 1632) and was likely written in the 1630s by the largely unknown writer Lu Renlong, "A Husband Leaves His Wife," 37.12b.

13. Grant, *Chinese Physician*, 103–54. *Stone Mountain Medical Cases* was the first collection of medical cases published. An influential medical text, often reprinted, it was also included in the *Complete Library of the Four Treasuries*.

14. *Jinping mei cihua*, 100.6b; *Zhang Zhupo piping diyi qishu*, 100.6b.

15. *Jinping mei cihua*, 100.12b; *Zhang Zhupo piping diyi qishu*, 100.13a.

16. Hanson, *Speaking of Epidemics*, 7.

17. Leung, *Leprosy in China*, 32–33.

18. Volkmar, "Concept of Contagion," 149–50.

19. Leung, *Leprosy in China*, 38.

20. Gong Tingxian, *Wanbing hui chun*, 966. The term "careless while traveling" probably refers to men carelessly seeking sexual pleasure during their travels. The consequence would be contagion by sexual intercourse or contact with materials contaminated by the sick.

21. Strickmann, *Chinese Magical Medicine*, 35–38.

22. Gong Tingxian, *Jishi quanshu*, 1066.

23. Zhibin and Unschuld, *Dictionary*, 639.

24. *Golden Mirror of the Medical Lineage, juan* 73.

25. Hanson, *Speaking of Epidemics*, 92–103.

26. See Kuriyama "Epidemics," 10.

27. The ideas in this section are largely taken from Leung, "Evolution."

28. Dikötter, *Sex, Culture, and Modernity*; Furth, *A Flourishing Yin*; Hanson, *Speaking of Epidemics*.

29. By the late Qing, *yangmei* was known to be sexually transmitted, though some still believed it to be caused primarily by transgression. One prescription in the Berlin medical manuscripts ("Good Recipes that Have Proved to Be Effective" [Yingyan liangfang], SBB Slg. Unschuld 8082, late nineteenth century) for treating "red bayberry toxin knot" (*yangmei jiedu*, presumably syphilis) is followed by the comment that it is "transmitted from a prostitute boat" (*changchuan chuanlai*), which is to say that professional groups transmitted certain relevant prescriptions among themselves, and that in this case the cure for syphilis was transmitted from the prostitutes to the doctor. In this case the prescription and the illness share a vector. Some medical manuscripts from the Republican period show a great deal of interest in syphilis and venereal disease but do not include antibacterial prescriptions.

30. Li, *Bencao gangmu*, 18.27.

31. Ibid.

32. Li, *Bencao gangmu*, 18.27. Li writes, in the same entry (*tufuling*), "Nowadays persons who love lewdness [*haoyin zhi ren*] often suffer from red bayberry poison sores [*yangmei du chuang*]."

33. Zeitlin, *Historian of the Strange*, 61–65.

34. Yi Ming, *Essentials of Domestic Living*, chapter on "protecting life" *weisheng*.

35. As Hanson notes, Chen exchanged the original 梅 *mei*, of *yangmei* and *meichuang*, meaning "Myrica berry" that rotting sores resemble, for the homonym *mei* 黴, meaning "damp" or "moldy," and subsequent publications wrote the title as *mei* 霉, or "rotten," pointing also to the meaning "corrupt" (*Speaking of Epidemics*, 88).

36. Chen Sicheng, *Meichuang milu*, 10. Based on the 1885 edition.

37. Ibid., 6.

38. Chen Sicheng, *Meichuang milu*, 10–11. Translation modified from Leung, *Leprosy in China*, 46.

39. Evil qi was pathogenic evil that could harm from outside or inside. Drugs used to treat it also treated demons, spirit beings, and *gu* poison. It was also related to "wind evil," "summer heat evil," "dampness evil," and so on.

40. Zhang Hong in Yang Bin, "Zhang on Chinese Southern Frontiers," 172–73.

41. Wu Qian et al., *Yizong jinjian*, 52.78.

42. The idea that *chuanran* contamination could be a factor in the spread of epidemic diseases began to be discussed in the seventeenth century. See Hanson, *Speaking of Epidemics*.

43. Xiao Xiaoting, *Fengmen quanshu*, 1:9a.

44. Kuriyama, "Epidemics," 9.

45. Ibid.

46. "The Bell Doctor's Handbook" (Lingyi shouce), SBB Slg. Unschuld 8253; Unschuld and Zheng, *Chinese Traditional Healing*, 1340.

47. "Hand-copied Miscellaneous Pharmaceutical Recipes" (Yaofang zachao), SBB Slg. Unschuld 8167. Syphilis becomes a topic of great interest to a wide variety of doctors in the late Qing and Republican periods. One manuscript ("Handcopied Miscellaneous Medical Recipes Transmitted through the Generations" [Shichuan yifang zachao], SBB Slg. Unschuld 8138), copied at the beginning of the Republican period, records seventy prescriptions, thirty of them for venereal diseases such as syphilis. Late Qing manuscripts often focus on opium smoking, syphilis, malaria, scrofula, and dysentery. Unschuld and Zheng, *Chinese Traditional Healing*, 1087.

48. Unschuld and Zheng, *Chinese Traditional Healing*, 64–65.

49. Few dispute the fact that the arrival of syphilis in Europe coincided with the return of Columbus's men from Hispanola in 1493, but whether the two events are connected is hotly debated. There is similarly no clear geography of the disease's transmission to China, but it was likely first introduced by (Portuguese?) traders to the ports of Guangdong in the sixteenth century, as a 1502 medical work recorded that it was called "boils of Guangdong" (*guangchuang*) by the people of the lower Yangzi region.

50. *Lai* was used to refer to a variety of contagious diseases, including leprosy and syphilis.

51. Quoted in Zhou Zuoren, "On Passing the Itch," 45.

52. Ibid.

53. Leung, in *Leprosy in China*, details how the concept of "selling the sickness" had a strong effect on medical theory.

54. Wu Jianren, *Ershi nian mudu*, 547–49.

55. Leung, *Leprosy in China*, 118.

56. Quoted in Leung, *Leprosy in China*, 116.

57. Quoted in Zhou Zuoren, "On Passing the Itch," 45.

58. It also points to a male anxiety toward female sexual activity, particularly outside of the bonds of marriage.

59. For the cult of female chastity, see Theiss, *Disgraceful Matters*.

60. Furth, "Androgynous Males," 1. Daily-use encyclopedias invariably had chapters on "foreigners" (*zhuyi, waiyi*) depicting a great variety of biological variation. Encyclopedias also always contained chapters on fertility and birth (*taichan*).

61. The Berlin medical manuscripts attest to this with their great variety of aphrodisiac recipes and prescriptions for conceiving.

62. The concept of the "stone maiden" persisted well into the modern period. Tsung writes, "Some naive girls are talked into having [premarital] sexual relations with men to prove that they are not 'stone girls' [*shinü*]" (*Moms, Nuns, and Hookers*, 44). Chai Fuyuan details the varieties of "stone maidens" in his *ABC of Sexology* (Xingxue ABC), 115–16.

63. Li, *Bencao gangmu*, 52.37.

64. The fifth or "pulse" is a woman with highly erratic menses, often the result of an emotional condition.

65. A variant of "stone maiden" (shinü) is "solid maiden" (*shinü*). Shen Yaofeng, author of *Master Shen's Essentials of Medicine for Women* (Shen-shi nüke qiyao, 1850, with preface by Wang Shixiong), suggests that "drums" can be cured in infancy by surgery (19).

66. Furth, "Androgynous Males," 20–22.

67. Ibid.

68. Li Yu, *Bian nü wei er*, in Li Yu, *Silent Operas*, 137–59.

69. All of the text in quotations is from the *Thousand Character Classic*. (*Peony Pavilion*, scene 17).

70. The locus classicus from Zhuangzi reads, "The emperor of the South Sea was called Swift, the emperor of the North Sea was called Sudden, and the emperor of the central region was called Chaos [*hundun*]. Swift and Sudden from time to time came together for a meeting in the territory of Chaos, and Chaos treated them very generously. Swift and Sudden, devising a way to repay Chaos' generosity, said, "Human beings all have seven openings through which they see, hear, eat, and breathe. Chaos alone is without them." They then attempted to bore holes in Chaos, each day boring one hole. On the seventh day, Chaos died. *Zhuangzi*, 98.

71. In *Li Yu quanji, juan* 9, 195–97.

72. Sommer discusses Qing court cases that center around "stone maidens," in which the woman not only symbolizes chaos but literally creates practical dilemmas for the marriage market and the legal system ("Gendered Body," 20–22).

73. Suchen recommends a similar treatment for the emperor, who suffers depletion from too much intercourse with women. He prescribes the emperor to lie down with one young boy hugging him from behind, and another hugging him from the front, thereby infusing him with *yang* energy. (Xia, *Yesou puyan*, chapter 96).

74. Xia, *Yesou puyan*, chapter 94. Quoted in McMahon, *Misers, Shrews, and Polygamists*, 160.

75. Xia, *Yesou puyan*, chapter 96, 1099. Huli Zheng points out that this is clearly a process of domestication, of taming barbarians, but it is also about restoring bodily order, curing non-Chinese sexual bodies with a Chinese sexual body (*Encountering the Other*, 102).

76. Xia, *Yesou puyan*, chapter 102, 1178.

77. Ibid.

78. Feng Menglong, "The Fan Tower Restaurant," 275–90. This story is also discussed by Zeitlin in *Phantom Heroine*.

79. Zeitlin, *Phantom Heroine*, 136.

80. Tang Xianzu, *Mudan ting*, 1. As Huang explains, in the late Ming, the term *qing* included "sexual desire," but was gradually divorced from this meaning in Qing-era fiction (*Desire and Fictional Narrative*, chapter 3).

81. When responding to the judge's question about Liniang's cause of death, the Flower Spirit explains, "She was tenderly entwined in a dream of a young scholar when a chance fall of petals startled her into wakefulness. Passionate longings brought about her death." See Tang Xianzu, *Peony Pavilion*, scene 23, "Infernal Judgment," 130. The phrase "to die from longing for sex/desire" appears in the title of the *huaben* story that was the probable source for the play.

82. Hua Wei, "How Dangerous Can the Peony Be?," 751.

83. Tang Xianzu, *Mudan ting*, *juan* 7 and 16. Phrases such as *hailin de*, *niniao qulai*, *huaming liulu*, and *nian huanong liulin* refer to dribbling urine, and thus sometimes are interpreted by medical historians as referring to the penile discharges associated with biomedical gonorrhea. The last phrase, though, can also point to dallying with women and becoming depleted through such dalliance. Appropriating a term for male behavior and applying it to virginal Du Liniang, even if it does not refer explicitly to biomedical syphilis (as Birch believes it does; see Tang Xianzu, *Peony Pavilion*, 28, 76), emphasizes her longing as a sexual one and its attendant maladies.

84. See Tang Xianzu, *Mudan ting*, 74n25.

85. Tang Xianzu, *Tang Xianzu quanji*, 644–45.

86. Ibid. I follow Huang, *Desire*, 5.

87. Elsewhere, Tang Xianzu even expressed his admiration for Tu's romantic lifestyle; see his poem "Huai Dai Siming xiansheng bingwen Tu Changqing" in Tang Xianzu, *Shiwen ji, juan* 7, 202–3.

88. Li, *Bencao gangmu*, 1.11. In at least one encyclopedia, too, *yangmei* is listed under the heading "good prescriptions for [diseases] of retribution [*yingyan liangfang*]." "Spitting blood and blood in the phlegm" is also listed under this category.

89. See Martinson, *Pao Order*, 136–218.

90. E.g., such commentaries include the following: "How could the retribution due a character as vicious as Ximen Qing be complete without his wife becoming a prostitute?" (*Zhang Zhupo piping diyi qishu*, chapter 18); "It is certainly fitting that the imperial commissioner's retribution [*huanbao*] should come in the form of Lady Lin's adultery with Ximen Qing"; ". . . . Clearly [Ying Bojue] is another Ximen Qing who will suffer a similar indescribable retribution for his own sins" (chapter 23); and "Ximen Qing does not have a single relative from his own family. The retribution [*baoying*] meted out by Heaven is cruel enough, but the author's hatred for him is also virulent" (chapter 86).

91. *Jinping mei cihua*, 3.1a.

92. *Jinping mei cihua*, 3.1a; *Plum in the Golden Vase*, 1.62. This poem is not in the Chongzhen or Zhang Zhupo editions, likely because of a change to most of the verse passages rather than any systematic attempt to eliminate references to venereal disease, since such mention is not excised from prose passages.

93. *Zhang Zhupo piping diyi qishu*, 1269.

94. Ibid., 1296.

95. Xu Dachun, "Bing you guishen lun," 1.38a–b.

96. Zeng Pu, *Niehai hua*, 343.

97. Berg suggests this major theme in *Carnival in China*, 112–14.

98. Ibid., 1–3.

99. The close homophones *tian bao chuang* and *tian pao chuang* (boils and chancre sent from heaven) were often used interchangeably. The former are discussed in *Marriage Destinies* in chapters 11, 153; 25, 337; and 93, 1136. "Retributory chancres" (*baoying chuang*) are mentioned in chapter 66.

100. Chapters 6, 7, 25, 39, and 93.

101. Chapter 39.

102. Xizhousheng, *Xingshi Yinyuan Zhuan*, chapter 39, 508–10.

103. *Xingshi Yinyuan Zhuan*, chapter 93, 1135.

104. Ibid., chapter 93, 1136. This description is similar to those of Ximen Qing's illness causing his bone marrow to dry up. The illness of "penis shrinkage" is not acknowledged by elite medicine but was apparently widely recognized among the general population. It is recorded in one medical manuscript as resulting from "excessive sexual intercourse." Unschuld and Zheng, *Chinese Traditional Healing*, 798.

105. *Xingshi Yinyuan Zhuan*, chapter 93, 1136. Cheng An exhibits venereal ulcers (*yukou*), a symptom also displayed by Li Ping'er in *Plum in the Golden Vase*.

106. Dohi, *Beitrage*, 32. While the use of mercury had moments of popularity and disrepute, the side-effects of taking it were often misdiagnosed as symptoms of syphilis itself.

107. *Xingshi Yinyuan Zhuan*, chapter 93, 1136.

5. DISEASES OF *QING*

1. *Plum in the Golden Vase*, 17.349.

2. Roy translates this as "a consumptive inflammation of the bones." *Plum in the Golden Vase*, 1:349–50; *Jinping mei cihua* edition, 17.7b–8a;

Chongzhen edition, 214. The Zhang Zhupo commentary (*Gaohetang pip-ing diyi qishu*, 17.8b) has "points to yin depletion leading to inner heat." The phrase that Dr. Jiang uses, "necessarily of the category of the family of [fatal] melancholic [disorders]" is taken from a story titled "The Story of Mr. Penglai" (Penglai xiansheng), which contains a similar plot scenario. The story is found in the *Emulative Frowns Collection* (Xiaopin ji), the postface to which is dated 1428. But the phrase in "Story of Mr. Penglai" refers to the deadliness of unrestrained emotion, and it was the author of the *Plum in the Golden Vase* who made it clear that it was "bone steaming" that was related to the six passions and the seven emotions, and in particular static conges-tion *yujie*. "The Story of Mr. Penglai" does suggest that the (fatal) melan-choly syndrome was contagious, with the suggestion to bury the clothes and gifts of the beloved dead for fear of infection or contagion (*ranji*).

3. *Plum in the Golden Vase*, 1.349; 363 (Roy).

4. Ibid., 1.351.

5. *Jinping mei cihua*, 59.15a.

6. *Plum in the Golden Vase*, 5.412.

7. In his survey of *kewu*, Cullen shows how what he terms the "non-ratio-nalistic discourse" of this children's illness persisted in certain contexts. Cul-len, "Threatening Stranger," 39–62.

8. *Plum in the Golden Vase*, 4.59.

9. Ibid., 4.33, 46.

10. Ibid., 4.49.

11. The authorship is uncertain, but it seems that Xue Ji (1487–1559) is the likeliest candidate. It contains entries on over three hundred medicinal substances and is illustrated by almost five hundred paintings in color.

12. *Shiwu bencao*, late Ming Wellcome Library, image number L0039387.

13. *Jinping mei cihua*, 17.4b.

14. *Plum in the Golden Vase*, 4.35.

15. Ibid., 4.50.

16. BCGM 12.31.

17. Ibid.

18. It is also made clear that white *jiguanhua* is to treat diseases with whitish discharge, and red flowers are to treat those with bloody discharge. BCGM 15.26.

19. Xifeng is approximately the same age when she dies, perhaps twenty-six.

20. *Plum in the Golden Vase*, 4.42.

21. Ibid., 4.46.

22. Ibid.

23. The *heishu* was a generic term for the esoteric numerological and divi-natory texts used by yin-yang masters and diviners to ascertain information about the past and future lives of the deceased, based on the dates of their birth and death.

24. This refers to cases in which the earthy branches that occur in a per-son's horoscope and the five phases that are correlated with them are thought to conflict with each other.

25. He also predicts that in her next life, she will die from a fit of anger at age forty-one. *Plum in the Golden Vase*, 4.76.

26. Ibid., 3.489.

27. Ibid., 3.340–42. *Jinping mei*, 54.18b–19a.

28. *Plum in the Golden Vase*, 3.346.

29. Hanan believes that chapter 55 was edited first, and then chapter 54 was edited by a different person. Hanan, "Text of the *Chin P'ing Mei*," 32.

30. "Five overstrains" can refer either to "overstrains of the five Viscera" (liver, heart, spleen, lungs, and kidneys), which can happen from exhaustion or excessive emotion, or, to the "five pathological conditions" (overstrained seeing, lying, sitting, standing, and walking, which will damage the blood, the vital energy, the muscle, the bone, and the tendons, respectively). The seven impairments are too much food, impairing the spleen; too much anger, causing adverse flow of vital energy and impairing the liver; prolonged sitting in a damp place, injuring the kidneys; cold weather or drinking of cold beverages, injuring the lungs; too much sorrow and anxiety, injuring the heart; excessive wind and rain, cold, and summer heat, impairing the constitution; and great shock, impairing thought.

31. BCGM 3.34. "Qi" in this context also refers to semen, as in the phrase "astringing primordial qi," or stopping seminal emission.

32. Grant finds that exhaustion (*lao*) is the leading factor in male illness, with 40 percent of male patients diagnosed with it, and 20 percent of female patients. Grant, *Chinese Physician*, 69–90.

33. Xu Dachun, *Huixi Yian*.

34. Furth, *Flourishing Yin*, 300.

35. Ibid., 48.

36. Zhu Zhenheng, *Additional Discourses on Extending Knowledge through the Investigation of Things* (Gezhi yulun, comp. 1347), "Seyu zheng," 8a.

37. Medical manuscripts sometimes refer to involuntary seminal emission as "to let down the white" (*diaobai*), and they were also quite concerned with this malady.

38. Shapiro, "Puzzle of Spermatorrhea," 557.

39. SBB Slg. Unschuld 48024.

40. E.g., Ms. 8138, 8747, 48024, and 8180.

41. Shapiro, "Puzzle of Spermatorrhea," 553.

42. Unschuld and Zheng, *Chinese Traditional Healing*, 922.

43. *Annals of Herbs and Trees*, play, scene 10.

44. "Treatise on Yang Being Abundant and Yin Being Insufficient" in Zhu Zhenheng, *Gezhi yulun, juan* 2, 4b–5a.

45. Quoted in Unschuld and Zheng, *Chinese Traditional Healing*, 2709.

46. Compiled by Wang Kentang (1549–1613). Shapiro, "Puzzle of Spermatorrhea," 557.

47. Zhu Zhenheng, *Danxi zhifa xinyao* (Danxi's Method from the Heart), *juan* 66.

48. Ibid.

49. Quoted in Shapiro, "Puzzle of Spermatorrhea," 558.

50. BCGM 3.52

51. One edition of the recension of *Sequel to Plum in the Golden Vase* is titled *Flower Shadows on the Curtain* [Demonstrating] *Retribution over Three Lives, Newly Engraved with Commentary.*

52. E.g., those who suffered from *yangmei* were being punished for their licentiousness. Smallpox, for instance, was surrounded by popular rituals that called attention to the uncleanliness of sex and of the female reproductive body. Parents were to abstain from intercourse during their child's illness, and menstruating women were to keep out of the sickroom. This ritual is observed (and violated) by Xifeng's husband, Jia Lian, in *Story of the Stone* (1.21.424). For more on retributory illnesses, see Schonebaum, "Medicine," 172–79.

53. *Story of the Stone*, 1.12.251. Eifring translates both as "lovesickness," but it is important to keep in mind that they also have implications of sin and retribution ("Psychology of Love," 300).

54. "Melancholy distempers" in Hawkes's translation (*Story of the Stone*, 1.8.189).

55. Hawkes translates it as "retributory illness" (*Story of the Stone*, 1.12.251). For a discussion of Jia Rui, see chapter 2 of this volume.

56. *Story of the Stone*, chapter 12.

57. Wang Ji cited in Grant, *Chinese Physician*, 112.

58. See Shapiro "Puzzle of Spermatorrhea," 560.

59. That is, except as the depleting object of man's uncontrolled desire and expenditure. Shapiro, "Puzzle of Spermatorrhea," 562.

60. E.g., BCGM 13.11, 52.29. Some drugs treat continual uterine bleeding as well as seminal emission (e.g., 9.29, 13.11, 14.21, 35.07, 51.15, 52.29). One drug, if overdosed, causes seminal emission in men and uterine bleeding in women (BCGM 20.03). Li claims of many drugs that they treat seminal emission due to consumptive disease (*laoji, chuanshi, guizhu*) and depleted states.

61. Unschuld and Zheng, *Chinese Traditional Healing*, 2746.

62. Furth, *Flourishing Yin*, 79.

63. Dai Yuanli, *Michuan zhengzhi yaojue, juan* 5.

64. Zhang Junfang, *Yunji qiqian, juan* 32, quotes *Medical Ethics Discussed by Doctors Throughout the Ages* (*Lidai* Mingyi lun Yide) to substantiate this claim.

65. BCGM 3.34.

66. Quoted in Furth, *Flourishing Yin*, 71–72.

67. Quoted in Furth, "Blood, Body, Gender," 304.

68. Ibid.

69. Ibid., 305.

70. Ibid.

71. Ibid., 306.

72. Yi-Li Wu has pointed out to me that some medical texts, such as the *Yizong jinjian*, may have used 蟲 *chong* (bug, worm) to write 爞 *chong*, meaning to be fumigated or steamed by hot qi, as noted in the *Kangxi Dictionary* (Kangxi cidian) and commentaries to the *Book of Songs*. Private correspondence.

73. *Zhong'e* is an early term used in pre-Tang works for symptoms of sudden pain and fullness in the abdomen, constipation, coma, etc., due to a

sudden attack of malignant, pathogenic factors. See Cullen and Lo, *Medieval Chinese Medicine*, 423.

74. Lin Daiyu's illness is a prominent exception, given her karmic "debt of tears." Yet her consumption is always discussed in the novel as being caused by her sadness or lovesickness.

75. This is also the case with the ailment known as "ghost fetus" (*guitai*). See Wu, "Ghost Fetuses," 184–95.

76. Consumption worms (*laochong*) were discussed by a broad group of healers well into the Republican period. For instance, one medical manuscript in the Berlin collections dating to the 1930s or 1940s presents a "technique of restoring to life patients suffering from consumption" (*laozhai huanzhe zhi huishengshu*). The author claims to be able to use drugs to detect if "consumption worms" are present inside the patient's body. Included is a detailed explanation of how to persuade an audience on the road to accept treatment. Ms, 8033, 786.

77. Wu, "Body, Gender and Disease," 101.

78. Wu Yi-Li, *Reproducing Women*, chapter 1. Chen Hsiu-fen examines this shift in the history of stagnation syndromes (*yuzheng*). Chen Hsiu-fen, "Between Passion and Repression," 51–82.

79. Ding Yaokang, *Xu Jinping mei*, 44.340.

80. Ibid., 44.8b–9b.

81. Furth, *Flourishing Yin*, 32. Another medieval work that instead of healing focused on the bedchamber arts, the *Secrets of the Jade Chamber* (Yufang mijue, six dynasties period), reiterated this medical view that sexual frustration and erotic thoughts often result in "having sex with demons." (Hsiu-fen Chen, "Between Passion and Repression," 52).

82. Sun Simiao, *Beiji qianjin yaofang*, 389.

83. Hsiu-fen Chen, "Between Passion and Repression," 59. The comparative difference is presumably related to women's more restricted access to sex.

84. Ibid., 62. *Yuzheng* might also be translated "depression disorder," since it was frequently linked to extreme melancholy.

85. Xue Ji (approximately 1488–1558), e.g., in *Annotations on Good Prescriptions for Women* (Jiaozhu furen liangfang), 6:16. See Chen Hsiu-fen, "Between Passion and Repression," 61.

86. In Chinese, "*gui*" generally refers to "the spirits or souls of a dead person" (e.g., deceased ancestors), which seems to be equivalent to "ghost" in English. However, the "*gui*" in "*meng yu guijiao*" as recorded in classic Chinese medical texts has more ambiguous connotations. It could refer to ghosts, evil spirits, devils, fox fairies, or a malignant supernatural being. I thus interpret "*gui*" as "demons" unless otherwise specified. As for the different meanings of "ghost," see Zeitlin, *Phantom Heroine*, 4–5.

87. Unschuld and Zheng, *Chinese Traditional Healing*, 1349. Another manuscript has a recipe to treat "bewitchment by coquettish fox spirits"; see chapter 2 of this volume.

88. Both trends are usually identified as beginning in the seventeenth century and peaking in the eighteenth. For the former, see Ko, *Teachers*; for the latter, see Theiss, *Disgraceful Matters*.

89. Furth, "Blood, Body and Gender," 61. Zhang Ji, *Jinkui yaolue lunzhu* (Commentaries and annotations on medical treasures of the golden casket), 6:90–91.

90. Feng Menglong, "Jiang Xingge chonghui zhenzhu shan" (Jiang Xingge reencounters his pearl shirt), 28.

91. Dating back to the great preface of the *Book of Songs*, "Poetry expresses what is intently in the heart" (*shiyan zhi*) is one of the earliest formulations of that genre.

92. For a more detailed argument about these characters, see Schonebaum, "Medicine." For Daiyu, see chapter 82, 2519, 2521, and 2523; chapter 96, 2913; and chapter 97, 2919. Qin Shi's deficiency of blood (*xinqi xu er sheng huo*) is discussed in chapter 10, 283. Adamantina's illness is "heat which allowed pathogenic influx" (*zou moru huo*), chapter 87. Aroma coughs blood from taxation (chapter 77). The actress Lingguan (Charmante) coughs blood (chapter 72).

93. See Theiss, *Disgraceful Matters*.

94. Schonebaum, "Medicine." *Honglou meng*, chapters 55, 69, and 74, respectively.

95. *Honglou meng*, chapters 93, 110, and 111, respectively.

96. Ibid., chapter 10.

97. The detailed prescription for Qin Shi bears out a condition of depletion. A textual crisis (that Qin Shi's death is foretold in chapter 5 to be one of suicide by hanging, and then she dies of depletion and blood loss in chapter 12) is explained by a red inkstone (actually "odd tablet") comment "that 'Qin Keqing dies in the Celestial Fragrance Pavilion because of her licentiousness [*yinsang*]' indicates the author's historiographical style ... [but] this Old Codger let her off the hook and ordered Xueqin and Meixi to delete [the incident of incest?] *pingyu*" (Cao Xueqin, *Xinbian Shitou ji Zhiyan zhai*, 253). The consequent illness is thus one that points to licentiousness / sexual transgression.

98. This formulation seems to be original to *Story of the Stone*.

99. *Story of the Stone*, 5:372; *Honglou meng*, 1602.

100. *Story of the Stone*, 4:343. Daiyu is told not to worry so much; on at least three occasions she is told that she is making herself ill. *Story of the Stone* 1:410, 2:134, 4:67.

101. A further aspect is that by this time Daiyu has decided to will her own death.

102. *Honglou meng*, chapter 34.

103. That *Story of the Stone* attempts to separate depletion disorders into those caused by desire or lust and those caused by passionate longing is reflective of what Martin Huang has identified as the unresolvable tension between *qing* and *yu* in *Story of the Stone*. *Story of the Stone* is held up as the most powerful synthesis achieved in the Chinese literature of desire, since it concludes in a way that avoids the desexualization of *qing* while fully acknowledging the difficulty of reconciling *qing* and *yu*. Carlitz, "Review," 52–158.

104. "The basic sinew" refers to the sexual organ, thought to be the meeting place of all sinews. "White overflow," according to the commentator

Wang Bing, refers to semen in men, and vaginal fluids in women. See Unschuld and Tessenow, Huang Di, *Nei jing su wen*, 658–59.

105. *Story of the Stone* labels Daiyu's illness with a term whose exact formulation is quite rare in any literature. "*Laoqie zhi zheng*" occurs very rarely in that exact that formulation, and "*laoqie*" only a few times in the *Complete Library of the Four Treasuries*. Of those occurrences, all are from Ming and Qing sources. This term seems to be borrowed from Ling Meng-chu's book of vernacular stories *Slapping the Table in Amazement* (Erke paian jingqi, 1628), *juan* 32.

106. Sun Simiao, *Hua Tuo shenfang, juan* 18, item 18012, 251.

107. Chen Hsiu-fen, "Between Passion and Repression," 60.

108. Zhang Jiebin, *Jingyue quanshu*, 16:346. Quoted in Chen Hsiu-fen, "Between Passion and Repression," 55.

109. Li Yanshi, *Maijue huibian*, 3:62.

110. *Zhulin nüke, juan* 1, cited in Wu, Yi-Li, *Reproducing Women*, 257.

111. Peng Dingqiu, *Quan Tang Shi*, 539:41; 802:9027.

112. *Plum in the Golden Vase*, 60.490.

113. For another example of a chaste, consumptive beauty, see Wu Jian-ren, *Ershi nian nudu zhi guai* (Strange events witnessed in the last twenty years), chapter 16.

114. Hanson, "Depleted Men," 303.

115. On the connections between hyperfemininity and masculinity, see Zeitlin, *Phantom Heroine*. See also Huang on *caizi* and femininity, *Negotiating Masculinities*, chapter 7.

116. Hanson, "Depleted men," 303. Unschuld and Zheng (*Chinese Traditional Healing*, 1816–17) note that restorative recipes are almost always found in texts that were written by city dwellers, and thus are not frequently found in the medical manuscripts, which tend to be written by itinerant physicians who travel through the countryside.

117. Hanson, "Depleted Men," 303–4. See Furth, *Flourishing Yin*, 145–51.

118. Grant's claim, in *Chinese Physician*, 134.

119. Hanson, "Depleted Men," 304.

120. Andrew Plaks's book *The Four Masterworks of the Ming Novel* famously makes the case for these novels to be seen as works of great complexity written by and for hyper-literate readers (3–55).

121. *Jinping mei*, 8.129.

122. And those readers, and the readers who were fascinated with them, created a market for depictions of sickly women.

6. CONTAGIOUS TEXTS

1. "A letter on [the courtesan] Lin Daiyu to the 'Master of Entertainment,'" *Youxi bao*, November 2, 1897. Quoted from Yeh, "Shanghai Leisure," 213.

2. In the 1870s, a courtesan surnamed Hu became known by the professional name Lin Daiyu. Another courtesan named Jinbao who admired Hu

took up the name Lin Daiyu and shortly afterward became one of the four most famous courtesans (*sida jingang*) of the late Qing and early Republic, discussed above by Li Boyuan. At least two other well-known courtesans of this period also took Daiyu's name for their own, Lu Daiyu and Su Daiyu. Yeh, *Shanghai Love*, 142.

3. See McMahon, "Eliminating Traumatic Antimonies," 104–7; Widmer, *Beauty and the Book*, 217–48. These sequels to and imitations of *Story of the Stone* were popular in the early modern era, such as *In the Shadow of the Story of the Stone* (Honglou meng ying, 1877), *Dream of the Green Chamber* (Qinglou meng, 1878); in the modern era, with its *True Dream of the Red Chamber* (Honglou zhen meng, 1939); and still are today, with works such as *Murder in the Red Mansion* (Honglou meng sharen shiqing, 2004) and *The Story of Tanchun* (Tanchun ji, 2007).

4. One sequel that is more properly identified as a parody, social satire, or science fiction, Wu Jianren's 1907 *New Story of the Stone* (Xin Shitou ji) finds Baoyu in modern Shanghai, where he learns of Lin Daiyu the courtesan.

5. See the descriptions of Daiyu's life and activities in Hershatter, *Dangerous Pleasures*, 145–52.

6. Yeh writes, "Popular papers … contained almost daily reports on fashion in the Shanghai courtesan world, including the minutest details about the color and cut of their newest outfits." An article titled "Lin Daiyu's Dress Most Extravagant" in *Youxi bao*, October 11, 1897, raves about courtesans' display of beauty and about their competition in fashion on the occasion of the Shanghai Derby's autumn race. *Youxi bao* ran a full-page article with a close-up of Lin Daiyu on May 4, 1899 that read, "Yesterday … Lin Daiyu wore a blue satin gown trimmed with pearls; she was riding in a four-wheeled carriage drawn by black horses, with her coachman dressed in a gray crepe de chine jacket and a black-rimmed straw hat." This detailed report about Lin Daiyu's pearl-embroidered coat helped to make this garment a rage among upper-class wives. One article reports on Lin Daiyu's choice of date to first appear wearing her winter hat for afternoon tea at the fashionable Zhang Garden, and another discusses her choice of auspicious day to open a business. Yeh, *Shanghai Love*, 54.

7. Hershatter, *Dangerous Pleasures*, 150; Chen Boxi, *Lao Shanghai*, 102. Her inspiration for this makeup might have come from her involvement in the stage world. Lin Daiyu was also an active and well-known opera singer who regularly performed at the theater in the Zhang Garden with the all-female Mao'er opera troupe Mao'er Xi (Yeh, *Shanghai Love*, 62).

8. Hershatter, *Dangerous Pleasures*, 150.

9. Hawkes, *Story of the Stone*, 16. Courtesan novels describe women asking the wives of men who frequent courtesan houses to share their knowledge of courtesan fashion and behavior. Yeh writes that some wives, concubines, and even daughters were driven by such curiosity about courtesan lives that they disguised themselves in men's clothes and accompanied their husbands or fathers to the courtesan establishments (*Shanghai Love*, 47).

10. Wang Liaoweng, *Shanghai liushinian huajie shi*, 50–51.

11. David Wang makes a similar claim when he writes of the figure of the courtesan in late Qing fiction that they "may well have prefigured the

emotionally and behaviorally defiant postures of the 'new woman'" portrayed in 1920s women's writing (*Fin-de-siècle Splendor*, 59).

12. For many examples of concepts that were supplanted by Western medicine, see Wong and Wu Lien-Tie, *History of Chinese Medicine*.

13. Zhou Zuoren, "On Passing the Itch," Pollard trans., 94.

14. Ibid.

15. Ibid., 93.

16. Ibid., 95.

17. Zhou essentially updates traditional fiction criticism by claiming that fiction should disseminate scientific knowledge, as opposed to moral messages.

18. Although as early as the 1840 scientists such as Allgemeines Krankenhaus, John Snow, Louis Pasteur, and Joseph Lister had theorized that microorganisms might have the potential to cause disease, it was not until 1876 that Robert Koch isolated the anthrax bacillus, the first bacterium identified as the cause of a disease.

19. Ge Hong, *Baopuzi neiwai pian, juan* 7.20.

20. In the chapter "Prescriptions for Treating Corpse Infestation and Ghost Infestation."

21. Strickmann, *Chinese Magical Medicine*, 25.

22. Unschuld and Zheng, *Chinese Traditional Healing*, 1171 and 166.

23. In China, *La Dame aux Camelias* was reprinted at least four times, rewritten in short story form, serialized, and made into a film by 1932. Committee for Research on Chinese Culture, *Shinmatsu Minsho shosetsu mokuroku*, 15.

24. One of the reasons for its popularity was that *La Dame aux Camelias* (and a year later the opera based on it, *La Traviata*), were not thought not only to be true to life but actually true. This may have appealed to modern Chinese authors and readers who were invested in rectifying the past and making fiction more about conveying truth than titillating with sex and romance (Coward, "Introduction," xv).

25. Lee, *Romantic Generation*, 167.

26. Sontag, *Illness as Metaphor*, 22, 13.

27. Zhang Gongrang, *Feibing ziyi ji*, 8.

28. Nietzsche, Baudelaire, Flaubert, and Maupassant were all famous syphilitic writers. For more on the metaphors and meanings ascribed to syphilis, see Hayden, *Pox*, 111.

29. Zhang Gongrang, *Feibing ziyi ji*, 8–9. See also Andrews, "Tuberculosis," 132. Again, Lin Daiyu is brought to life, this time treated as a "real" poet with a disease from which historical people suffered.

30. This is Rey Chow's observation (*Woman and Chinese Modernity*, 74).

31. Ibid., 75.

32. Dumas, *La Dame aux Camélias*, Lin Shu trans., 139.

33. Ibid.

34. *Boming* is the classical term used to describe unlucky beauties—particularly Lin Daiyu. In the Ming, this term encompassed lusty men too, e.g., "Let the reader take note: there is a limit to one's energies, but desires are

without bound. He whose lusts go deep has a shallow fate [*boming*]. Ximen Qing gave himself up to licentious ways, ignoring [the fact that] when the oil is used up the lamp is extinguished and that when the marrow is exhausted a man dies" (*Jinping mei cihua*, 79.8a–b).

35. Dumas fils, *La Dame aux Camélias*, David Coward trans., 106, 118.

36. Ibid., 119.

37. Ibid., 124.

38. Roland Barthes focuses on the objective gaze that Marguerite seeks to gain and control through her love and illness, arguing that "Marguerite is never anything more than an alienated awareness: she sees that she suffers, but imagines no remedy which is not parasitic to her own suffering; she knows herself to be an object but cannot think of any destination for herself other than that of ornament in the museum of the masters" ("*The Lady of the Camellias*," 103–5).

39. Dumas fils, *Chahua nü*, Lin Shu trans., 89, 131.

40. Ibid., 9.

41. Dumas, *La Dame aux Camélias*, David Coward trans., 10.

42. Ibid., 11.

43. Dumas, *Chahua nü*, Lin Shu trans., 130.

44. Ibid., 39.

45. See Lai Douyan's comments in note 103 below.

46. "Because I have had happiness in my life, I am now paying for it twice over." Dumas, *La Dame aux Camélias*, Lin Shu trans., 141.

47. *The Predestined Affinity of Sickness and Jade* was based on Xuan Ding's (1832–1880) short piece "Story of Qiu Liyu, the *Mafeng* [Leper] Girl" (Mafeng nü Qiu Liyu chuanqi, 1877), and also known by the name "Story of the Leper Girl." Several actresses were famous for their portrayal of Qiu Liyu. For more on *The Predestined Affinity of Sickness and Jade*, see Leung, *Leprosy in China*, 124–31.

48. Viper wine, a treatment for *mafeng*, was found in both medical texts and fiction since the Tang. Leung, *Leprosy in China*, 33.

49. Leung makes this point in *Leprosy in China* (127).

50. Ibid., 129.

51. Modengxianzhai zhuren, *Bing yu yuan chuanqi*, 31.

52. The title change was made to thwart censors. See Shang Wei, "*Stone Phenomenon*." *Bing yu yuan* could also be translated "[Drama of] the Love Story of the Sick Beauty."

53. Translated by Lau as "consumption," and by Barlow as "TB." This is the term used by Xiao Hong in "Hands" (Shou, 1936) and Ba Jin in *Cold Nights* (Hanye, 1947) as well. Lu Xun used the older term *laobing* in "Medicine."

54. Ding, *I Myself Am a Woman*, 78.

55. Ibid., 52.

56. "Shafei nüshi de riji" was published in *Xiaoshuo Yuebao* in 1928, less than three years after Lin Daiyu's highly publicized death. Courtesans re-refigured Daiyu (from the Confucian wish-fulfilling refigurations of the many *Story of the Stone* sequels) to be not only beautiful, sensitive, and gifted, but the emblem of the modern romantic female to be loved and pitied.

57. See Leung, *Leprosy in China*, 84–131.

58. Ding, *I Myself Am a Woman*, 58; Ding, "Shafei nüshi de riji," 340.

59. Ding, *I Myself Am a Woman*, 90.

60. Dumas, *Chahua nü*, Lin Shu trans., 50.

61. Feuerwerker, *Ding Ling's Fiction*, 44.

62. Ding, "Shafei nüshi de riji," 352, 354.

63. Feuerwerker, *Ding Ling's Fiction*, 44.

64. Ding, *I Myself Am a Woman*, 53.

65. Li Jianmin, "Contagion and Its Consequences," 5.

66. Ibid., 20.

67. Ding, *I Myself Am a Woman*, 79.

68. Keaveney, *Subversive Self*, 101.

69. Tang Xiaobing, *Chinese Modern*, 158.

70. From *The Trick of Succeeding on the Literary Scene* (Wentan denglong shu, 1933), quoted in Lee, *Romantic Generation*, 39.

71. *Xulao* is defined in the 1587 *Myriad Ailments Return to Spring*: "Fire surges and burns up 'true yin' [a term for the source of vital energy and reproductive functions], thereby producing coughs, shortness of breath, phlegm, fever, vomiting of blood, bleeding, spontaneous sweating, and nocturnal semen emission." Gong Tingxian, *Wanbing huichun*, 20.

72. Yu Dafu, while writing stories about love denied by national movements, and himself suffering from tuberculosis, felt he was a kindred spirit with Huang Zhongze (Huang Jingren, 1749–1783), the Qianlong-period poet. Yu liked to think that Huang and his wife suffered from tuberculosis, as he himself did (Tang, *Chinese Modern*, 99).

73. Guo Moruo's 1926 novel *Fallen Leaves* (Luoye) is a notable exception, but one that also connects syphilis and tuberculosis.

74. *Chong* can refer to bugs, insects, worms, and their demonic variations. The breadth of this category is indicated in the earliest etymology of *chong*, first used as a name for the viper and then expanded as a general term for anything small that crawls or flies, is hairy or naked, or has shell-like plates or scales (Harper, *Early Chinese Medical Literature*, 74).

75. See Strickmann, *Chinese Magical Medicine*, chapters 1 and 2. Unschuld and Zheng, *Chinese Traditional Healing*, 9–11.

76. They emphasize "bugs as natural and demonic agents of destruction," a concept that can be traced to Shang inscriptions. See Unschuld and Tessenow, *Huang Di nei jing su wen*, 180–83; and Harper, *Early Chinese Medical Literature*, 74.

77. Li Jianmin, "Contagion and Its Consequences," 3. For more on *sha* and "killer demons," "dark afflictions" (*heiqi*), and the epidemic of rumor attending them in the seventeenth and eighteenth centuries, see Haar, *Telling Stories*, chapter 5. On *sha* in *jiezhu wen*, see Liu Zhaoru, "Tan kaogu faxian de Daojiao jiezhu wen," 51–57.

78. Trans. Li Jianmin, "Contagion and Its Consequences," 24.

79. Consumption was caused by or related to conditions called flying corpse (*feishi*), transmission by corpse (*chuanshi*), corpse influx (*shizhu*), ghost pouring (*guizhu*), corpse worm (*shichong*), taxation worm (*laochong*).

Refer to fig. 5.2. All of these terms also appear in the medical manuscripts:
e.g., *chuanshi* is found in BSS Slg. Unschuld, 8420, 8346, 8125; *feishi* in
8385, 8381; *shiqi* in 8453; *guizhu* in 8645; *laochong* in 8559, etc.

80. Quoted in Li Jianmin, "Contagion and Its Consequences," 8.

81. *Plum in the Golden Vase*, 62.61, 62.73.

82. Cao Xueqin, *Honglou meng*, 2:1077; Hawkes, *Story of the Stone*,
78.563.

83. Wang Dao, *Waitai miyao, juan* 13.

84. Hong Mai, Yijian *jiazhi, Chicheng guang zhou* section.

85. Li Jianmin, "Contagion and Its Consequences," 18.

86. Tang Yiji, *Wei Jin nanbei chao*, 361–73.

87. Yang, "Concept of Pao," 299.

88. Strickmann, *Chinese Magical Medicine*, 25.

89. Quoted in Li Jianmin, "Contagion and Its Consequences."

90. Ibid.

91. Andrews, "Tuberculosis," 128. See also Li Jianmin, "Contagion and
Its Consequences," 203.

92. Wu Qian et al., *Yizong jinjian*, 4.485.

93. Gong Tingxian, *Wanbing huichun*, 200.

94. Lei, "Habituating Individuality," 262. A manuscript copied in the
1930s includes a "technique of restoring to life patients suffering from consumption" (*laozhai huanzhe zhi huishengshu*) that was likely copied from
the records of an itinerant healer. The author claims to be able to employ
pharmaceutical drugs to detect whether or not "consumption worms" (*laochong*) are present inside the patient's body. Unschuld and Zheng, *Chinese
Traditional Healing*, 786.

95. Ge Chenghui, "Zhongguoren yu jiehebing," 589.

96. Lei, "Habituating Individuality," 262.

97. Zhang and Elvin, "Environment and Tuberculosis," 523.

98. Ibid., 521.

99. See Andrews, "Tuberculosis," 116–22. We are concerned here with
perceptions, and not with "reality," since creation of statistics for illness and
death at this time was either educated guesswork or the careful collection of
flawed data (e.g., incidence of TB in a hospital taken as reflective of incidence
of TB in the population at large).

100. Unschuld and Zheng, *Chinese Traditional Healing*, 1170–71 and
166.

101. Andrews, "Tuberculosis," 133.

102. Lei, "Habituating Individuality," 260.

103. For instance, Lai Douyan, a graduate from the University of Chicago
and a professor of Public Health at the National Medical College of Shanghai wrote in 1934, "The rich people in our country are quite different from
those in Europe and America. They prefer to congregate in large numbers,
dislike outdoor activities, and call the kind of woman threatened by a gust of
wind a paragon of beauty. The rich, as a result, are more likely than the poor
laboring masses to be infected with tuberculosis. That is the crucial difference between China and the West" (Lei, "Habituating Individuality," 260).

104. According to Sean Lei, in the 1930s, even in the capital of Nanjing, one-third of the city's dying received no medical care at all ("Habituating Individuality," 261).

105. Wong and Wu, *History of Chinese Medicine*, 757–58.

106. China Medical Commission of the Rockefeller Foundation, *Medicine in China*, 2.

107. According to Ott, American medical writers began to associate tuberculosis with poverty and the "dangerous classes" in the 1890s. This reconfigured the identity of the Western consumptive patient and resulted in permanent stigmatization (*Fevered Lives*, 70).

108. Lei, "Habituating Individuality," 261.

109. Li Boyuan, *Guanchang xianxing ji*, 578.

110. Fitzgerald points out that ever since Lord McCartney visited Beijing in 1793, spitting was seen as the trademark of "John Chinaman." The prevalence of this racist stereotype among Westerners and its impact on Chinese national pride was even more evident over a century later when Sun Yatsen (1866–1925), the founding father of the Republic of China and a Western-trained physician, interrupted the last of his public lectures on the "three principles of the people" to counsel his audience against spitting and burping in public "because this habit revealed to Westerners that Chinese people had no control even over their own bodies" (9–12).

111. Lei, "Habituating Individuality," 261.

112. This, even though statistics indicate that from one-third to one-half of Chinese households had only two generations. Lei, "Habituating Individuality," 267.

113. For a detailed account of the antituberculosis movement, see Lei, "Habituating Individuality," 256–52.

114. "In the classics of Chinese medicine, winds [*feng*] cause chills and headaches, vomiting and cramps, dizziness and numbness, loss of speech. And that is but the beginning. 'Wounded by Wind' [*shangfeng*], a person burns with fever. 'Struck by Wind' [*zhongfeng*], another drops suddenly senseless. Winds can madden, even kill.... Chinese doctors traditionally suspected [wind's] ravages in nearly all. 'Wind is the chief of the hundred diseases,' the *Neijing* declared. And again, 'The hundred diseases arise from wind.'" (Kuriyama, "Epidemics, Weather and Contagion," 234).

115. See, e.g., Lu Xun, "Fuqin de bing," 53–57.

116. Zhou, *Bingzhu Houtan*, 96. Zhou is referring to *Unorthodox Observations from Liu Ya* (Liuya waibian), published in 1791, in which Xu Houshan (erroneously) describes the phenomenon of the "winter insect, summer grass" (actually a fungus that grows as a parasite on small insects). Zhou quotes his claim, "With the onset of winter the grasses gradually wither. The insect then pulls itself out of the ground and wriggles along, its tail still swishing the grass attached to it," and derides him for believing that summer grass really did spring from the winter insect.

117. Ibid., 96.

A. Ying 阿英. *Wanqing wenxue congchao: Xiaoshuo xiqu yanjiujuan* 晚清文學叢鈔: 小說戲曲研究卷. Shanghai: Zhonghua Shuju, 1960.

Andrews, Bridie J. "Tuberculosis and the Assimilation of Germ Theory in China, 1895–1937." *Journal of the History of Medicine and Allied Sciences* 52, no. 1 (Jan. 1997): 114–57.

Anonymous. "Cao Xueqin kanbing" 曹雪芹看病 and "Minjian yanfang jiu xianglin" 民間驗方就鄉鄰. In *Zhongguo chuanqi* 中國傳奇, edited by Jiang Tao薑濤 et al., 4:283–96. Taipei: Huayan, 1995.

Anonymous. "Han hua'an suibi" 寒花盦隨筆. In *Jinping mei ziliao huibian* 金瓶梅資料彙編, edited by Hou Zhongyi 侯忠義 and Wang Rumei 王汝梅, 475–76. Beijing: Beijing Daxue Chubanshe, 1985.

Anonymous. *Shanhai jing quanyi* 山海經全譯. Edited and annotated by Yuan Ke袁珂. Guizhou: Guizhou Renmin Chubanshe, 1991.

Anonymous. "Shuang Dou Yi" 雙鬥醫. In *Guben yuanming zaju* 孤本元明雜劇, edited by Wang Shifu 王實甫 and Wang Jilie 王季烈. Taipei: Taiwan Shangwu Yinshuguan, 1977.

Barnes, Linda L., and T. J. Hinrichs, eds. *Chinese Medicine and Healing: An Illustrated History*. Cambridge, MA: Belknap / Harvard, 2013.

Barthes, Roland. "*The Lady of the Camellias*." In Roland Barthes and Annette Lavers. *Mythologies*. New York: Hill and Wang, 1972.

Bartholomew, Terese Tse. "One Hundred Children: From Boys at Play to Icons of Good Fortune." In *Children in Chinese Art*, edited by Ann Elizabeth Barrott Wicks, 57–83. Honolulu: University of Hawai'i, 2002.

Benedict, Carol. *Bubonic Plague in Nineteenth-century China*. Stanford: Stanford University Press, 1997.

Berg, Daria. *Carnival in China: A Reading of the Xingshi Yinyuan Zhuan*. Leiden: Brill, 2002.

———. *Women and the Literary World in Early Modern China: 1580–1700*. New York: Routledge, 2013.

Bréard, Andrea. "Knowledge and Practice of Mathematics in Late Ming Daily Life Encyclopedias." In *Looking at It from Asia: The Processes that Shaped the Sources of History of Science*, edited by Florence Bretelle-Establet, 305–29. New York: Springer, 2010.

Brokaw, Cynthia. *Commerce in Culture: The Sibao Book Trade in the Qing and Republican Periods*. Cambridge, MA: Harvard Asia Center, 2007.

———. *Ledgers of Merit and Demerit: Social Change and Moral Order in Late Imperial China*. Princeton, NJ: Princeton University Press, 1991.

Burton, Robert. *Anatomy of Melancholy*. 1620. New York: New York Review of Books, 2001.

Cao Xueqin 曹雪芹. *Bajia pingpi Honglou meng* 八家評批紅樓夢. Edited by Feng Qiyong 馮其庸 and Chen Qixin 陳其欣. Beijing: Wenhua Yishu Chubanshe 1991.

———. *Honglou meng* 紅樓夢. Beijing: Renmin Chubanshe, 2005.

———. *Honglou meng yibai ershi hui* 紅樓夢一百二十囘. Qianlong period. Call number D8653500. University of Tokyo Library.

———. *The Story of the Stone*. Edited and translated by David Hawkes and John Minford. Vols. 1–5. New York: Penguin, 1973–86.

———. *Xinbian Shitou ji Zhiyan zhai pingyu jijiao* 新編石頭記脂硯齋評語輯校. Edited by Chen Qinghao 陳慶浩. Taipei: Lianjing, 1986.

Carlitz, Katherine. "The Conclusion of the *Jin Ping Mei*." *Ming Studies*, no. 1 (1980): 23–29.

———. "Review of Martin Huang *Desire*." *Harvard Journal of Asiatic Studies* 64, no. 1 (Jun. 2004): 152–58.

———. *The Rhetoric of* Chin P'ing Mei. Bloomington: Indiana University Press, 1986.

Cass, Victoria B. *Dangerous Women: Warriors, Grannies, and Geishas of the Ming*. New York: Rowman and Littlefield, 1999.

Chai Fuyuan 柴福沅. *Xingxue ABC* 性學. Shanghai: ABC Congshu, 1928.

Chao, Yüan-ling. "The Ideal Physician in Late Imperial China: The Question of *Sanshi* 三世." *East Asian Science, Technology, and Medicine*, no. 17 (2000): 66–93.

Chen Boxi 陳伯熙. *Lao Shanghai* 老上海. 2 vols. Shanghai: Shanghai Taidong Tushuju, 1919. Reprinted as *Shanghai Yishi Daguan* (上海軼事大觀). Shanghai: Shanghai Shudian, 2000.

Chen Hongmou. [1742]. *Xunsu yigui* 訓俗遺規. In *Wuzhong yigui* 五種遺規. 1828. Vol. 1. Sibu beiyao edition. 四部備要. Taipei: Zhonghua Shuju, 1984.

Chen Hsiu-fen. "Between Passion and Repression: Medical Views of Demon Dreams, Demonic Fetuses and Female Sexual Madness in Late Imperial China." *Late Imperial China* 32, no. 1 (Jun. 2011): 51–82.

———. "Medicine, Society, and the Making of Madness in Imperial China." PhD thesis, School of Oriental and African Studies, University of London, 2003.

Chen Jiongzhai 陳炯齋. "Liyang chuanran" 癘瘍傳染. In *Nanyue youji* 南越遊記. N.p., 1850.

Chen Sicheng 陳思成. *Meichuang milu* 黴瘡秘錄. Beijing: Xueyuan Chubanshe, 1994.

Chen Yiting. 陳貽庭. "Cong Jinghua yuan kan Li Ruzhen de yiyao yangsheng guan" 從鏡花緣看李汝珍的醫藥養生觀. *Zhonghua yishi zazhi* 中華醫史雜誌 35, no.3 (2005): 165–69.

Chen Yong 陳鏞. "Chusanxuan congtan" 樗散軒叢談. In *Honglou meng ziliao huibian* 紅樓夢資料彙編, edited by Yi Su 一粟, 349–50. Beijing: Zhonghua Shuju, 2003.

Chen Yuanpeng 陳元朋. "Liang Song de 'shang yi shiren' yu ruyi': Jian lun qi zai Jin Yuan de liubian" 兩宋的尚醫士人與儒醫—兼論其在金元的流變. In *Guoli Taiwan daxue wenshi congkan* 國立臺灣大學文史叢刊, 104. Taipei: Guoli Taiwan Daxue Chuban Weiyuanhui, 1997. Chen Ziming 陳自明. *Furen Daquan Liangfang* 婦人大全良方. Beijing: Renmin Weisheng, 1985.

Chia, Lucille. *Printing for Profit*. Cambridge, MA: Harvard University Asia Center, 2002.

China Medical Commission of the Rockefeller Foundation. *Medicine in China*. Chicago: University of Chicago Press, 1914.

Chong Huai 沖懷, ed. *Xinke yejia xincai wanbao quanshu* 新刻鄴架新裁萬寶全書. University of California Berkeley Library, 1614.

Chow, Rey. *Woman and Chinese Modernity: The Politics of Reading between West and East*. Minneapolis: University of Minnesota Press, 1991.

Chu Ping-yi 祝平一. "Song, Ming zhi ji de yishi yu ruyi" 宋、明之際的醫史與儒醫. In *The Bulletin of the Institute of History and Philology, Academia Sinica* 77, part 3 (2006): 401–49.

Chu Renhuo 褚人獲. *Xiuxiang Sui Tang yanyi* 繡像隋唐演義. 1675. Shanghai: ShangwuYinshuguan, [between 1911 and 1949].

Committee for Research on Chinese Culture. *Shinmatsu Minsho shōsetsu mokuroku* 清末民初小說目錄. Osaka: Chūgoku Bungei Kenkyūkai, 1988.

Coward, David. Introduction to *La Dame aux Camelias*, by Alexandre Dumas fils, Oxford: Oxford University Press, 1986. vii–xx.

Cullen, Christopher. "The Threatening Stranger: *Kewu* 客悟 in Pre-modern Chinese Paediatrics." In *Contagion: Perspectives from Pre-Modern Societies*, edited by Lawrence I. Conrad and D. Wujastyk, 39–52. Farnham, UK: Ashgate, 2000.

Cullen, Christopher, and Vivienne Lo, eds. *Medieval Chinese Medicine: The Dunhuang Medical Manuscripts*. New York: Routledge, 2013.

Dai Yuanli 戴元禮. *Michuan zhengzhi yaojue* 秘傳證治要訣. Taipei: Yiwen, 1967.

Dikötter, Frank. *Sex, Culture, and Modernity in China: Medical Science and the Construction of Sexual Identities in the Early Republican Period.* Honolulu: University of Hawai'i Press, 1995.

————. "Sexually Transmitted Diseases in Modern China: A Historical Survey." *Genitourin Med* 69 (1993): 341–45.

Ding Ling 丁玲.—"Miss Sophia's Diary." In Ding Ling, *I Myself Am a Woman*, translated by Tani E. Barlow and Gary J. Bjorge, 49–81. Boston: Beacon Press, 1989.

————. "Shafei nüshi de riji" 莎菲女士的日記. In *Xiandai Zhongguo xiaoshuo xuan* 現代中國小說選, edited by Zheng Shusen 鄭樹森, 1:339–91. Taipei: Gongfan Shudian, 1989.

Ding, Naifei. *Obscene Pleasures: Sexual Politics in Jinping mei.* Durham, NC: Duke University Press, 2002.

Ding Yaokang. *Gelian huaying* 隔簾花影. Shanghai: Shanghai Guji Chubanshe, 1990.

————. *Xu Jinping mei* 續金瓶梅. In *Ding Yaokang quanji* 丁耀亢全集, edited by Li Zengpo 李增坡. Zhengzhou: Zhongzhou Guji Chubanshe, 1999.

————. *Xu Jinping mei* 續金瓶梅. Edited by Ziyang Daoren 紫陽道人. Shanghai: Shanghai Guji Chubanshe, 1990.

Dohi, Keizo. *Beitrage zur Geschichte der Syphilis: Insbesondere Uber Ihren Ursprung und Ihre Pathologie in Ostasien.* Leipzig: Akademische Verlagsgesellschaft, 1923.

Dong Xiaoping 董曉萍, ed. 紅樓夢的傳說 Beijing: Xinhua Shudian, 1990.

Du Ji 杜稷. *Caomu chunqiu yanyi xu* 草木春秋演義序. [China]: Zuile Tang, n.d.

Dumas, Alexandre, fils. *Chahua nü yishi* 茶花女遺事. Translated by Lin Shu 林紓. Shanghai: Shanghai Zhixinshu Sheyingxing, 1933.

————. *La Dame aux Camélias.* Paris: Michel Lévy Frères, 1852.

————. *La Dame aux Camélias.* Translated by David Coward. Oxford: Oxford University Press, 1986.

Eifring, Halvor. "The Psychology of Love in *Story of the Stone*." In *Love and Emotions in Traditional Chinese Literature*, edited by Halvor Eifring, 271–324. Leiden: Brill, 2004.

Elman, Benjamin A. *From Philosophy to Philology: Intellectual and Social Aspects of Change in Late Imperial China.* Cambridge, MA: Harvard University Press, 1984.

Esherick, Joseph W. *Ancestral Leaves: A Family Journey through Chinese History.* Berkeley: University of California Press, 2011.

Fang Yizhi 方以智. *Fushan wenji qianbian* 浮山文集前編. 1671? Shanghai: Shanghai Guji Chubanshe, 2002.

Feng Menglong 馮夢龍. "The Fan Tower Restaurant as Witness to the Love of Zhou Shengxian." In *Stories to Awaken the World*, translated by Shuhui Yang and Yuqin Yang, 275–90. Seattle: University of Washington Press, 2009.

———. "Jiang Xingge chonghui zhenzhu shan" 蔣興哥重會珍珠衫. In *Yushi mingyan* 喻世明言, 1–34. Beijing: Renmin Wenxue Chuban She, 1958.

———. *"Jiang Xingge Reencounters His Pearl Shirt."* In *Stories Old and New*, translated by Shuhui Yang and Yuqin Yang, 9–47. Seattle: University of Washington Press, 2000.

———. *Nao Fanlou duoqing Zhou Shengxian* 鬧樊樓多情周勝仙. In *Xingshi hengyan* 醒世恆言, edited by Liu Shide 劉世德 et al. Guben xiaoshuo congkan 古本小說叢刊, 30. Beijing: Zhonghua Shuju, 1991.

Feuerwerker, Yi-tsi Mei. *Ding Ling's Fiction: Ideology and Narrative in Modern Chinese Literature*. Cambridge, MA: Harvard University Press, 1982.

Fitzgerald, John. *Awakening China: Politics, Culture, and Class in the Nationalist Revolution*. Stanford: Stanford University Press, 1996.

Flueckiger, Joyce Burkhalter. *In Amma's Healing Room: Gender and Vernacular Islam in South India*. Bloomington: Indiana University Press, 2006.

Foucault, Michael. *The History of Sexuality.*Vol. 1, *An Introduction*. New York: Pantheon 1978.

———. *The History of Sexuality*. Vol. 3, *The Care of the Self*. New York: Pantheon, 1986.

Furth, Charlotte. "Androgynous Males and Deficient Females: Biology and Gender Boundaries in Sixteenth- and Seventeenth-Century China." *Late Imperial China* 9, no. 2 (1988): 1–31.

———. "Blood, Body and Gender: Medical Images of the Female Condition in China, 1600–1850." *Chinese Science* 7 (1986): 43–66.

———. *A Flourishing Yin: Gender in China's Medical History, 960–1665*. Berkeley: University of California Press, 1999.

———. "The Physician as Philosopher of the Way: Zhu Zhenheng (1282–1358)." *Harvard Journal of Asiatic Studies* 66, no. 2 (2006): 423–59.

———. "Producing Medical Knowledge through Cases: History, Evidence, Action" In *Thinking with Cases*, edited by Charlotte Furth, Judith T. Zeitlin, and Ping-chen Hsiung, 125–51. Honolulu: University of Hawai'i Press, 2007.

Gai Qi 改琦. *Honglou meng tuyong* 紅樓夢圖詠. N.p. Early eighteenth century. Waseda University Library, Japan.

Ge Chenghui 葛成慧. "Zhongguoren yu jiehebing" 中國人與結核病. *Kexue* 科學 10, no. 5 (1925): 587.

Ge Hong 葛洪. *Baopuzi neiwai pian* 抱樸子內外篇. Taibei: Taiwan Zhonghua Shuju, 1965.

Goldschmidt, Asaf. *The Evolution of Chinese Medicine: Song Dynasty, 960–1200*. New York: Routledge, 2009.

Gong Tingxian 龔廷賢. *Jishi quanshu* 濟世全書. Beijing: Zhongyi Guji, 1987.

———. *Wanbing huichun* 萬病回春. Beijing: Renmin Weisheng Chubanshe, 1984.

Grant, Joanna. *A Chinese Physician: Wang Ji and the Stone Mountain Medical Case Histories*. London: Routledge Curzon, 2003.

Hanan, Patrick. *The Chinese Vernacular Story*. Cambridge, MA: Harvard University Press, 1981.

———. "The Early Chinese Short Story: A Critical Theory in Outline." In *Studies in Chinese Literary Genres*, edited by Cyril Birch. Berkeley: University of California Press, 1974.

———. "The *Sources* of the Chin P'ing Mei." *Asia Major* 10 (1963): 60ff.

———. "The Text of the *Chin P'ing Mei*." *Asia Major* 9 (1962):1–57.

Handlin-Smith, Joanna. *The Art of Doing Good: Charity in Late Ming China*. Cambridge, MA: Harvard Asia Center, 2009.

Hanson, Marta, "Depleted Men, Emotional Women: Gender and Medicine in the Ming Dynasty." *Nan Nü* 7, no. 2 (2005): 287–304.

———. "Robust Northerners and Delicate Southerners: The Nineteenth Century Invention of a Southern Medical Tradition." In *Innovation in Chinese Medicine*, edited by Elisabeth Hsu, 297–324. Cambridge: Cambridge University Press, 2001.

———. *Speaking of Epidemics in Chinese Medicine: Disease and the Geographic Imagination in Late Imperial China*. New York: Routledge, 2011.

Harper, Donald J. *Early Chinese Medical Literature: The Mawangdui Medical Texts*. New York: Kegan Paul, 1997.

Hawkes, David. Introduction to *The Story of the Stone*, by Cao Xueqin, 1:15–46. London: Penguin Classics, 1974.

Hay, Johnathan. *Sensuous Surfaces: The Decorative Object in Early Modern China*. Honolulu: University of Hawai'i Press, 2010.

Hayden, Deborah. *Pox: Genius, Madness, and the Mysteries of Syphilis*. New York: Basic Books, 2003.

Hegel, Robert. *Reading Illustrated Fiction in Late Imperial China*. Stanford: Stanford University Press, 1998.

Hershatter, Gail. *Dangerous Pleasures: Prostitution and Modernity in Twentieth-Century Shanghai*. Berkeley: University of California Press, 1997.

Hinrichs, T. J. "Pragmatism, Rationalism, and their Resistance in Southern Song Medicine." Conference paper for The (After) Life of Traditional Knowledge: The Cultural Politics and Historical Epistemology of East Asian Medicine, August 20–21, 2010, University of Westminster.

Hong Mai 洪邁. *Yijian jiazhi* 夷堅甲志. Beijing: Beijing Airusheng Shuzihua Jishu Yanjiu Zhongxin, 2009.

Hsia, C. T. *The Classic Chinese Novel: A Critical Introduction*. New York: Columbia University Press, 1968.

———. "The Scholar-Novelist and Chinese Culture: A Reappraisal of *Ching-hua Yuan*." In *C. T. Hsia on Chinese Literature*, 188–222. New York: Columbia University Press, 2004.

Hsiung, Ping-chen. "Facts in the Tale: Case Records and Pediatric Medicine in Late Imperial China." In *Thinking with Cases*, edited by Charlotte Furth, Judith T. Zeitlin, and Ping-chen Hsiung, 152–68. Honolulu: University of Hawai'i Press, 2007.

Hu Hsiao-chen. "In the Name of Correctness: Ding Yaokang's *Xu Jinping mei* as a Reading of *Jinping mei*." In *Snakes Legs: Sequels, Continuations, Rewritings and Chinese Fiction*, edited by Martin Huang, 75–97. Honolulu: University of Hawai'i Press, 2004.

Hu Shi 胡適. *Xingshi yinyuan zhuan kaozheng* 醒世姻緣轉考證. Taipei: Yuanliu Chubanshe, 1986.

Hua, Wei. "How Dangerous Can the 'Peony' Be? Textual Space, 'Caizi Mudan Ting,' and Naturalizing the Erotic." *Journal of Asian Studies* 65, no. 4 (2006): 741–62.

Huai Yuan 懷遠 "Yizhen." In *gujin yiche* 古今醫徹. Shanghai: Shanghai Kexuejishu Chubanshe, 1985.

Huang, Martin, *Desire and Fictional Narrative in Late Imperial China*. Cambridge, MA: Harvard University Asia Center, 2001.

———. *Negotiating Masculinities in Late Imperial China*. Honolulu: University of Hawai'i Press, 2006

———, ed. *Snakes' Legs: Sequels, Continuations, Rewritings, and Chinese Fiction*. Honolulu: University of Hawai'i, 2004.

———. "*Xiaoshuo* as 'Family Instructions': The Rhetoric of Didacticism in the Eighteenth- Century Chinese Novel *Qilu Deng*." *Tsing Hua Journal of Chinese Studies, New Series* 30, no. 1 (Mar. 2000): 67–91.

Huayue chiren 花月癡人. *Honglou huanmeng* 紅樓幻夢. Beijing: Beijing Daxue Chubanshe, 1990.

Hucker, Charles O. *A Dictionary of Official Titles in Imperial China*. Stanford: Stanford University Press, 1985.

Hymes, Robert. "Not Quite Gentlemen? Doctors in Sung and Yuan." *Chinese Science*, no. 8 (Jan. 1987): 9–76.

Jiang Hong 江洪. *Caomu chunqiu yanyi* 草木春秋演義. Eighteenth or nineteenth century. East Asian Special Collection, Columbia University
Library, 5765 3138.

———. *Huitu caomu chunqiu yanyi* 繪圖草木春秋演義. Taibei: Fenghuang
Chubanshe, 1974.

Idema, Wilt. "Diseases and Doctors, Drugs and Cures: A Very Preliminary
List of Passages of Medical Interest in a Number of Traditional Chinese
Novels and Related Plays." *Chinese Science* 2 (1977): 37–63.

Idema, Wilt L., and Beata Grant. *The Red Brush: Writing Women of Imperial China*. Cambridge, MA: Harvard University Asia Center, 2004.

Idema, Wilt, and Lloyd Haft. *A Guide to Chinese Literature*. Ann Arbor:
Center for Chinese Studies, University of Michigan, 1997.

Jia Zhizhong 賈治中. "Caomu zhuan zuozhe kao bian zhiyi" 草木傳作者考辨
質疑. *Zhongyi wenxian zazhi* 中醫文獻雜誌 3 (1995): 26–27.

Jia Zhizhong 賈治中 and Yanfei Yang 楊燕飛. *Qingdai yaoxing ju* 清代藥性
劇. Beijing: Xueyuan Chubanshe, 2013.

Jiang Guan 江瓘 (1503–1565). *Mingyi lei'an* 名醫類案. Electronic resource.
Beijing: Beijing Airusheng Zhuzihua Jishu Yanjiu Zhongxin, 2009.

Keaveney, Christopher T. *The Subversive Self in Modern Chinese Literature:
The Creation Society's Reinvention of the Japanese Shishosetsu*. New
York: Macmillian, 2004.

Ko, Dorothy. *Teachers of the Inner Chambers: Women and Culture in Seventeenth-Century China*. Stanford: Stanford University Press, 1994.

Kuhn, Philip. *Soulstealers: The Chinese Sorcery Scare of 1768*. Cambridge,
MA: Harvard University Press, 1990.

Kuriyama, Shigehisa. "Epidemics, Weather and Contagion in Traditional
Chinese Medicine." In *Contagion: Perspectives from Pre-Modern Societies*, edited by Lawrence I. Conrad and Dominik Wujastyk, 3–22. Alder-
shot, Hampshire: Ashgate, 2000.

Lam, Ling Hon. "The Matriarch's Private Ear: Performance, Reading, Cen-
sorship, and the Fabrication of Interiority in 'The Story of the Stone.'"
Harvard Journal of Asiatic Studies 65, no. 2 (Dec. 2005): 357–415.

Lee, Leo Ou-fan. *The Romantic Generation of Modern Chinese Writers*.
Cambridge, MA: Harvard University Press, 1973.

Lei, Sean Hsiang-lin. "Habituating Individuality: The Framing of Tuberculosis and Its Material Solutions in Republican China." *Bulletin of the History of Medicine* 84, no. 2 (Summer 2010): 248–79.

———. "Moral Community of *Weisheng*: Contesting Hygiene in Republican
China." *East Asian Science, Technology, and Society: An International
Journal* 3 (2009): 475–504.

Leung, Angela Ki Che. "The Evolution of the Idea of *Chuanran* Contagion in Imperial China."

In *Health and Hygiene in Chinese East Asia: Policies and Publics in the Long Twentieth Century*, edited by Angela Ki Che Leung and Charlotte Furth, 25–50. Durham, NC: Duke University Press, 2011.

———. *Leprosy in China: A History*. New York: Columbia University Press, 2009.

———. "Medical Ethics in China." In *Encyclopaedia of the History of Science, Technology, and Medicine in Non-Western Cultures*, edited by H. Selin, 667–69. Dordrecht, Netherlands: Kluwer Academic Publishers, 1997.

———. "Medical Instruction and Popularization in Ming-Qing China." *Late Imperial China* 24, no. 1 (2003): 130–52.

———. "Medical Learning from the Song to the Ming." In *The Song-Yuan-Ming Transition in Chinese History*, edited by Paul Jakov Smith and Richard von Glahn, 374–98. Cambridge, MA: Harvard University Press, 2003.

———. "The Yuan and Ming Periods." In *Chinese Medicine and Healing: An Illustrated History*, edited by Linda L. Barnes and T. J. Hinrichs, 129–60. Cambridge, MA: Harvard University Press, 2013.

Levy, Dore. *The Ideal and Actual in the Story of the Stone*. New York: Columbia University Press, 1999.

Li, Wai-yee. *Enchantment and Disenchantment: Love and Illusion in Chinese Literature*. Princeton: Princeton University Press, 1993.

Li Boyuan 李伯元 (Baojia 寶嘉). Guanchang *xianxing ji*官場現形記. 1906. Taipei: Sanmin Shuju, 2008.

Li Jianmin. "Contagion and Its Consequences: The Problem of Death Pollution in Ancient China." In *Medicine and the History of the Body: Proceedings of the 20th, 21st, and 22nd International Symposium on the Comparative History of Medicine—East and West*, edited by Yasuo Otsuka, Shizu Sakai, and Shegehisa Kuriyama, 201–22. Tokyo: Ishiyaku Euro America, 1999.

Li Liangsong 李良松. *Zhongguo chuantong wenhua yu yixue* 中國傳統文化與醫學. Xiamen: Xiamen Daxue Chubanshe, 1990.

Li Ruzhen 李汝珍. *Jinghua yuan* 鏡花緣. Beijing Renmin Wenxue Chubanshe, 1990.

———. N. P. Xu Qiaolin 許喬林. Preface, 1832 edition. Waseda University Library, Japan.

Li Shizhen. 李時珍 *Bencao gangmu* 本草綱目. Annotated and edited by Liu Hengru 劉衡如 et al. Beijing: Huaxia Chubanshe, 2002.

———. *Compendium of Materia Medica* [Bencao gangmu]. Translated by Luo Xiwen. Beijing: Foreign Languages Press, 2003.

Li Yanshi 李延是. *Maijue huibian* 脈訣彙辨. Shanghai: Shanghai Guji Chubanshe, 2002.

Li Yu 李漁. "Benxing kuhao zhi yao" 本性酷好之藥. In *Xianqing Ouji* 閑情偶寄. Annotated and edited by Jiang Jurong 江巨榮 and Lu Shourong 盧壽榮 318–19. Shanghai: Shanghai Guji Chubanshe, 2000.

———. "Bian nü wei er pusa qiao" 變女為兒菩薩巧. In *Wusheng xi* 無聲戲 in *Liyu quanji* 李漁全集, edited by Helmut Martin, 8.173–89. Taipei: Chengwen Chubanshe, 1970.

———. "A Daughter Is Transformed into a Son through the Bodhisattva's Ingenuity." In *Silent Operas* (Wusheng xi), translated by Patirck Hanan, 137–59. Hong Kong: Research Centre for Translation, Chinese University of Hong Kong, 1990.

———. *The Carnal Prayer Mat* (Roupu tuan). Translated by Patrick Hanan. Honolulu: University of Hawai'i Press, 1990.

———. Nü Chenping jisheng qichu 女陳平計生七出. "The Female Chen Ping Saved Her Life with Seven Ruses." In *Wusheng xi* 無聲戲 in *Li Yu Quanji* 李漁全集, edited by Helmut Martin, 8.93–106. Taipei: Chengwen Chubanshe, 1970.

———. *Rou putuan* 肉浦團. Qing edition. Waseda University Library, Japan.

———. *Shijinlou* 十卺樓. "The Hall of the Ten Weddings." In *Li Yu Quanji* 李漁全集, edited by Helmut Martin, 195–97. Taipei: Chengwen Chubanshe, 1970.

Liang Qichao 梁啟超. "Lun xiaoshuo yu qunzhi zhi guanxi." 論小說與群治之關係. Xin Xiaoshuo, 1902.

———. "On the Relationship between Fiction and the Government of the People." In *Modern Chinese Literary Thought: Writings on Literature, 1893–1945*, edited and translated by Kirk Denton, 74–81. Stanford: Stanford University Press, 1996.

Liu Chun 劉純. *Yuji weiyi* 玉機微義. In *Liu Chun yixue quanshu* 劉純醫學全書, edited by Jiang Dianhua 姜典華. Beijing: Zhongguo Zhongyiyao Chubanshe, 1999.

Liu Dabai 劉大白. *Du He Dian* 讀何典. 1926. Republished in Zhang Nanzhuang 張南莊, *He Dian: Xinzhu ben* 何典新注本, edited by Cheng Jiang 成江, 211–18. Shanghai: Xuelin Chubanshe, 2000.

Liu E 劉鶚. *Lao Can Youji* 老殘遊記. Taipei: Sanmin Shuju, 1986.

———. *The Travels of Lao Can*. Translated by Harold Shadick. New York: Columbia University Press, 1990.

Liu Shuangsong 劉雙松, ed. *Xinban quanbu tianxia bianyong wenlin miaojin wanbao quanshu* 新版全補天下便用文林妙錦萬寶全書. 1612. Edited by

Sakai Tadao 酒井忠夫, Sakade Yoshinobu 阪出祥伸, and Ogawa Yoichi 小川陽一. 3 vols. Tokyo: Kyuko Shoin 汲古書院, 2003.

Liu Zhaorui 劉昭瑞. "Tan kaogu faxian de Daojiao jiezhu wen" 談考古發現的道教解注文. *Dunhuang Yanjiu* 敦煌研究 1991: 4, 51–57.

Lu, Tina. *Persons, Roles, and Minds: Identity in Peony Pavilion and Peach Blossom Fan.* Stanford: Stanford University Press, 2001.

Lu Renlong 陸人龍. "Xi'an fu fu bie qi, Heyang xian nan hua nü" 西安府夫別妻, 郃陽縣男化女. In *Xingshi yan* 型世言, 490–502. Beijing: Zhonghua Shuju, 1993.

Lu Xun 魯迅. *A Brief History of Chinese Fiction.* Translated by Yang Hsien-yi and Gladys Yang. Beijing: Foreign Languages Press, 1976.

———. "Fuqin de bing" 父親的病. In *Zhaohua xi shi* 朝花夕拾, 53–57. Beijing: Renmin Wenxue, 1997.

———. *Lu Xun quanji* 魯迅全集. Beijing: Renmin Wenxue Chubanshe, 1981.

———. *Zhongguo xiaoshuo shilüe* 中國小說史略. Taipei: Fengyun Shidai Chubanshe, 1995.

Lu Yitian 陸以湉. *Lenglu yihua* 冷廬醫話. Shanghai: Shanghai Zhongyi Xueyuan Chubanshe, 1993.

Luo Guanzhong 羅貫中 and Shi Naian 施耐庵. *Outlaws of the Marsh.* Translated by Sidney Shapiro. Beijing: Foreign Languages Press, 1980.

———. *Li Zhuowu xiansheng piping zhongyi shuihu zhuan* 李卓吾先生批評忠義水滸傳. Shanghai: Shanghai Guji, 1995.

———. *Shui Hu Zhuan* 水滸傳. Beijing: Renmin Wenxue Chubanshe, 2010.

Mair, Victor, ed. *The Hawai'i Reader in Traditional Chinese Culture.* Honolulu: University of Hawai'i Press, 2005.

Mao Dun 矛盾. "Xianzai wenxuejia de zeren shi shemne" 現在文學家的責任是什麼. *Xiaoshuo yuebao* 小說月報, October 1920.

Martinson, Paul Varo. *Pao Order and Redemption: Perspectives on Chinese Religion and Society Based on a Study of the Chin P'ing Mei.* Diss., University of Chicago Divinity School, 1973.

McMahon, Keith. "Eliminating Traumatic Antimonies: Sequels to *Honglou meng.*" In *Snakes' Legs: Sequels, Continuations, Rewritings, and Chinese Fiction*, edited by Martin W. Huang, 98–115. Honolulu: University of Hawai'i Press, 2004.

———. *Misers, Shrews, and Polygamists: Sexuality and Male-Female Relations in Eighteenth- Century Chinese Fiction.* Durham, NC: Duke University Press, 1995.

Medical Manuscript. "Chengfangyao juan" 成方藥卷, late Qing or early Republican era. East Asia Department, Berlin State Library, Prussian

Cultural Heritage Foundation (Staatsbibliothek zu Berlin—Preussischer Kulturbesitz). Slg. Unschuld 8429.

———. "Jianbian qifang" 簡便奇方, early Republican era. East Asia Department, Berlin State Library, Prussian Cultural Heritage Foundation (Staatsbibliothek zu Berlin—Preussischer Kulturbesitz). Slg. Unschuld 8217.

———. "Liangfang zalu," 良方雜錄, late Qing. East Asia Department, Berlin State Library, Prussian Cultural Heritage Foundation (Staatsbibliothek zu Berlin—Preussischer Kulturbesitz). Slg. Unschuld 8823.

———. "Lingyi shouce" 鈴醫手冊, late Qing. East Asia Department, Berlin State Library, Prussian Cultural Heritage Foundation (Staatsbibliothek zu Berlin—Preussischer Kulturbesitz). Slg. Unschuld 8253.

———. "Mai gaoyao shu" 賣膏藥書, 1909. East Asia Department, Berlin State Library, Prussian Cultural Heritage (Staatsbibliothek zu Berlin—Preussischer Kulturbesitz). Slg. Unschuld 8011.

———. "Minjia zachao" 民家雜抄, late Qing or early Republican era. East Asia Department, Berlin State Library, Prussian Cultural Heritage Foundation (Staatsbibliothek zu Berlin—Preussischer Kulturbesitz). Slg. Unschuld 8288.

———. "Neiwai ke" 內外科, early Republican era. East Asia Department, Berlin State Library, Prussian Cultural Heritage Foundation (Staatsbibliothek zu Berlin—Preussischer Kulturbesitz). Slg. Unschuld 8467.

———. "Quan Yaoshu" 全藥書, 1859. East Asia Department, Berlin State Library, Prussian Cultural Heritage Foundation (Staatsbibliothek zu Berlin—Preussischer Kulturbesitz). Slg. Unschuld 8071.

———. "Shibing lun. Beiyong zhufa" 時病論. 備用諸法, 1882. East Asia Department, Berlin State Library, Prussian Cultural Heritage Foundation (Staatsbibliothek zu Berlin—Preussischer Kulturbesitz). Slg. Unschuld 8315.

———. "Shichuan yifang zachao" 世傳醫方雜抄, early Republican period. East Asia Department, Berlin State Library, Prussian Cultural Heritage Foundation (Staatsbibliothek zu Berlin—Preussischer Kulturbesitz). Slg. Unschuld 8138.

———. "Souji Shenxiaofang" 搜集神效方, 1930s to 1950s. East Asia Department, Berlin State Library, Prussian Cultural Heritage Foundation (Staatsbibliothek zu Berlin—Preussischer Kulturbesitz). Slg. Unschuld 8033.

———. "Wanyao bu" 丸藥簿, late Qing. East Asia Department, Berlin State Library, Prussian Cultural Heritage Foundation (Staatsbibliothek zu Berlin—Preussischer Kulturbesitz). Slg. Unschuld 8670.

———. "Xiabu shanqi" 下部疝氣, early Republican era. East Asia Department, Berlin State Library, Prussian Cultural Heritage Foundation (Staatsbibliothek zu Berlin—Preussischer Kulturbesitz). Slg. Unschuld 8180.

———. "Yangchong yaoyin" 洋蟲藥引, late Qing or early Republican era. East Asia Department, Berlin State Library, Prussian Cultural Heritage Foundation (Staatsbibliothek zu Berlin—Preussischer Kulturbesitz). Slg. Unschuld 8503.

———. "Yangsheng shu" 養生書, 1848. East Asia Department, Berlin State Library, Prussian Cultural Heritage Foundation (Staatsbibliothek zu Berlin—Preussischer Kulturbesitz). Slg. Unschuld 8799.

———. "Yaofang shouchao ben" 藥方手抄本, 1937 or later. East Asia Department, Berlin State Library, Prussian Cultural Heritage Foundation (Staatsbibliothek zu Berlin—Preussischer Kulturbesitz). Slg. Unschuld 8157.

———. "Yaofang zachao" 藥方雜抄, early Republican era. East Asia Department, Berlin State Library, Prussian Cultural Heritage Foundation (Staatsbibliothek zu Berlin—Preussischer Kulturbesitz). Slg. Unschuld 8167.

———. "Yifang bianlan" 醫方便覽, late Qing. East Asia Department, Berlin State Library, Prussian Cultural Heritage (Staatsbibliothek zu Berlin—Preussischer Kulturbesitz). Slg. Unschuld 8453.

———. "Yilun" 醫論, early Republican period. East Asia Department, Berlin State Library, Prussian Cultural Heritage Foundation (Staatsbibliothek zu Berlin—Preussischer Kulturbesitz). Slg. Unschuld 48024.

———. "Yingyan liangfang" 應驗良方, late Qing. East Asia Department, Berlin State Library, Prussian Cultural Heritage Foundation (Staatsbibliothek zu Berlin—Preussischer Kulturbesitz). Slg. Unschuld 8082.

———. "Yixue zachao" 醫學雜抄, late Qing. East Asia Department, Berlin State Library, Prussian Cultural Heritage (Staatsbibliothek zu Berlin—Preussischer Kulturbesitz). Slg. Unschuld 8484.

———. "Yiyao biji" 醫藥筆記, 1940s. East Asia Department, Berlin State Library, Prussian Cultural Heritage Foundation (Staatsbibliothek zu Berlin—Preussischer Kulturbesitz). Slg. Unschuld 8480.

———. "Yuxia ji" 玉匣記, Daoguang (1821–50) period. East Asia Department, Berlin State Library, Prussian Cultural Heritage Foundation (Staatsbibliothek zu Berlin—Preussischer Kulturbesitz). Slg. Unschuld 8649.

———. "Zashu" 雜書, late Qing. East Asia Department, Berlin State Library, Prussian Cultural Heritage Foundation (Staatsbibliothek zu Berlin—Preussischer Kulturbesitz). Slg. Unschuld 8747.

———. "Zhongguo xinwen zhidao quanshu" 中國新聞指導全書, early Republican era. East Asia Department, Berlin State Library, Prussian Cultural Heritage Foundation (Staatsbibliothek zu Berlin—Preussischer Kulturbesitz). Slg. Unschuld 8145.

Metailie, Georges, and Elizabeth Hsu. "The *Bencao gangmu* of Li Shizhen: An Innovation in Chinese Natural History?" In *Innovation in Chinese Medicine*, edited by Elizabeth Hsu, 221–61. Cambridge: Cambridge University Press, 2001.

Ming-Qing xiaoshuo yanjiu zhongxin. *Zhongguo Tongsu Xiaoshuo Zongmu Tiyao.* 中國通俗小說總目提要 Beijing: Zhongguo Wenlian Chuban Gongsi, 1991.

Modengxianzhai Zhuren 莫等閒齋主人. *Bing yu yuan chuanqi* 病玉緣傳奇. Shanghai: Zhonghua Shuju, 1932.

Murray, Julia K., and Suzanne E. Cahill. "Recent Advances in Understanding the Mystery of Ancient Chinese "Magic Mirrors."" *Chinese Science* 8 (1987): 1–8.

Nappi, Carla. *The Monkey and the Inkpot: Natural History and Its Transformations in Early Modern China.* Cambridge, MA: Harvard University Press, 2010.

Nienhauser, William, ed. *The Indiana Companion to Traditional Chinese Literature.* Bloomington: Indiana University Press, 1986–98.

Oki Yasushi 大木康. "Minmatsu Konan ni okeru shuppan bunka no kenkyu" 明末江南出版文 化研究. Special issue. *Hiroshima Daigaku Bungakubu kiyō* 廣島大學文學部紀要 50, no. 1 (Jan. 1991): 103–7.

Ōtsuka Hidetaka 大塚秀高, ed. *Zōho chūgoku tsūzoku shōsetsu shomoku* 增補中國通俗小說書. Tokyo: Kyūko Shoin, 1987.

Ott, Katherine. *Fevered Lives: Tuberculosis in American Culture since 1870.* Cambridge, MA: Harvard University Press, 1996.

Pan Guangdan 潘光旦. *Feng Xiaoqing xing xinli biantai jiemi* 馮小青性心理變態揭秘. Beijing: Wenhua Yishu Chubanshe, 1990.

Pan Jianguo. "Metal Typography, Stone Lithography and the Dissemination of Ming-Qing Popular Fictions in Shanghai between 1874 and 1911." *Frontiers of Literary Studies in China* 2, no. 4 (Dec. 2008): 561–82.

Peng, Dingqiu 彭定球, et al., eds. *Quan Tang Shi* 全唐詩. Beijing: Zhonghua Shu Ju, 1960.

Peterson, Willard J. *The Cambridge History of China.* Vol. 9, part 1, *Ch'ing Empire to 1800.* Cambridge: Cambridge University Press, 2008.

Plaks, Andrew H. *The Four Masterworks of the Ming Novel: Ssu-ta Ch'i-shu.* Princeton, NJ: Princeton University Press, 1987.

Porter, Roy. *Quacks: Fakers and Charlatans in English Medicine.* Charleston, SC: Tempus, 2001.

Pu Songling 蒲松齡. *Liaozhai zhiyi* 聊齋志異. Beijing: Renmin Wenxue Chubanshe, 2012.

Qi Zhongfu 齊仲甫. *Nüke Baiwen* 女科百問. 2 *juan.* Original preface 1220. Facsimile reprint of the Zongbutang edition of 1735. Shanghai: Shanghai Guji Shuju, 1983.

Rolston, David L., ed. *How to Read the Chinese Novel.* Princeton, NJ: Princeton University Press, 1990.

———. *Traditional Chinese Fiction and Fiction Commentary: Reading and Writing between the Lines*. Stanford: Stanford University Press, 1997.

Ropp, Paul. "The Price of Passion in Three Tragic Heroines of the Mid-Qing: Shuangqing, Lin Daiyu, and Chen Yun." In *From Skin to Heart: Perceptions of Emotions and Bodily Sensations in Traditional Chinese Culture*, edited by Paolo Santangelo, 203–28. Weisbaden: Verlag, 2006.

Rulin Yiyin 儒林醫隱. *Weisheng xiaoshuo: Yijie jing* 衛生小說: 醫界鏡. Shanghai: Shangwu Yinshuguan, 1908.

Santangelo, Paolo. *Sentimental Education in Chinese History: An Interdisciplinary Textual Research on Ming and Qing Sources*. Leiden: Brill, 2003.

Satyendra, Indria. "Metaphors of the Body: The Sexual Economy of the *Jinping mei cihua*." *Chinese Literature: Essays, Articles, and Reviews* 15 (1993): 85–97.

Scheid, Volker. *Currents of Tradition in Chinese Medicine, 1626–2006*. Seattle: Eastland Press, 2007.

Schonebaum, Andrew. "Medicine in *The Story of the Stone*: Four Cases." In *Approaches to Teaching the Story of the Stone (Dream of the Red Chamber)*, edited by Andrew Schonebaum and Tina Lu, 164–86. New York: Modern Languages Association, 2012.

Shahar, Meir. *Crazy Ji: Chinese Religion and Popular Literature*. Cambridge, MA: Harvard University Press, 1998.

———. "Vernacular Fiction and the Transmission of Gods' Cults in Late Imperial China." In *Unruly Gods: Divinity and Society in China*, edited by Meir Shahar and Robert P. Weller, 184–211. Honolulu: Hawai'i University Press, 1996.

Shang Wei. "*Jinping mei* and Late Ming Print Culture." In *Writing and Materiality in China*, edited by Judith Zeitlin and Lydia H. Liu, 187–238. Cambridge, MA: Harvard University Press, 2003.

———. "The Making of the Everyday World: *Jinping mei Cihua* and Encyclopedias for Daily Use." In *Dynastic Crisis and Cultural Innovation: From the Late Ming to the Late Qing and Beyond*, edited by David Wang and Wei Shang, 63–92. Cambridge, MA: Harvard Asia Center, 2006.

———. "The *Stone* Phenomenon and Its Transformation from 1791 to 1919." In *Approaches to Teaching the Story of the Stone*, edited by Andrew Schonebaum and Tina Lu, 390–412. New York: MLA, 2012.

Shang Zhijun 尚志鈞, Lin Qianliang 林乾良, and Zheng Jinsheng 鄭金生. *Lidai zhongyao wenxian jinghua* 歷代中藥文獻精華. Beijing: Kexue Jishu Wenxian Chubanshe, 1989.

Shapiro, Hugh. "The Puzzle of Spermatorrhea in Republican China." *Positions* 6, no. 3 (1998): 551–596.

Shen Defu 沈德符. *Wanli Ye Huo Bian* 萬曆野獲編. In *Jinping mei Ziliao*

Huibian, 金瓶梅資料彙編, edited by Hou Zhongyi 侯忠義 and Wang Rumei 王汝梅, 222. Beijing: Beijing Daxue Chubanshe, 1985.

Shen Jin 沈津. "Mingdai fangke tushu zhi liutong yu jiage" 明代坊刻圖書之流通與價格. *Guojia tushuguan guankan* 國家圖書館館刊 85, no. 1 (1996): 101–18.

Shen Yaofeng 沈堯封. *Chenshi nüke qiyao* 沈氏女科輯要. 1850. Reprint, Shanghai: Shanghai Weisheng Chubanshe, 1958.

Sima Qian 司馬遷. *Shiji* 史記. Edited by Gu Jiegang 顧頡剛 et al. Beijing: Zhonghua Shuju, 2011.

Sivin, Nathan. "Emotional Counter-Therapy." In *Medicine, Philosophy, and Religion in Ancient China: Researches and Reflections*, 2:1–19. Brookfield, VT: Variorum, 1995.

Smith, Richard J. *Chinese Almanacs*. Hong Kong: Oxford University Press, 1992.

Sommer, Matthew. "The Gendered Body in the Qing Courtroom." *Journal of the History of Sexuality* 22, no. 2 (May 2013): 281–311.

Sontag, Susan. *Illness as Metaphor*. New York: Farrar, Strauss and Giroux, 1978.

Starr, Chloe. *Red-light Novels of the Late Qing*. Leiden: Brill, 2007.

Strickmann, Michael. *Chinese Magical Medicine*. Stanford: Stanford University Press, 2002.

Struve, Lynn A., ed. *The Qing Formation in World-Historical Time*. Cambridge, MA: Harvard University Asia Center, 2004.

Sun Dianqi 孫殿起. *Fanshu ouji xubian* 販書偶記續編. Shanghai: Shanghai Guji Chubanshe, 1980.

Sun Jiaxun 孫佳訊. *Jinghua yuan gongan bianyi* 鏡花緣公案辨疑. Shandong: Qilu Shushe, 1984.

Sun Simiao 孫思邈. *Beiji qianjin yaofang* 備急千金藥方. Comp. 650/659. Beijing: Huaxia Chubanshe, 1999.

———, comp. *Hua Tuo shenfang* 華佗神方. Beijing: Zhongyi Guji Chubanshe, 1992.

Sutton, Donald S. "Shamanism in the Eyes of Ming and Qing Chinese Elites." In *Heterodoxy in Late Imperial China*, edited by K. C. Liu and Richard Shek, 209–37. Honolulu: University of Hawai'i Press, 2004.

Swatek, Catherine Crutchfield. *Peony Pavilion Onstage: Four Centuries in the Career of a Chinese Drama*. Ann Arbor: Center for Chinese Studies, University of Michigan, 2002.

Tang Xianzu 湯顯祖. "Huai Dai Siming xiansheng bingwen Tu Changqing" 懷戴四明先生並問屠長卿. In *Tang Xianzu shiwen ji*, 湯顯祖詩文集, edited by Xu Shuofang 徐朔方, 7:202–3. Shanghai: Shanghai Guji Chubanshe, 1982.

———. "Ku Loujiang nüzi" 哭婁江女子. In *Tang Xianzu shiwen ji* 湯顯祖詩文集, edited by Xu Shuofang 徐朔方, 1:654–56. Shanghai: Shanghai Guji Chubanshe, 1982.

———. *Mudan ting* 牡丹亭. Beijing: Renmin Wenxue Chubanshe, 1997.

———. *The Peony Pavilion*. Translated by Cyril Birch. Bloomington: Indiana University Press, 1980.

Tang Xiaobing. *Chinese Modern: The Heroic and the Quotidian*. Durham, NC: Duke University Press, 2000.

Tang Yijie 湯一介. *Wei Jin nanbei chao shiqi de Daojiao* 魏晉南北朝時期的道教. Taibei: Dongda Tushu Gongsi, 1988.

Tao Hongjing 陶弘景. *Yangxing yanming lu* 養性延命錄. Jinan: Shandong Huabao Chubanshe, 2004.

ter Haar, Barend J. *Telling Stories: Witchcraft and Scapegoating in Chinese History*. Leiden: Brill, 2006.

Theiss, Janet. *Disgraceful Matters: The Politics of Chastity in Eighteenth-Century China*. Berkeley: University of California Press, 2004.

Thompson, Laurence G. "Medicine and Religion in Late Ming China." *Journal of Chinese Religions* 18 (1990): 45–59.

Tian Zhiwen 田志文. "*Caomu chunqiu yanyi*" 草木春秋演義. In *Zhongguo gudai xiaoshuo zongmu: Baihua juan* 中國古代小說總目: 白話卷, edited by Shi Changyu 石昌渝, 25. Taiyuan: Shanxi Jiaoyu Chubanshe, 2004.

Tsung, Shiu-kuen Fan. *Moms, Nuns, and Hookers: Extrafamilial Alternatives for Village Women in Taiwan*. PhD diss., University of California, San Diego, 1978.

Unschuld, Paul U. "Chinese Retributive Recipes: On the Ethics of Public and Secret Health Care Knowledge." *Monumenta Serica* 52 (2004): 325–43.

———. *Forgotten Traditions of Ancient Chinese Medicine: A Chinese View from the Eighteenth Century*. Brookline: Paradigm Publications, 1998.

———. *Medical Ethics in Imperial China: A Study in Historical Anthropology*. Berkeley: University of California Press, 1979.

———. *Medicine in China: A History of Ideas*. Berkeley: University of California Press, 1985.

———. *Medicine in China: A History of Pharmaceutics*. Berkeley: University of California Press, 1986.

———. "Plausibility of Truth? An Essay on Medicine and World View." *Science in Context* 8, no. 1 (1995): 9–30.

Unschuld, Paul U., and Hermann Tessenow, in collaboration with Zheng Jingsheng, translator. *Huang Di nei jing su wen: An Annotated Translation of Huang Di's Inner Classic Basic Questions*. Berkeley: University of California Press, 2011.

Unschuld, Paul U., and Jinsheng Zheng. *Chinese Traditional Healing: The Berlin Collections of Manuscript Volumes from the 16th through the Early 20th Century*. Leiden: Brill, 2012.

Unschuld, Ulrike. "Traditional Chinese Pharmacology: An Analysis of Its Development in the Thirteenth Century." *Isis* 68 no. 2 (Jun., 1977): 224–48.

Van Gulik, R. H. *Sexual Life in Ancient China: A Preliminary Survey of Chinese Sex and Society from Ca. 1500 B.C. till 1644 A.D.* Leiden: E. J. Brill, 1961.

Volkmar, Barbara. "The Concept of Contagion in Chinese Medical Thought: Empirical Knowledge *versus* Cosmological Order." *History and Philosophy of the Life Sciences* 22 (2000): 147–65.

Wang, Cheng-hua. "Art in Daily Life: Knowledge and Practice in Late-Ming Riyong Leishu." Paper presented at Discourses and Practices of Everyday Life in Imperial China. New York: Department of East Asian Languages and Cultures, Columbia University, October 25, 2002.

Wang Ji 汪機. *Shishan yian* 石山醫案. Beijing: Zhonghua Shuju, 1991.

Wang Kentang 王肯堂. *Zhengzhi zhunsheng* 證治準繩. 1589. Reprint, Beijing: Renmin Weisheng Chubanshe, 1991.

Wang Dao 王燾. *Waitai miyao* 外臺秘要.Beijing: Renmin Weisheng Chubanshe, 1955.

Wang, David Der-wei. *Fin-de-siècle Splendor: Repressed Modernities of Late Qing Fiction, 1849–1911*. Stanford, CA: Stanford University Press, 1997.

Wang Liaoweng. *Shanghai liushinian huajie shi*上海六十年花界史 (A sixty-year history of the Shanghai flower world). Shanghai: Shixin Shuju, 1922.

Wang Qi 汪淇, ed. *Chidu xinyu chubian* 尺牘新語初編. Taipei: Guangwen Shuju, 1971

Wang Qingyuan 王清原 et al., eds. *Xiaoshuo shufang lu* 小說書坊錄. Beijing: Beijing Tushuguan Chubanshe, 2002.

Wang Qiongling 王瓊玲. *Qingdai de sida caixue xiaoshuo* 清代的四大才學小說. Taipei: Taiwan Shangwu Yinshuguan, 1997.

Wang Shifu 王實甫. *Jiping jiaozhu xixiang ji* 集評校注西廂記. Edited by Wang Jisi 王季思 and Zhang Renhe 張人和. Shanghai: Shanghai Guji Chubanshe, 1987.

———. *The Story of the Western Wing*. Edited and translated by Stephen West and Wilt Idema. Berkeley: University of California Press, 1995.

Wang Wenmo 王文謨. "Michuan shenxian qiaoshu gese qifang" 秘傳神仙巧術各色奇方. In *Xinqie Wang shi jiachuan jishi suijin fang* 新鍥王氏家傳濟世碎金方, *juan* 4. Beijing: Zhongyi Guji Chubanshe, 2002.

Wang Yongjian 王永健. "Lun Wu Wushan sanfu heping ben *Mudan ting* ji qi piyu" 論吳吳山三婦合評本牡丹亭及其批語. *Nanjing daxue xuebao* 南京大學學報 4 (1980): 18–26.

Wei Yilin 危亦林. *Shiyi de xiaofang* 世醫得效方. Taipei: Taiwan Shangwu Yinshuguan, 1983.

West, Stephen H., and W. L. Idema. *The Orphan of Zhao and Other Yuan Plays: The Earliest Known Versions*. New York: Columbia University Press, 2014.

Widmer, Ellen. *The Beauty and the Book: Women and Fiction in Nineteenth-Century China*. Cambridge, MA: Harvard University Asia Center, 2006.

———. "The Huanduzhai of Hangzhou and Suzhou: A Study in Seventeenth-Century Publishing." *Harvard Journal of Asiatic Studies* 56, no.1 (Jun. 1996): 77–122.

———. "Modernization without Mechanization: The Changing Shape of Fiction on the Eve of the Opium War." In *From Woodblocks to the Internet: Chinese Publishing and Print Culture in Transition, circa 1800 to 2008*, edited by Cynthia Brokaw and Christopher Reed, 59–77. Leiden: Brill, 2010.

———. "Xiaoqing's Literary Legacy and the Place of the Woman Writer in Late Imperial China." *Late Imperial China* 13, no.1 (June 1992): 111–55.

Wile, Douglas. *Art of the Bedchamber: The Chinese Sexual Yoga Classics Including Women's Solo Meditation Texts*. Albany: State University of New York Press, 1992.

Wong, K. Chimin. "Notes on Chinese Medicine: Origin of Syphilis in China." *China Medical Journal* 27 (1913): 379–83.

Wong, K. Chimin, and Wu Lien-Tie. 中國醫史 *History of Chinese Medicine*: *Being a Chronicle of Medical Happenings in China from Ancient Times to the Present Period*. 2nd ed. Shanghai, 1936.

Wu Bing 吳炳 (*jinshi* 1619). "Liaodu geng" 療妒羹. Reprinted in *Huike chuanju* 彙刻傳劇, edited by Liu Shiheng 劉世珩. Yangzhou : Guangling Guji Keyinshe, 1919.

Wu Cheng'en 吳承恩. *The Journey to the West*. Translated by Anthony Yu. Rev. ed. Chicago: University of Chicago Press, 2012.

———. *Juanxiang guben Xiyou zhengdao shu* 鐫像古本西遊證道書. Edited and commentary by Wang Qi 汪淇. Shanghai: Shanghai Guji Chubanshe, 1990.

———. *Li Zhuowu pingben Xiyou ji* 李卓吾評本西遊記. Reprint of *Li Zhuowu Xiansheng piping Xiyou ji* 李卓吾先生批評西遊記, 1620–27. Shanghai: Shanghai Guji Chubanshe, 1994.

———. *Xinshuo xiyouji* 新說西遊記. Annotated by Zhang Shushen 張書紳. Shanghai: Shanghai Guji Chubanshe, 1990.

———. *Xiyou ji* 西遊記 (Journey to the West). Beijing: Renmin Wenxue Chubanshe, 2005.

Wu Huifang 吳慧芳. "Minjian Riyong leishu de yuanyuan yu fazhan" 民間日用類書的淵源 與發展." *Guoli Zhengzhi daxue lishi xuebao* 國立政治大學歷史學報 18 (May 2001): 1–27.

Wu Jianren 吳趼人 (Wu Woyao 吳沃堯). *Ershi nian mudu zhi guai xianzhuang* 二十年目睹 之怪現狀. Shanghai: Shanghai Guji Chubanshe, 2001.

Wu Jingzi 吳敬梓. *Rulin Waishi* 儒林外史. Taipei: Lianjing, 1991.

———. *Rulin Waishi*. Photo reprint ed. Beijing: Renmin Wenxue Chubanshe, 1975. 4 vols. Woxian Caotang ed., 1803.

———. *The Scholars*. Edited and translated by Yang Hsien-yi and Gladys Yang. New York: Columbia University Press, 1992.

Wu Kun 吳崑. *Yifang kao* 醫方考. Jiangsu: Jiangsu Kexue Jishu Chubanshe, 1985.

Wu Liande 伍聯德. "Jiehebing" 結核病. *Zhonghua yixue zazhi* 20, no. 1 (1934): 84–115.

Wu Qian 吳謙 et al., eds. *Yizong jinjian* 醫宗金鑑. 1742. 2 vols. Reprint, Beijing: Renmin Weisheng Chubanshe, 1990.

Wu Yi-Li. "The Bamboo Grove Monestary and Popular Gynecology in Qing China." *Late Imperial China* 21, no. 1 (Jun. 2000): 41–76.

———. "The Qing Period." In *Chinese Medicine and Healing: An Illustrated History*, edited by Linda L. Barnes and T. J. Hinrichs, 160–207. Cambridge, MA: Belknap / Harvard, 2013.

———. *Reproducing Women: Medicine, Metaphor, and Childbirth in Late Imperial China*. Berkeley: University of California Press, 2010.

Xia Jingqu 夏敬渠. *Yesou Puyan* 野叟曝言. Jilin: *Jilin* Wenshi Chubanshe, 1994.

Xiao Guanlan 蕭觀瀾. *Sang ji sheng zhuan* 桑寄生傳. Taizhong: Changhan, 1988.

Xiao Jing 蕭京. *Xuan Qi jiuzheng lun* 軒岐救正論. Beijing: Zhongyi Guji Chubanshe, 1983.

Xiao Xiaoting 蕭曉亭. *Fengmen quanshu* 瘋門全書. Beijing: Renmin Weisheng Chubanshe, 1990.

Xiaoxiaosheng 笑笑生. *Jinping mei cihua* 金瓶梅詞話. 1618. Reprint, Tokyo: Daian, 1963.

———. *The Plum in the Golden Vase or Chin P'ing Mei*. Translated by David Tod Roy. 5 vols. Princeton, NJ: Princeton University Press, 1993–2013.

———. *Xinke xiuxiang piping Jinping mei* 新科修像批評金瓶梅. "Chongzhen" ed. Originally published ca. 1628–1644. Modern print ed. Taipei: Xiaoyuan Chubanshe, 1990.

———. *Zhang Zhupo piping diyi qishu Jinping mei* 張竹坡批評第一奇書金瓶梅. 2 vols. Edited by Zhang Zhupo 張竹坡 and Wang Rumei 王汝梅. Jinan: Qiru Sushi, 1991.

Xie Yi 謝頤. "*Jinping mei Xu*." 金瓶梅序 In *Jinping mei Ziliao Huibian* 金瓶梅資料彙編, edited by Zhu Yi Hai, 197. Nankai: Nankai Daxue Chubanshe, 1985.

Xizhousheng 西周生. *Xingshi yinyuan zhuan* 醒世姻緣傳. Taipei: Tianyi Chubanshe, 1985.

Xu Dachun 徐大椿. *Huixi Yian* 洄溪醫案. Shanghai: 上海古籍, 2002.

———. *Xu Lingtai yi xue quan shu* 徐靈胎醫學全書 (Complete medical works of Xu Lingtai). Edited by Liu Yang 劉洋 et al. ed. Beijing: Zhongguo Zhongyiyao Chubanshe, 1999.

———. *Yixue yuan liu lun* 醫學源流論. Taipei: Shang Wu, 1978.

———. *Yiguan bian* 醫貫砭. N.p. Bansongzhai, early eighteenth century. Call no. 09 00170 0005. Waseda University Library, Japan.

Xu Fuming 徐扶明. *Mudan ting yanjiu ziliao kaoshi* 牡丹亭研究資料考釋. Shanghai: Shanghai Guji Chubanshe, 1987.

Xu Qilong 徐企龍, ed. *Xinke quanbu shimin beilan bianyong wenlin huijin wanshu yuanhai* 新刻全補士民備覽便用文林彙錦萬書淵海. 1610. Edited by Sakai Tadao 酒井忠夫, Sakade Yoshinobu 阪出祥伸, and Ogawa Yōichi 小川陽一. 2 vols. Tokyo: Kyuko Shoin, 2001.

———. *Xinke souluo wuche hebing wanbao quanshu* 新刻搜羅五車合併萬寶全書. 1614. Edited by Sakai Tadao 酒井忠夫, Sakade Yoshinobu 阪出祥伸, and Ogawa Yōichi 小川陽一. 2 vols. Tokyo: Kyuko Shoin, 2001.

Xu Sanyou 徐三友 et al. *Wuche bajin* 五車八錦. Edited by Sakai Tadao 酒井忠夫, Sakade Yoshinobu 阪出祥伸, and Ogawa Yōichi 小川陽一. 2 vols. Tokyo: Kyuko Shoin, 2001.

Xuan Ding 宣鼎. "Mafeng nü Qiu Liyu chuanqi" 痲瘋女邱麗玉傳奇. Reprinted in *Bing yu yuan chuanqi*. Shanghai: Zhonghua Shuju, 1932.

Yang Bin. "The Zhang on Chinese Southern Frontiers: Disease Constructions, Environmental Changes, and Imperial Colonization." *Bulletin of the History of Medicine* 84, no. 2 (Summer 2010): 163–92.

Yang Yu-Chun. "Re-orienting *Jinping mei: The Moralizing Tales of Xingshi Yinyuan Zhuan and Xu Jinping Mei*." Diss., Princeton University, 2003.

Yao Kecheng 姚可成. *Shiwu bencao* 食物本草, late Ming. Wellcome Library, London.

Yeh, Catherine Vance. "Shanghai Leisure, Print Entertainment, and the Tabloids" *xiaobao* 小報. In *Joining the Global Public: Word, Image, and City in Early Chinese Newspapers, 1870–1910*, edited by Rudolf G. Wagner, 201–33. Albany: State University of New York Press, 2007.

———. *Shanghai Love: Courtesans, Intellectuals, and Entertainment Culture, 1850–1910*. Seattle: University of Washington Press, 2006.

Yi Ming 佚名, ed. *Jujia biyong shilei quanji* 居家必用事類全集. Shanghai: Shanghai Guji Chubanshe, 2002.

Yim, Chi-hung. "The 'Deficiency of Yin in the Liver': Dai-yu's Malady and Fubi in *Dream of the Red Chamber*." *Chinese Literature: Essays, Articles, and Reviews* 22 (2000): 85–111.

Yu, Anthony. *Rereading the Stone: Desire and the Making of Fiction in Dream of the Red Chamber*. Princeton: Princeton University Press, 1997.

Yu Wentai 余文台 (Yu Xiangdou 餘象鬥), ed. *Jianqin Chongwenge huizuan shimin wanyong zhengzong bu qiu ren qianbian* 鼎鍥崇文閣彙纂士民萬用正宗不求人全編. 1609. Edited by Sakai Tadao 酒井忠夫, Sakade Yoshinobu 阪出祥伸, and Ogawa Yōichi 小川陽一. 2 vols. Tokyo: Kyuko Shoin, 2001.

Yu Xiangdou 餘象鬥, ed. *Xinke tianxia simin bianlan santai wanyong zhengzong* 新刻天下四民便覽三台萬用正宗. 1599. Edited by Sakai Tadao 酒井忠夫, Sakade Yoshinobu 阪出祥伸, and Ogawa Yōichi 小川陽一. 2 vols. Tokyo: Kyuko Shoin, 2001.

Yu Yaohua 餘耀華. *Zhongguo jiageshi* 中國價格史. Beijing: Zhongguo Wujia Chubanshe, 2000.

Yuan Hongdao 袁宏道. *Yuan zhonglang quanji* 袁中郎全集. Taipei: Shijie Shuju, 1990.

Yuan Ke 袁珂, ed. and annot. *Shanhai jing quanyi* 山海經全譯. Guizhou: Guizhou Renmin, 1991.

Yue Jun 樂鈞. "Chi nüzi" 癡女子. In Ershi lu 耳食錄二編*Honglou meng ziliao huibian* 紅樓夢資料彙編, edited by Yi Su 一粟, 347. Beijing: Zhonghua Shuju, 2003.

Zeitlin, Judith. *Historian of the Strange: Pu Songling and the Chinese Classical Tale*. Stanford: Stanford University Press, 1997.

———. "The Literary Fashioning of Medical Authority: A Study of Sun Yikui's Case Histories." In *Thinking with Cases: Specialist Knowledge in Chinese Cultural History*, edited by Charlotte Furth, Judith Zeitlin, and Ping-chen Hsiung, 169–204. Honolulu: University of Hawai'i Press, 2005.

———. *The Phantom Heroine: Ghosts and Gender in Seventeenth-Century Chinese Literature*. Honolulu: University of Hawai'i Press, 2007.

———. "Shared Dreams: The Story of the Three Wives' Commentary on *The Peony Pavilion*." *Harvard Journal of Asiatic Studies* 54, no. 1 (Jun. 1994): 127–79.

Zeng Pu 曾樸, *Niehai hua* 孽海花. Beijing: Huaxia Chubanshe, 2013.

Zhang Chao 張潮. "Shu bencao" 書本草 in *Tanji congshu* 檀幾叢書. Qing edition. Xiaju Tang, 1754. Waseda University Library, Japan.

Zhang Congzheng 張從正. *Rumen Shiqin* 儒門事親. Beijing: Zhonghua Shuju, 1991.

Zhang Gongrang 張公讓. *Feibing ziyi ji* 肺病自醫記 [Record of self-treatment for lung disease]. Canton: Zhang Gongrang Zhensuo, 1943.

Zhang Hong, "Pingmian lu," quoted in Wang Shuwu, "Nanyishu zhanzhu bing kaoyi." *Yunnan minzuyueyuan xuebao* 3 (2001): 58–72.

Zhang Ji, comp., Xu Bin, annot. *Jinkui yaolue lunzhu* 金匱要略論注. Beijing: Renmin Weisheng Chubanshe, 1993.

Zhang Jiading 張嘉鼎. *Cao Xueqin chuanshuo gushi* 曹雪芹傳說故事. Beijing: Guangming Ribao Chubanshe, 1987.

Zhang Jiebin 張介賓 (ca. 1563–1640). *Jingyue Quanshu: Yuzheng Mo* 景岳全書:鬱証謨. Edited by Wang Dachun 王大淳. Beijing: Zhongguo Renmin Daxue Chubanshe, 2010.

Zhang Jun 張俊. *Qingdai xiaoshuo shi* 清代小說史. Zhejiang: Zhejiang Guji Chubanshe, 1997.

Zhang Junfang 張君房. *Yunji qiqian*. 雲笈七簽. Beijing: Huaxia Chubanshe, 1996.

Zhang Lu 張潞. *Zhangshi yitong* 張氏醫通. 1695. Shanghai: Shanghai Kexue Jishu Chubanshe, 1990.

Zhang Yanhua. *Transforming Emotions with Chinese Medicine: An Ethnographic Account from Contemporary China.* Albany: SUNY, 2007.

Zhang, Yixia, and Mark Elvin. "Environment and Tuberculosis in Modern China." In *Sediments of Time: Environment and Society in Chinese History*, edited by Mark Elvin and Ts'ui-jung Liu, 520–43. Cambridge: Cambridge University Press, 1998.

Zhang Zhibin and Paul Unschuld. *Dictionary of the Ben Cao Gang Mu.* Vol. 1, *Chinese Historical Illness Terminology.* Berkeley: University of California Press, 2015.

Zhang Zhongjing 張仲景 (Zhang Ji 張機). *Jingui yaolue* 金匱要略. Beijing: Xinshijie Chubanshe, 2007.

Zhang Zhupo 張竹坡. "How to Read *Jinping mei*" (Jinping mei dufa). Translated by David Tod Roy. In *How to Read the Chinese Novel*, edited by David L. Rolston 202–41. Princeton, NJ: Princeton University Press, 1990.

Zhao Bi 趙弼. "Peng-lai xiansheng zhuan" 蓬萊先生傳 (The story of Mr. Penglai). In *Xiaopin ji* 效顰集, 69–76. Shanghai: Gudian Wenxue Chubanshe, 1957.

Zhao Chunhui 趙春輝. "*Caomu chunqiu* zuozhe chutan" 草木春秋作者初探. *Guji zhengli yanjiu xuekan* 古籍整理研究學刊 3 (May 2011): 83–84.

Zhao Xuemin 趙學敏. *Chuanya quanshu* 串雅全書. Beijing: Zhongguo Zhon-gyiyao Chubanshe, 1998.

Zheng, Huli. *Encountering the Other: Identity, Culture, and the Novel in Late Imperial China*. PhD diss., University of California, Irvine, 2010.

Zheng Yunchai 鄭雲齋, ed. *Quanbu tianxia simin liyong bianguan wuche bajin* 全補天下四民利用便觀五車拔錦. 1597. Edited by Sakai Tadao 酒井忠夫, Sakade Yoshinobu 阪出祥伸, and Ogawa Yōichi 小川陽一. 2 vols. Tokyo: Kyuko Shoin, 1999.

Zhou Yimou, ed. *Lidai Mingyi Lun Yide*. Changsha: Hunan Kexue Jishu Chubanshe, 1983.

Zhou Zuoren 周作人. *Bingzhu Houtan* 秉燭後談, 89–96. Hebei: Hebei Jiaoyu Chubanshe, 2001.

———. "On Passing the Itch." In *The Chinese Essay*, translated and edited by David Pollard, 139–49. New York: Columbia University Press, 2000.

Zhu Xi 朱熹, ed. *Sishu Jizhu* 四書集注. Taipei: Xuehai, 1988.

Zhu Yixuan 朱一玄et al., eds. *Zhongguo gudai xiaoshuo zongmu tiyao* 中國古代小說總目提 要. Beijing: Renmin Wenxue, 2005.

Zhu Zhenheng 朱震亨. *Danxi xinfa* 丹溪心法. Shenyang: Liaoning Kexue Jishu Chubanshe, 1997.

———. *Gezhi yulun* 格致餘論. In *Zhu Danxi yixue quanshu*朱丹溪醫學全書, edited by Tian sisheng 田思勝 et al. Beijing: Zhongguo Zhongyiyao Chubanshe, 2006.

Zhuangzi, *Chuang-tzu: The Inner Chapters*. Translated by A. C. Graham. Indianapolis: Hackett, 2001.

Zhulinsiseng 竹林寺僧, eds. *Zhulin nüke* 竹林女科. Beijing: Huaxia Chuban-she, 1999.

INDEX

accounts of the strange (*zhiguai*), 20, 40
almanacs, 25–27, 194
ancestors, 127, 132, 177, 193
Annals of Herbs and Trees (the novel)
    (Caomu chunqiu yanyi), 73–75,
    96–109
Annals of Herbs and Trees (the play)
    (Caomu chunqiu), 81–96
aphrodisiacs, 31, 66–70, 94, 110, 112
apotropaic medicine, 8, 34–38

Badou Dahuang (*badou dahuang*),
    97–107
Baochai. *See* Xue Baochai
Baoyu. *See* Jia Baoyu
*Bencao gangmu. See Systematic
    Materia Medica*
bian du (bian poison [sore]), 123–24
"Biblio Materia Medica" (Shu bencao),
    70–72
"The Bitterness of Filial Piety" (Kuxiao
    shuo), 57–58
black gold pills, 103–04
blood: definitions, 15–16; coughing of,
    158, 169; and essence, 50, 155, 161;
    loss of, 148–55
bone steaming (*guzheng*), 79, 124–25,
    150, 161, 165–66

Cao Xueqin, 22, 119–20
case histories, 9, 38–40, 49–50
Chahua nü. See La Dame aux Camelias
chuanran (contagion), 125–137, 177,
    181, 193–94
chuanshi (corpse-transmission), 79, 162,
    190–95
Classic of Mountains and Seas (Shanhai
    jing), 35–43
consumption (*lao, xulao*), 17, 123–26,
    159–200
Corpse worms, 191–93

Cui Yingying, 77–81

Dai-yu. *See* Lin Daiyu
demons, 17, 32–38, 161–68, 177–78,
    190–94
depletion, 17, 31–32, 49–51, 62, 124–
    27, 148–72
depression. *See* melancholy
desire. *See* qing
doctors, 5–13, 30–40, 100–04, 127–37
Dream of the Red Chamber (Honglou
    meng). *See The Story of the Stone*
Du Fu, 33
Du Liniang, 48, 52, 141

emotions, 49–51, 61–66, 133, 148–72
epidemics, 30, 125, 128
encyclopedia, 15, 23–29, 75–77, 110–12

fangshu (formularies, medical recipes),
    12, 17, 45, 86–88
fei jiehe (tuberculosis), 185
feng. See wind. *See also* leprosy
fertility, 67–70, 137–39
Flower Shadows behind the Screen
    (Gelian huaying). *See Sequel to
    Jinping mei*
Flowers in the Mirror (Jinghua yuan),
    3–4, 30, 112–20
foxes, fox spirits, 17, 31, 42–45, 140,
    170

Gautier, Marguerite, 178–90
germ theory, 176, 178, 190, 200
ghosts, 19, 30, 36–43, 108, 123–25,
    140–44
*The Golden Mirror of the Medical
    Lineage*, 11, 29
gender, 53, 64, 125, 165–71
gu poison (*gudu*), 58–61, 126
gui. See ghosts.

healing (contradistinction from
    medicine), 7–12
The Heart Sutra, 49, 146
Humble Words of an Old Rustic (Yesou
    puyan), 30, 139
hun. See soul

involuntary seminal emission, 55, 65,
    95, 154–59, 165–68

Jia Baoyu, 37–38, 47–48, 53, 63–64,
    168–69
Jia Rui, 36, 53–55, 158–9
Journey to the West, 80, 93, 101–11

karma, 158, 182, 197
King of Medicine (*Yao wang*), 83

laozhai. See consumption
La Dame aux Camelias, 178–84
leishu. See encyclopedia
leprosy (*li, mafeng*, numbing wind),
    126–35
Li Ping'er, 143, 148–54, 164–70, 192
Li Ruzhen, *Flowers in the Mirror*
    (Jinghua yuan), 3–4, 114–16
Li Shizhen, see *Systematic Materia
    Medica* (Bencao gangmu), 18
Liaozhai's Records of the Strange
    (Liaozhai zhiyii), 41, 185
Lin Daiyu, 38, 51–53, 160–61, 167–71,
    173–84
Lin Shu, 178–82
lineage, 195–200
Listing the Elegant Practice (Chuanya),
    9, 43, 116
literary logic, 8, 13, 18, 33–35, 41, 100,
    108
literati, 5–10, 20–23, 31–33, 50–51,
    62–64
lovesickness, 31–32, 48, 54, 141, 157–
    58, 164–68, 185

Madame Zhou, 3–4
magic, 13, 32–38, 54
*Marriage Destinies to Awaken the
    World* (Xingshi yinyuan zhuan), 28,
    109–11, 120, 144–46
meichuang (Bayberry sores, rotting
    sores). *See* syphilis
Meichuang milu (*Secret Account of the
    Rotting Sores Disorder*), 130
melancholy, 53, 62–72, 109, 150
memory, mnemonics, 75, 91–92
miasma, 7, 19, 50, 130–33, 181
Mirror for the Romantic (Fengyue
    baojian). *See The Story of the Stone*

"Miss Sophie's Diary," 184–90
Miss Yu (Yu Niang), 51–53
Mituo (Mituo seng), 85–89, 94, 99–102

Peony Pavilion (Mudan ting), 47–52,
    138–39, 140–42. *See also* Du
    Liniang
Pharmaceutical Plays, 81–96
Physicians. *See* doctors
Plum in the Golden Vase (Jinping mei),
    27, 55–63, 70, 80, 110–12, 122–25,
    150–63
poetry, 18–21, 33–34, 51, 110, 166
pollution, 187, 192
popular knowledge, 7–8, 12, 28, 80,
    100
*The Predestined Affinity of Sickness
    and Jade* (Bing yu yuan chuanqi),
    182–84
pregnancy, 19, 25–26
prompt notes, 9

retribution, 30–31, 67–70, 122–47, 154,
    157–59, 191–200
The Romance of the Three Kingdoms,
    61
ruyi. See scholar-physician

scholar-physician, 10–12
*Seeking No Help from Others for Myriad
    Things* (Wanshi buqiuren), 28, 111
Sequel to Plum in the Golden Vase (Xu
    Jinping mei), 57, 109–12, 120,
    144–46, 163
sequels, 23, 173
"song on natures of medicines" (*yaoxing
    ge*), 91–92
soul loss, 19, 37, 50
The Soul's Return (Huanhun ji). *See The
    Peony Pavilion*
static congestion (*yu*), 160–69
Stone Mountain Medical Cases (Shishan
    yi'an), 124, 170
stone woman, 137–40
The Story of the Stone (Shitou ji), 22,
    36–37, 47–54, 75–77, 158–84
The Story of the Western Wing (Xixiang
    ji), 64, 70, 77, 81, 93–95
Sun Wukong ("Monkey"), 101–05, 111
syphilis, 16, 17, 42, 123–34, 144–46,
    174, 179, 197
Systematic Materia Medica (Bencao
    gangmu), 4, 8, 18–19, 33–37, 107–
    08, 113–14

talisman, 13, 19, 26, 37, 42–43, 158, 190
Tang Ao, 4, 114–19

Tang Xianzu, 51, 141
Tu Long, 141–42
tuberculosis. *See* consumption and *fei
    jiehe*

venereal disease, 16, 19, 40, 129–47
vernacular fiction, 5, 7, 48, 51, 140, 165
vernacular knowledge. *See* popular
    knowledge

Wang Xifeng, 53–54, 158–61, 167
wenren. See literati
wind, 19, 61, 130–33
word games, 75, 96
worms, 7, 58, 98–100, 159–68,
    190–200

Xiaoqing, 48–52

xiaoshuo, 19–23
Ximen Qing, 122–47
Xu Dachun , 35, 40, 50, 114–16, 155,
    158
Xue Baochai, 120, 161, 184

Yan Shifan, 57, 80
yangmei. See syphilis
yi'an. See medical cases
yinyang, 15, 22, 127, 133, 152, 156,
    171, 190
Yingying. *See* Cui Yingying
yixue. See medicine

zhang. See miasmas
Zhang Zhupo, 57, 60, 143–44, 152
Zhou Zuoren, 175, 200
Zhu Zhenheng, 26, 51, 6, 155–57, 170